DATE DUE

SEP 2 8 2007		
OCT 1 9 2007		
DEC 2 9 2011		

PROTECTING THE SELF

Protecting the Self
Defense Mechanisms in Action

PHEBE CRAMER

THE GUILFORD PRESS
New York   London

©2006 The Guilford Press
A Division of Guilford Publications, Inc.
72 Spring Street, New York, NY 10012
www.guilford.com

Printed in the United States of America

This book is printed on acid-free paper.

Last digit is print number: 9   8   7   6   5   4   3   2   1

Library of Congress Cataloging-in-Publication Data

Cramer, Phebe.
    Protecting the self : defense mechanisms in action / Phebe Cramer.
        p. cm.
    Includes bibliographical references and index.
    ISBN-13: 978-1-59385-298-6 (hard cover : alk. paper)
    ISBN-10: 1-59385-298-3 (hard cover : alk. paper)
    1. Defense mechanisms (Psychology) 2. Defense mechanisms (Psychology)—Testing.
    3. Psychology, Pathological. I. Title.
    BF175.5.D44C735   2006
    155.2—dc22
                                                    2006005148

About the Author

Phebe Cramer, PhD, is a clinical psychologist and Professor of Psychology at Williams College in Williamstown, Massachusetts. She is also on the editorial boards of the *Journal of Research in Personality,* the *Journal of Personality Assessment,* and the *European Journal of Personality.* Dr. Cramer is the author of a number of research articles and books, including *Storytelling, Narrative, and the Thematic Apperception Test.* Her research takes a developmental approach to the study of defense mechanisms and personal identity.

Preface

In 1991, I published a book titled *The Development of Defense Mechanisms: Theory, Research, and Assessment*. In that book, I presented a theory of defense mechanism development in which defenses were characterized as becoming predominant at different chronological periods of development, and in which each defense was characterized as having its own developmental history.

This theory, now supported by empirical research, focuses on three defense mechanisms chosen to represent three different developmental periods. Of the three, denial, a cognitively simple mental operation, is used most frequently by young children but declines in predominance as the child grows older. Projection, a defense of greater cognitive complexity, increases in use during late childhood and becomes predominant by adolescence. The third defense, identification, of even greater complexity, increases slowly throughout childhood and becomes most important during late adolescence when issues of identity development are central to the individual. Each of these defenses has its own developmental history, and the way in which each defense is manifest may change with increasing maturity. A full discussion of the developmental trajectory of the three defenses is provided in Chapters 3, 4, and 5 of the present book.[1]

In the earlier book, I also reviewed the existing research studies of defenses. While my thinking about the developmental theory has changed very little, the research literature from the past 15 years has burgeoned; more than 2000 empirical studies of defense mechanisms were published between 1990 and today. A recent review of research with the Defense Style Questionnaire (Bond, 2004) cites more than 60 studies that have focused

vii

on the use of this single assessment method to study the role of defenses in psychopathology and therapy.

The concept of defense mechanisms has a rich history, from the earliest papers of S. Freud (1894, 1896, 1915, 1926), who described defense as a mental operation that kept painful thoughts and emotions out of awareness, through the work of A. Freud (1936) and Fenichel (1945), who focused on defenses as mechanisms for "warding off" anxiety and guilt feelings. Subsequent theorizing of Loewenstein (1967), Lampl-de Groot (1957), Van der Leeuw (1971), and Wallerstein (1967) stressed that the use of defenses is part of normal mental development and not necessarily an indication of pathology.[2]

While the theory of defense mechanisms was being developed in psychoanalytic writings, academic psychologists were attempting to create experimental paradigms to study defense mechanisms in the laboratory. From 1930 to 1960, these studies focused on the defenses of repression and projection, using experiments involving learning, memory, and perception. Eventually, this work was strongly criticized. What had initially appeared as experimental support for the concept of repression was challenged as being due to processes of attention and response suppression, while apparent support for projection was relabeled as the process of attribution.

Although this criticism brought an end to the experimental study of defenses until fairly recently, clinicians were not swayed by the negative critiques. Rather, they considered the experimental studies to lack ecological validity.[3] Further attempts to create paper-and-pencil self-report measures of defenses (e.g., Byrne, 1961; Gleser & Ihilevich, 1969; Haan, 1965; Joffee & Naditch, 1977) were unfortunately limited by both conceptual and psychometric problems (see Cramer, 1991a; Davidson & MacGregor, 1998).

More recently, there has been a significant change in the methods used to study defense mechanisms. Reliance on the earlier questionnaires that asked for direct self-report on the use of defense behaviors has been supplanted by methods that rely on clinical observation and ratings. Also new questionnaire methods have been developed and refined, resolving some of the earlier problems with self-report approaches.

Given the very large number of new research studies, I have limited my discussion in the present book to those investigations that study defense mechanisms, as contrasted with defensiveness, which is better considered a personality or response style. I focus primarily on those investigations using observational ratings, including my own method for coding defenses from narrative material, and the interview-based Defense Mechanism Rating Scale (Perry, 2001). I have also included research using the very popular Defense Style Questionnaire (Bond, 1992; Andrews, Singh, & Bond, 1993). In a few cases, because of an interesting or little researched topic, I have included studies using other methods to assess defenses. The details of these measures, including advantages and disadvantages, are discussed in Chapter 16.

Within the topic of each chapter, I have generally grouped studies by these methods of investigation and then have determined whether different methods lead to the same or different conclusions. Given the developmental focus of my thinking about defense mechanisms, I discuss research carried out with children and adolescents separately from that carried out with adults. Among other reasons, this organization reflects the understanding that defense immaturity is a concept relative to the age of the person being studied; thus denial is an immature defense for a 20-year-old but not for a 5-year-old.

Since my earlier book reviewed defense studies published prior to 1990, the current book focuses on investigations published since 1990. In a few cases, research published prior to this time is included, either because it was inadvertently omitted from the previous book or because it is essential for understanding the more recent work.

When the earlier book was published, I had already been working in this area of scholarly study for more than 10 years. But, in another way, I was just beginning my exploration of defense mechanisms. Since that time, empirical studies of defenses—my own and those of others—have expanded into new areas of inquiry. I have also had the good fortune to be able to carry out several longitudinal investigations of how defenses influence personality development over time. These latter opportunities occurred through the gracious sharing of information from the Block and Block (1980) longitudinal study of children from age 3 to age 23 and from the Institute of Human Development Intergenerational longitudinal study of development from early childhood to late adulthood (Eichorn, Clausen, Haan, Honzik, & Mussen, 1981). In both cases, Thematic Apperception Test stories had been collected but had remained largely unexamined. I was able to code these stories and thus obtain measures of defense use that could be examined in conjunction with the extensive longitudinal data that existed for these individuals. As you will see from the work reported in this book, there is still much to be learned and understood about defense mechanisms. I hope this gathering together of current knowledge will contribute to further investigation.

I thank colleagues and students who have expressed interest in my work on defenses. They have contributed to the growing body of knowledge showing that the analysis of narrative material through the use of the Defense Mechanism Manual is an informative and valid method for assessing defenses. This has been a source of continuing motivation for my own work. I am especially grateful to Dr. Sarah Hampson and Dr. Rainier Riemann, whose invitation to be a keynote speaker at the 11th European

Conference on Personality, held in Jena, Germany in July of 2002, served as the catalyst to write this new book.

Finally, the production of the book was handled skillfully by the staff at The Guilford Press. I thank especially Senior Editor Jim Nageotte and Senior Production Editor Anna Nelson for their many helpful suggestions in bringing this book to completion.

Contents

xi

PART I

Defenses in Everyday Life

*I*n this first part of the book the theory of defense mechanisms is discussed, with particular attention to defense mechanism development. Chapter 1 introduces the concept of the defense mechanism and its importance in normal development. The features that distinguish defense mechanisms, defensiveness, and coping mechanisms are explained. Several frequently used measures of defense are described. The chapter ends with a statement of six theoretical premises that may be put to empirical test.

Chapter 2 describes the theory of defense mechanism development and provides empirical support for this theory. Change in defense use, as related to stage of development, is demonstrated. Although the chapter focuses on defense development in children and adolescents, it also includes studies showing defense use to be related to adult age.

Together, these two chapters set the stage for the material that follows. They provide a general orientation to the area, and they explain the particular orientation that guides my own work in the study of defense mechanisms.

1

CHAPTER 1

Introduction

Whether 'tis nobler in the mind to suffer
The slings and arrows of outrageous fortune
Or to take arms against a sea of troubles
And by opposing end them . . .
    —SHAKESPEARE, *Hamlet* (Act III, Scene 1)

*I*n this soliloquy Hamlet raises the question of how we are to handle the "slings and arrows of outrageous fortune" that besiege us, that make us feel powerless. With psychological astuteness, Shakespeare sets out the options for reaction: either strike out on a physical level or manage the distress through mechanisms of the mind. The first is the primary option available to the infant, but with development, mental mechanisms may replace physical reactions.

The need for such protective reaction begins early in life; babies and children suffer innumerable mishaps and defeats as they begin to make their way in the world. In order to move forward, the baby at first falls backward. The infant who is learning to sit topples sideways, waiting for someone to reinstate her to an upright position. Attempts to locomote with two, rather than four, supports are frequently followed by tumbles to the ground. Early attempts at communication are met with puzzled adult reactions. Yet these disappointments, these "defeats," do not immobilize the infant. Later, artistic efforts to create a portrait of the family dog, only to have the work misperceived as a picture of a horse, is a blow to self-esteem. The child endures these and endless other reminders of being little, weak, and inept in the world of adults.

In the peer world the preschool child encounters children who are egocentric—that is, who lack interest in, or understanding of, his feelings,

3

hopes, and wishes. In the school years, the child may or may not be success-ful in academic pursuits, social relationships, or athletic endeavors. He may or may not have some special talent in music or art. But it is the rare child who is continually successful in every area, in every endeavor. Disappoint-ment, rejection, missed opportunities, and lost friendships are all part of the growing child's life.

Yet children survive—not unscathed, but not destroyed. Most children develop ways to protect themselves—that is, to protect their sense of self and their self-esteem. And they develop ways to control their expression of emo-tions, especially "negative" emotions such as anger, jealousy, and sadness. Especially as children grow older, they learn different strategies for control-ling emotions through specific instruction or by observing others. Learning these "coping strategies" is part of the process of socialization. In addition to these consciously learned and employed strategies, there are other mecha-nisms the developing child uses to control emotions and protect self-esteem. These operations, with their origins in the earliest reflex behaviors of the child, are known as the ego mechanisms of defense.

This is a book about these defense mechanisms—about the mental ma-neuvers in which we all engage to maintain our psychological equilibrium and protect our self-esteem. In this first chapter I make some distinctions between defense mechanisms and other mechanisms used for psychological adaptation. Then I present a developmental theory of defense mechanisms, stressing that defenses are part of normal development and are important to understand if we want to comprehend that development. I also consider the issue of how defenses are studied. Finally, I present six premises that are part of defense mechanism theory and indicate the chapters in the book that provide evidence relevant to these hypotheses.

WHY STUDY DEFENSES?

The phrase "in denial" is common parlance today. The student is said to be "in denial" that his failure to study will result in failing the course. The al-coholic is "in denial" that he has a problem and needs treatment. A country is "in denial" that it will be invaded by a rival nation. People are "in de-nial" that their government is committing atrocities toward other human beings. In these and other ways, we acknowledge that others make use of defenses in their everyday life.

Defenses change the way in which we perceive "reality" and think about ourselves. Particularly in our pragmatic American culture that values objectivity, rationality, and unbiased reporting—a culture that has produced an abundance of books on self-improvement through self-understanding—knowing about the ways in which we manage to deceive ourselves seems especially important. These self-deceptions are the work of defense mechanisms.

In addition to this opportunity for greater understanding of human nature, mental health practitioners and scholars are interested in defense mechanisms for other reasons. Defense use may be helpful in formulating clinical and differential diagnoses. Knowledge of defense mechanisms may also guide the type of therapeutic intervention selected by clinicians, as may knowledge of the specific relations between defenses and symptoms (Andrews, Singh, & Bond, 1993; Shaw, Ryst, & Steiner, 1996). Identifying defense mechanisms may be useful for targeting groups of individuals who are at risk for developing psychopathology, as well as for understanding why some individuals are vulnerable to pathology, whereas others, in the same environment, are resilient. For example, Vaillant (2000), in his longitudinal study of college men, found that the occurrence of a major depressive disorder occurred only among men who had experienced a large number of severe life stressors. However, not all men who were severely stressed became depressed. Within this group the use of adaptive defenses was a significant linear predictor of the *absence* of depression. Likewise, the incidence of posttraumatic stress disorder symptoms in World War II veterans was significantly lower in those who used the most adaptive defenses, as compared to those who had similar combat exposure but used less adaptive defenses (Vaillant, 2000). Other research has shown a difference in the well-being of people who are, and are not, aware of their unconscious strivings. Those whose explicit, conscious goals agree with their implicit, unconscious goals have been found to report greater emotional well-being than people whose implicit and explicit goals were inconsistent (Brunstein & Schultheiss, 1998; Schultheiss & Brunstein, 2001). One reason for this discrepancy is that implicit goals are kept out of awareness through the use of defense mechanisms.

The study of defense mechanisms is important for these reasons, but there is a problem: Defenses are effective because we are unaware of their functioning, and this absence of awareness creates a dilemma. How are we to study an important aspect of our inner life that colors our perception of reality and affects our adaptation but functions at a level that precludes our awareness? In short, how are we to learn about something that we can't know about? We will see how this dilemma has been addressed.

DEFENSES OCCUR EVERY DAY

Now you see it, now you don't.

We are all fascinated by magicians and their capacity to make us "not see" that which we just did see. How can magicians change reality—or, rather, change our perception of reality—so that what just existed appears to no longer exist? The magician's maneuvers accomplish for a group of people what a defense mechanism, such as denial, accomplishes for the individual.

I was introduced to this idea that we could change the perception of reality rather early in my life. When I was a child, there were three wooden monkeys that hung on the wall of our breakfast room, their curlicue tails connecting one to the next. The hands of the three monkeys were placed, first, to cover the eyes, then to cover the ears, and lastly to cover the mouth. My mother explained the moral to me: See no evil, hear no evil, speak no evil. Never mind if evil exists: The point is to protect the senses, protect the self from acknowledging what exists. In iconic form, these monkeys represented the capacity for self-protection through denial.

The occurrence of denial is not confined to wooden monkeys. My 4-year-old daughter received a lovely, decorative papier-mâché hand mirror as a gift from her aunt. The mirror was kept on a shelf in her bedroom. One afternoon she brought it to me, the long, elegant handle broken in two. With a look of considerable puzzlement on her face, she said, unprompted, "I didn't break it." Although it seemed likely that she had been responsible for the breakage, the expression on her face suggested to me that her statement "I didn't break it" was not an effort at conscious deception—that is, was not a lie. Rather, I think she was demonstrating her (likely) misconstrual of reality. To protect herself from self-reproach and, perhaps, an anticipated reproach from her parent, she had used the unconscious mental operation of denial.

On the playground of any school can be found children who are rejected by their peers. These "rejected" children are often trapped in a self-perpetuating cycle: Typically they attribute, or project, their own hostility onto others and then anticipate that the others will be hostile toward them—an anticipation that is sometimes validated (Crick & Dodge, 1994). However, through this use of projection, rejected children are able to attribute their difficulties to others rather than to themselves. In this way, they protect the self.

By adolescence, the teenager is beginning to struggle with issues of identity and the associated areas of personal values and goals. A frequent way to find security in this period of confusion is by adopting the clothes, hairstyle, and manners of the "in" group at school or of a current media star. In this way, for the time being, the adolescent knows who he is, or at least what he should look like, on the outside. His sense of self is protected through the use of the defense of identification.

Another example of defense use in everyday life comes from the story of the king who, on receiving a letter telling him that one of his cities had been lost in battle, burned the letter and had the messenger killed. By destroying the upsetting letter, he could deny that such an upsetting event had taken place. By projecting the cause of the upset onto the messenger, the king himself was absolved from any responsibility for the great loss.

WHAT IS A DEFENSE MECHANISM?

Thus far, I have been using the term *defense mechanism* in a rather loose, colloquial sense. Now I provide a more formal definition.

As presented by Freud in 1894, the original definition of a defense mechanism was that of a counterforce directed against the expression of drives and impulses. The idea here was that defenses served to control or modulate impulse expression so as to protect the individual from being overwhelmed by the anxiety that would result from conscious recognition of unacceptable impulses. This conception was subsequently expanded to include the use of defenses as reactions to external sources of stress as well as to internal forces (i.e., drives).

In current psychoanalytic theory of defenses, some emphasis has been placed on interpersonal factors in defense use and development (Cooper, 1998). A child may learn that the expression of certain feelings or needs would arouse a negative reaction in the caregiver; as a result, these feelings "go underground." Keeping the unacceptable feelings out of awareness helps maintain a relationship with the caregiver. This operation of putting thoughts and feelings out of awareness by keeping them "underground" is classically referred to as the defense of repression; its result is the development of a "false self," as described by Winnicott (1965) and Miller (1981).

Thus defenses operate both in reaction to internal pressures, as described in classical psychoanalytic theory, and as a reaction to external pressures, including those that emanate from significant adults. Especially important in this regard is the empathic failure of caregivers: The child mobilizes defenses to avoid recognizing these failures.

In contemporary theory, defenses also are understood to have another function: to protect the self and the sense of self-esteem (e.g., Kohut, 1977).[1] Here defenses are understood to protect the self from the negative effects of disappointment, including the disappointment of empathic failures that are experienced during childhood.

Thus defenses may be defined as unconscious mental mechanisms that are directed against both internal drive pressures and external pressures, especially those that threaten self-esteem or the structure of the self, as might occur when friends or family fail to be empathic or in some other way are "lost" to the individual. The function of the defense mechanism is twofold: to protect the individual from experiencing excessive anxiety, and to protect the integration of the self.

There are different opinions about how many defenses exist. Vaillant (1992) provided a list of 18 defense mechanisms about which there is some agreement across investigators, but others have listed up to 44 different defenses (Bibring, Dwyer, Huntington, & Valenstein, 1961). As I discuss below, different measures of defense assess different numbers of defenses.

DISTINCTION FROM COPING MECHANISMS

Using defense mechanisms is one way that people protect themselves from psychological upset. However, other strategies are available for this purpose, and people can usually describe these methods. When experiencing stress, an individual may consciously try to ignore it, focus on something else, find a solution, or seek assistance from others. These and other conscious attempts to reduce anxiety are referred to as *coping mechanisms*. Although they are similar to defense mechanisms in their purpose, there are important theoretical differences between the two concepts.

I have suggested (Cramer, 1998c, 2000a) that there are two critical differences between coping and defense mechanisms.[2] First, coping mechanisms involve a conscious, purposeful effort, whereas defense mechanisms occur without conscious effort and without conscious awareness (i.e., they are unconscious). Second, coping strategies are carried out with the intent of managing or solving a problem situation, whereas defense mechanisms occur without conscious intentionality. In this way, defenses function to change an internal psychological state but may have no effect on external reality and so may result in nonveridical perception—that is, in reality distortion.[3]

Both defense mechanisms and coping strategies are aroused by situations involving psychological disequilibrium. In this sense they are similar in that both are adaptational processes. Further, if the purpose of coping mechanisms is to (1) decrease negative affect, (2) return to baseline functioning as quickly as possible, and (3) solve or manage the problem (Aldwin, Sutton, & Lackman, 1996), then defense mechanisms may be seen as similar with regard to points 1 and 2. Defense mechanisms function (1) to ward off excessive anxiety or other disruptive negative affect, so as (2) to restore a comfortable level of functioning. It is with the third purpose of coping—to solve or manage a problem—that differences between coping and defense are seen. Coping strategies intentionally engage in activity that will address the problem (which includes diminishing negative affect). Defense mechanisms also function to diminish negative affect, but they do so without the conscious intent or awareness of the person. In addition, coping strategies sometimes address the problem by acting directly on the problematic situation, thereby reducing negative affect, whereas defenses are focused on changing internal states (negative affect) rather than external reality.

Three other differences between coping and defense mechanisms should also be considered, although these are not so much critically defining differences as they are a matter of emphasis. The first of these differences involves the question of whether the use of these mechanisms is best explained by situational or dispositional factors. Coping mechanisms are commonly thought of as reactions to situations, whereas defenses are generally conceptualized as dispositions that are part of the individual's enduring personality. Despite this theoretical difference, there is little empirical evidence that clearly supports the distinction. Clearly, situational factors are important for influencing defense use; under conditions of stress, more defenses should be used. Likewise, coping strategies have been found to be related to stable personality traits, suggesting that coping choice is to some degree dispositional (Watson & Hubbard, 1996).

Another factor that has been suggested to differentiate between coping and defense is the idea that defenses are related to psychopathology, whereas coping is part of normal psychological functioning. This idea likely stems from the original work of Freud (1894) in which the idea of a defense mechanism was identified within the context of understanding disturbed patients. However, this idea was forever changed by Anna Freud in 1936, when she wrote that the use of defense mechanisms is a part of *normal* development; this idea has been an integral part of psychoanalytic defense theory since that time. Nevertheless, as with any psychological function, a normal process may come to serve pathological ends if overused or if age or situationally inappropriate. However, the distinction between defense and coping on the basis of pathology or normality is not well founded. Empirically, the association of pathology or health with defenses or coping has shown that each of the two adaptational mechanisms may be related to either pathology or health, depending on which level of defense or which type of coping strategy is being considered. Mature defenses are related to psychological health (e.g., Vaillant, 1993, 2000; see also Chapters 11 and 12), whereas emotion-focused coping strategies are associated with psychological distress (e.g., Carver & Scheier, 1994; Watson & Hubbard, 1996).

In sum, the distinction between defense and coping mechanisms is based on theoretical differences in the two constructs rather than on whether they are situationally versus dispositionally determined, or on differences in their relation to health and pathology. A more detailed discussion of the criteria for distinguishing between defense and coping mechanisms is provided in an article devoted to this topic (Cramer, 1998c).

DISTINCTION FROM DEFENSIVENESS

Another source of difficulty in studying this area has been an occasional confusion between the terms *defense mechanism* and *defensiveness*. The term *defense mechanism* is a theoretical construct that describes a cognitive operation that occurs on an unconscious level, the function of which is to modify the conscious experience of thought or affect. Specific defense mechanisms are defined by the specific cognitive operations that bring about this modification, as discussed below. *Defensiveness* is a more general term and refers to behaviors that protect the individual from anxiety, loss of self-esteem, or other disrupting emotions. Defensiveness may thus be served by defense mechanisms, but there are other mechanisms that support defensiveness, such as the conscious decision to act differently from how one feels, or to suppress a disturbing idea. A critical distinction between the concept of defense mechanism and defensive behavior is that the former is always unconscious whereas the latter may be consciously recognized by the individual. Thus defensiveness is the broader category, including both defense mechanisms as well as other behaviors that are designed to reduce anxiety. (For further discussion of this issue, see Cramer, 1991a.) Both defensiveness and the use of defense mechanisms have been shown to distort people's self-report of their emotional state.

DEFENSES AS PART OF NORMAL DEVELOPMENT

As indicated above, defense mechanisms are part of normal development— in fact, are essential to normal development. Although Freud wrote about the connection between pathology and defenses, he also wrote that defense mechanisms are necessary as part of normal development, adding that it is "doubtful whether the ego could do without them altogether during its development" (1937, p. 237).

Although unusually heavy reliance on defense mechanisms may signal psychopathology, the use of defenses within a normative frequency is essential for daily healthy adaptation. Similarly, some forms of defense fall outside of the range of normality, whereas other forms are normatively appropriate. These distinctions apply equally to physical functioning: A heartbeat that is too rapid or too irregular may signal cardiac pathology, but *having* a heartbeat is a requirement for everyday living.

Yet the idea that defense mechanisms are an integral aspect of development that influence psychological functioning from childhood through adulthood is a novel idea to some researchers. In 1998 I published a paper with Jack Block in which we showed that psychological upset at age 3 predicted defense use at age 23. A reviewer of that paper was amazed that such a topic would even be considered for investigation, that anyone would even consider the idea that early childhood characteristics could be related to defense use in adulthood. I was as amazed by the reviewer's doubt as the reviewer must have been by my idea and by the positive findings that we reported in the paper. In reaction to the reviewer's remark, I thought, "Who could *not* think that this might be the case?" Clearly, anyone who holds a developmental, psychodynamically oriented view might expect to find a relation between early life experiences and later development.

All of which is to say, our theoretical orientations frame the kinds of questions we ask as well as the method we use to answer the questions. If you don't think there is developmental continuity from earlier to later life, you are unlikely to look for it. If you don't think that defense mechanisms exist, you are unlikely to find them.

THE DEVELOPMENTAL THEORY OF DEFENSES

In my previous book I discussed the theory of defense mechanism development in some detail. This continues to be an important way to conceptualize defenses because it makes clear that whether or not a defense is considered to be immature depends on the age of the person using the defense. For example, the defense of denial, when used by a 25-year-old, is immature, but when used by a 5-year-old is age appropriate. Defense maturity is relative to the age of the defender.

Two basic tenets are critical parts of defense development theory. The first is that different defenses become predominant at different ages, and that there is a developmental pattern for the emergence and decline of defenses. The second tenet is that each defense has its own developmental history, beginning as a motor reflex and ending as a mental mechanism that increases and then decreases in prominence. The theoretical model of defense mechanism development is shown in Figure 1.1 for the three defenses that I have studied most closely.

There is considerable empirical evidence for this theory. Both cross-sectional and longitudinal studies of defense mechanisms have shown that different defenses become predominant at different ages (Cramer, 1991a, 1997b; Cramer & Gaul, 1988; Cramer & Brilliant, 2001; Porcerelli, Thomas, Hibbard, & Cogan, 1998; Smith & Danielsson, 1982; Laor, Wolmer, & Cicchetti, 2001). In early childhood the defense of denial is predominant but by age 7 its use declines and remains at a relatively low level in future years. As denial decreases, the use of projection increases so that by age 7, denial and projection are used equally often. As children grow older, projection continues to increase in use and becomes predominant throughout late childhood and early adolescence, remaining important during late adolescence. A third defense, identification, is used very little in early childhood; its use increases slowly across childhood and early adolescence, until it becomes predominant in late adolescence. Thus, by late adolescence, denial is used infrequently, whereas projection and identification remain as important mechanisms for control and adaptation. Recent work (Cramer, 2003b, 2004) suggests that, under normal circumstances, the use of identification declines after late adolescence.

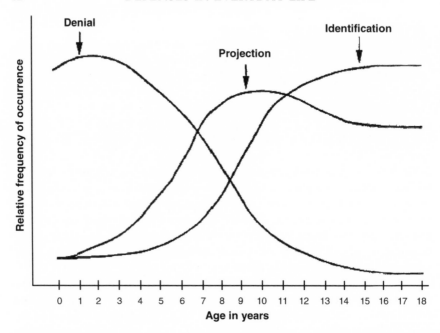

FIGURE 1.1. Hypothetical model of defense mechanism use. From Cramer (1991a). Copyright 1991 by Phebe Cramer. Reprinted by permission.

THE IMPORTANCE OF UNDERSTANDING
WHAT DEFENSES ARE AND HOW THEY FUNCTION

To understand how defense mechanisms function, it helps to believe that such motivated cognitive processes exist. It also helps to have some knowledge of psychodynamic theory, unconscious mental processes, and developmental theory. For these reasons I strongly suggest reading Chapters 3, 4, and 5, in which I present a theoretical description of the nature and development of three major defenses: denial, projection, and identification. Although some of this theorizing is summarized in Chapter 2, your thinking about the research reported will be enhanced by a greater understanding of the theory associated with the three defenses.

When approaching the study of defense mechanisms, it also helps to understand that human thinking is not always "logical," not always reality based, and not always objective. Even the most conscientious, intelligent person may sometimes deceive himself—that is, may not recognize the motives that guide his behavior—whereas an outsider, looking at the same behavior but without the need to protect the self-image of that person, can identify its defensive nature. It is this latter difference between the person displaying the defense and the person observing the defense—that is, the need, or not, to protect the self—that makes possible the assessment of defenses.

To recognize defenses it also helps to have a "third ear" with which to sense a disjunction, disruption, or nonsequitur in the flow of discourse—something that hovers on the edge of illogicality or disbelief. It is also important to recognize that defense mechanisms occur within a context, and that context will help determine whether a particular remark reflects a defense mechanism or not. For example, although it is true that the defense of denial may be schematically summarized as having an idea or feeling to which a negative marker (*no, not, doesn't*) is attached, this cannot be mechanically translated into a computer program that can identify the presence of denial in samples of text. This is because the defense of denial, or negation, involves more than the presence of the negative. Whether or not it is an example of a defense depends on the motivation, or intent, of the speaker who uses the negative marker. And here I do not refer to the conscious intent of the speaker but to sources of motivation that are likely unknown to her—that is, to unconscious motivation. It is the listener who must evaluate the nature of the statement and the intent of the speaker—that is, the context in which the remark occurs—in order to determine the presence of a defense mechanism.

PROBLEMS OF DEFENSE ASSESSMENT

This topic leads us into the important question of how to assess the use of defenses. Clearly, from what I have written, it does not make sense to directly ask a person if she reacts to stress or anxiety by using a mechanism that operates outside of awareness. As is shown later in the book, once a person understands the connection between motive and the mental mechanism of defense, she gives up the defense because its adaptive purpose is no longer functional.

However, it has been argued that it is possible to ask questions about behavior in stressful situations in such a way that the unconscious intent of the mechanism can be circumvented, allowing the individual to report on the mechanism without understanding its function. Measures of this type ask questions about behaviors that are derivatives of the defenses, assuming that these will be reported without being distorted by the work of the defense. Although it is possible that this approach may obviate the problem of asking people to report on a mechanism that operates outside of awareness, this is not clearly obvious. If the defense functions to disguise the connection between the unconscious motive and the behavior, then the response given to the questionnaire may deny the link made in the question.

On the other hand, some people may have some understanding that their behavior is influenced by defense mechanisms, and they may be able to report on these derivative behaviors. For others, such awareness is lacking. Equally likely is the case in which the very defenses under study are in use while responding to the self-report measure, such that, for example, the respondent denies that he uses denial as a defense.[4] Thus the question remains as to whether these self-report measures yield an assessment of defense use that corresponds with that obtained from clinical observation. There is little information on this issue.[5]

An alternative approach to asking people to self-report on their use of defense mechanisms is to give people free rein to express their thoughts and feelings while a trained observer closely follows what they say and how they say it. The expressions may be coded subsequently to indicate the use of different defenses. For the purpose of such coding, clear criteria for evidence of defense use are developed and applied to the narrative material.

These observer-based methods—which clearly rely on the acumen of the observer—include approaches in which the individual is given a standard "prompt" to which he crafts a perceptual or narrative response, as well as approaches based on verbal prompts to which the individual responds in a clinical interview.

The two most commonly used standard prompts are the Thematic Apperception Test (TAT; discussed in subsequent chapters) and the Rorschach Ink Blot assessment procedure.[6] The Rorschach consists of 10 abstract pictorial prompts. The viewer describes what she sees and provides a justification for that response. The use of various defense mechanisms in these descriptions may be assessed through the application of previously developed coding rules, which are applied to both the content and formal characteristics of the response. The most widely used methods of this type are the Lerner Defense Scales (Lerner & Lerner, 1980) and the Rorschach Defense Scales (Cooper, Perry, & Arnow, 1988). I discussed research using these methods in my previous book (Cramer, 1991a).

The second observer-based method to assess defense mechanism use is the clinical interview. Several scales have been developed for use in coding the interview material obtained.[7] The most widely used of the interview methods are Vaillant's clinical vignette method (Vaillant, 1976, 1977, 1993) and the Defense Mechanism Rating Scales (DMRS; Perry, 1990; Perry & Ianni, 1998). In the former approach, life vignettes are taken from more extensive interviews and rated for the presence of 18 defense mechanisms, based on the definitions of those defenses. In the DMRS interviews are rated for the presence or absence of 27 defenses, which are then grouped into seven defense levels, representing increasing levels of defense maturity, which may be additionally combined into an Overall Defensive Functioning (ODF) score, again indicating level of defense maturity.

As was true for self-report measures, there are also limitations associated with observer-based approaches. For one, they are time and labor intensive. Generally, they are conducted one-on-one; every subject hour requires an examiner hour,[8] and then numerous hours are required to code the material obtained. Further, considerable training and clinical sensitivity are required for the administration of the procedure and the coding of the material obtained. Coders who lack a clinical "ear" that is sensitive to the manifestation of defenses are unlikely to use this approach with success. In addition, although some of these approaches allow for the coding of many different defenses, the results obtained with these coding schemes indicate that many of the defenses are coded very infrequently. Moreover, as is repeatedly shown in the measures discussed in Chapter 16, when extended lists of defenses are factor analyzed, they are reduced to three or four factors. Grouping the defenses into three or four levels (e.g., Bond, 1992; Vaillant, 1976) or seven levels (Perry, 1990), based on defense maturity, produces more stable results and provides meaningful relations with personality variables and psychopathology. Perhaps due to low incidence, many of the defenses in the extended list fail to reach acceptable levels of reliability and do not relate to personality and psychopathology.

There is another type of problem associated with the assessment of defenses from clinical interviews, if these interviews are also used to make other ratings of psychological functioning, such as diagnosis, adjustment, or life satisfaction. As suggested by Bond (1990),[9] knowledge of the overall content of the interview, including diagnostic material, may influence the coding of defenses. In fact, this does happen, as noted by Busch, Shear, Cooper, Shapiro, and Leon (1995); when psychiatric interviews were being used to code the DMRS, "it was not possible to prevent discussion of symptoms that revealed the diagnosis" (p. 302). When this conflation happens, there is a clear confound, or bias, in the defense rating. This important problem is avoided when defense assessment is made entirely separate from other knowledge of the patient.

THE PRESENT BOOK

The research studies reviewed in this book are based primarily on three measures of defense mechanisms, two of which are observational and one self-report.[10] The Defense Mechanism Manual (DMM; Cramer, 1991a) assesses the use of defenses by coding narrative material, primarily stories told in response to the TAT, but also material from clinical interviews. The DMRS (Perry, 1992) assesses defense use by coding information obtained from clinical interviews and is most similar to the method used by Vaillant in his long-term study of defense use in men (Vaillant, 1975, 1983, 1993).

In contrast to these observational methods, the Defense Style Questionnaire (DSQ; Bond, 1992; Andrews et al., 1993) relies on the self-report responses of individuals to a series of structured questions. A detailed description of the DMRS and DSQ is provided in Chapter 16; the rationale for, and description of, the DMM is given in Chapters 15.

In addition to the DMM, DMRS, and DSQ, research based on several other measures is occasionally reported in the chapters to follow, including the Life Style Index (LSI; Conte & Plutchik, 1993), the Defense Mechanism Inventory (DMI; Gleser & Ihilevich, 1969), the Defense-Q (Davidson & MacGregor, 1997), the Ego Defense Scale (Pfeffer, 1986), the Comprehensive Assessment of Defense Style (CADS; Laor et al., 2001), and the Response Evaluation Measure (REM-71; Steiner, Araujo, & Koopman, 2001). A description of each of these measures is provided in Chapter 16.

As indicated above, the DMM, DMRS and DSQ differ in being either an observational (DMM, DMRS) or self-report (DSQ) measure. They also differ in the number of defenses assessed. The DMRS and the DSQ have individual measures for more than 20 defenses. The DMM, on the other hand, yields scores for only three defenses (denial, projection, and identification), although each of the three DMM defense measures is composed of seven subscales, several of which may be considered to represent individual defenses. For example, the Denial measure includes subscales for Negation, Reversal, Reaction Formation, Repression, Minimization, Disavowal, Distortion, and Fantasy. Projection includes Displacement, Magical Thinking, and Falling Ill, and Identification includes Introjection, Idealization, Controlling, Compliance, along with Identification with the Aggressor, with the Loved Object, with the Lost Object, and Out of Guilt (see Bibring et al., 1961).

An obvious question in comparing the three measures, then, is whether the multiscaled DMRS and DSQ yield more usable information than the DMM. Significantly, in research studies, the larger number of DMRS and DSQ scales are typically grouped into a smaller number of defense categories. In the case of the DSQ, factor analysis has been used to identify these more stable, underlying dimensions of the larger number of scales. Repeatedly, these analyses find three (or sometimes four) underlying factors, designated as Immature, Neurotic, and Mature. It is these summary categories that are typically used in research and clinical studies. In the case of the DMRS, the individual defense scales are grouped into seven categories or hierarchical levels. Although the results of selected individual defenses from both of these measures are sometimes also reported, the low incidence and low reliability of the individual defense scales reduce their likelihood of providing significant findings. Thus, for practical purposes, the DSQ and DMRS provide three or seven defense scales. Sometimes these are further collapsed into a single measure of defense maturity (ODF; Hersoug, Sexton, & Hoglend, 2002). Similarly, the 18 defenses assessed from Vaillant's (1993) clinical vignettes are grouped into four levels—Psychotic, Immature, Neurotic, and Mature—with the Psychotic level ignored when studying nonclinical samples, because this type of defense occurs so rarely in normal people. Again, it is three defense levels that are most often used to relate defenses to other aspects of personality, pathology, and life functioning. Sometimes the defenses are collapsed into two levels: Mature present (defenses coded at levels 1–3), and Mature absent (defenses coded at levels 4–9) (Vaillant & Mukamal, 2001). Thus, despite the coding of 18 defenses, the research findings are based on two defense scales. Furthermore, as with the DSQ and DMRS, Vaillant's defense measure is often collapsed into a single dimension of defense maturity.

The finding that defense measures with multiple scales are often reduced to three-factor scales has also been demonstrated in recent measures developed to assess children's defenses (CADS; Laor et al., 2001) and adolescents' defenses (REM-71; Steiner et al., 2001). Factor analysis of the 28 defenses of the CADS yielded three factors. The first factor is defined by Projection (the defense with the highest factor loading). The second factor is defined by Reaction Formation; Denial has the second highest loading on this factor. The highest loadings on the third factor are for Humor and Identification. Similarly, factor analysis of the 21 defense scales of the REM-71 yielded three factors.[11] The first is defined by Projection, the second by Denial, and the third by Altruism (the defense of identification is not assessed in the REM-71).

Thus, in the defense measures that include multiple defense scales, factor analyses consistently indicate the presence of three underlying dimensions. Conceptually, these dimensions are similar to the three defense measures of the DMM, indicating either increasing levels of developmental maturity or defense styles defined by denial, projection, and identification. Looked at in this way, the information provided by the DMM and the multidefense measures such as the DMRS or the DSQ is not so different.

The major difference between the DMM and the multidefense measures such as the DRMS and DSQ is not, I think, the number of defenses assessed, but rather the psychological range. Both the DMRS and the DSQ include defenses that are "healthy" or adaptive in adults. The expansion of these defense lists to include mechanisms such as suppression, humor, altruism, and sublimation follows from Vaillant's earlier studies of defense maturity in adult men. The DMM, which was originally devised to study defense development in children, does not include defenses that are more characteristic of adulthood. The DMRS and DSQ also include defenses that are characteristics of severely disturbed patients, such as splitting and projective identification. The DMM, which was originally designed to be used with healthy children and adolescents, does not include the most primitive defenses.

For many purposes, then, the use of three or four broader defense measures, rather than multiple individual defenses, is advantageous. Although some studies do show that an individual defense within one of the three factors is differentially related to some outcome variable, this is not a typical finding. More often, it is one of the three factor scores that is the successful predictor of behavior or pathology. Scores based on these three or four factors have shown adequate reliability, whereas many of the individual defense scales have not. This problem may well be due to the fact that the individual scales generally consist of only two or three items.

In thinking about this question of defense assessment, the words of Anna Freud are relevant. Referring to defense mechanisms, she noted:

> If you look at [defenses] microscopically, they all merge into each other. . . . You will find five or six defenses compressed into one attitude. The point is, one should not look at them microscopically, but macroscopically, as big and separate mechanisms, structures, events. [Then] the problem of separating them theoretically becomes negligible. You have to take off your glasses to look at them, not put them on. (Sandler & Freud, 1985, p. 176)

GENERAL ISSUES TO BE ADDRESSED

The theory of defense mechanisms includes several premises that may be tested empirically. The theoretical assumptions examined in this book are listed below. Evidence relevant to these assumptions is presented in the following chapters.

1. The theory of defense mechanism development asserts that the use of defenses changes with age. As a corollary, the implication of using any particular defense may change at different ages. (See Chapters 2 and 10.)
2. Defense mechanism theory says that the use of defenses increases under conditions of stress and anxiety caused either externally or internally. (See Chapters 6 and 7.)
3. Defense mechanism theory says that the use of defenses should reduce the subjective experience of anxiety. (See Chapters 6 and 7.)
4. Defenses are effective because they function outside of awareness— that is, they are unconscious; the awareness of the functioning of a defense should render it ineffective. (See Chapter 2.)
5. Excessive use of defenses—that is, greater than that found in

nonclinical community and student samples—is associated with psychopathology. (See Chapters 11, 12, and 13.)

6. Use of age-inappropriate, immature defenses is associated with psychopathology; use of mature defenses is associated with healthy adaptation. (See Chapters 11, 12, 13, and 14.)

In addition to these issues that relate directly to defense mechanism theory, other intriguing issues are considered in the following chapters. One of these is the question of whether different environmental stressors elicit the use of different defenses (see Chapter 7). Second is the question of whether different defenses are related to different aspects of personality and personality change (see Chapters 8 and 10). Third is the question of whether the implications of defense use differ for men, as compared to women, or for psychologically healthy, as compared to seriously disturbed, individuals (see Chapters 9 and 13).

CHAPTER 2

Development of Defenses

Defenses are phenomena serving to protect the integrity of
the ego organization. Thus their function is implicitly one
of adaptation.
—LOEWENSTEIN (1967, p. 800)

We can regard the defense mechanisms as being directed
towards the maintenance of well-being, rather than
specifically directed against the emergence of anxiety.
—SANDLER AND JOFFE (1967, p. 513)

*I*t seems clear that defense mechanisms play a useful and necessary
role in our everyday life; we find evidence that most people do use these
mental maneuvers to deal with disappointment, anger, and other stressful
emotions. But how do these mental operations come about? Are they
learned in the same way that we learn other mental skills, or are they part
of the innate developmental plan, unfolding over time as do many other
mental capacities, such as understanding causality, conservation, perspective taking, and the use of abstract logic.

This distinction between learned and unlearned mechanisms for adaptation is an important one. Failure to understand these two kinds of mechanisms as distinct has resulted in some confusion in psychology between
coping strategies and defense mechanisms (Cramer, 1998c). As discussed in
Chapter 1, coping strategies are intentionally used to manage, solve, or
bring about a change in a problem situation, or in our reaction to that situation, whereas defense mechanisms occur without conscious effort and operate outside of our awareness. Defense mechanisms work by changing our
internal psychological state—the way we feel, see, or interpret a situation—
but they do not change external reality. However, when defense mecha-

nisms are successful, they often result in a distorted perception of reality. Both coping strategies and defense mechanisms are used for adaptation to life stressors: whereas the former may be learned, the latter unfold as part of normal development.

The distinction between involuntary and volitional mechanisms of adaptation was made quite early by Freud (1905, 1925). Defense mechanisms were described as an intermediate step between innate, unlearned physiological reflexes that serve to protect the organism and learned behaviors that are consciously used to protect the individual.

A conceptually similar idea is that the immature defenses used in infancy and childhood are linked to innate temperament, which is "a biological predisposition to react to the environment in characteristic and predictable patterns" (Shaw et al., 1996, p. 107). In this view the early defenses are later modified as a result of interaction with the environment, resulting in more mature defenses that are less closely associated with innate temperament.

BIOLOGICAL ORIGINS OF DEFENSE MECHANISMS

The infant has available certain innate or reflex behaviors with which to protect herself from excessive, unsettling stimulation. Some of these reflex behaviors persist into adulthood. For example, an object moving rapidly toward your face will cause you to blink, thereby protecting your eyes from harm and, mentally, removing the offending object. Or the ingestion of a foul-tasting substance may spontaneously provoke spitting, to get that bad experience out of your mouth. In other cases the psychological derivative of the early reflex may be seen. When hungry, infants reflexively suck nourishment into their bodies. Later in life, in moments of feeling personally challenged, we may unknowingly call on sustenance acquired from someone else—his gestures, words, or style—to bolster a threatened self. Each of these involuntary, unintentional behaviors have their origins in infantile reflexes. These reflexes—shutting out the offending world, expelling unpleasant sensations, ingesting sustenance—are the antecedents of the subsequent development of three different defense mechanisms—denial, projection, and identification.[1]

This conception of defenses as originating in biologically given motor reflexes leads us to look among the infant's early motor behaviors for the prototypes and precursors of defense mechanisms. For each defense we should expect to find a common pattern of development: a biologically given defensive reflex which then comes under the conscious control of the child, becoming a voluntary motor behavior. Subsequently, this motor behavior is internalized and represented in ideational form, which allows the defense mechanism to come into existence. This sequence of development, from innate motor reflex to mental operation, has been explained at some length by Piaget, in his discussion of the child's cognitive development (Piaget, 1952).

It should be noted here that it is not the defense mechanisms that are believed to be innate but rather the child's capacities for using neurophysiological givens as a basis for developing ways to cope with stressful conditions[2] (Dorpat, 1985; Spitz, 1961). The specific pathways from reflex to mental defense mechanism for the three defenses of denial, projection, and identification are discussed in Chapters 3, 4, and 5.

A THEORY OF DEFENSE MECHANISM DEVELOPMENT

The idea that innate reflexes are the beginning step in a chain of events that eventually results in a functioning defense mechanism provides a developmental perspective on the origin of defenses. This perspective includes two key assumptions. The first is that different defenses emerge into prominence at different points in development. The timing is determined, at least in part, by the cognitive capacities that are available to the child at each age. Defenses that are cognitively simple in form will require less cognitive development and so will be available to the child earlier in life. Defenses that are cognitively complex, requiring greater cognitive capacity, will not emerge until later, when those capacities are in place. Thus, just as we may identify periods or stages of cognitive development in which new mental operations are available to the child, so we may identify points in development in which new defenses emerge and become prominent.

The second assumption in the theory of defense mechanism development is that each defense has its own developmental "history." The idea here is that every defense has its origin in some constitutionally given reflex-like reaction, and that in many cases this physiological prototype may be identified. It further assumes that voluntary motor reactions—derivatives of the inborn reflex—serve as precursors of defense mechanisms, and that different defenses have different motor precursors. The next step on this developmental path consists of the internalization and transformation of the motor precursors into ideational form, at which point a defense mechanism comes into existence. From that point, the defense may continue to evolve; more advanced forms of each defense may come into being. When the development of the defense is complete, the potential for its use continues to exist. Whether or not it is used will depend on (1) the relative strength of other available defenses (the chronology of defense development), (2) individual temperament and character style, and (3) the degree of stress being experienced.

Early on, I decided to study three specific defenses: denial, projection, and identification. Briefly, denial may be defined as the failure to see, recognize, or understand the existence or the meaning of an internal or external stimulus, so as to avoid the anxiety that would occur if the stimulus were recognized. Projection may be defined as attributing one's own unacceptable thoughts, feelings, or intentions to others, so as to avoid the anxiety associated with harboring them. Identification is the process of taking on as one's own (internalizing) the attitudes, beliefs, values, or behaviors of another, so as to protect oneself from feelings of weakness or helplessness. Whereas denial and projection tend to distort reality, identification functions by bringing about a change in the self.

I chose these three defenses to study because they represent, theoretically, different degrees of complexity and maturity. Denial is a simple defense, accomplished by the single operation of negating a thought, feeling, or perception, as in "It didn't happen." Because of its cognitive simplicity, it is also considered an "immature" defense. Projection is more complex; it requires the individual to differentiate between what is inside the self and what is outside, and it assumes the establishment of a set of standards regarding what is acceptable to the self and what is not. This defense operates by attributing the internal, unacceptable thought or feeling to something or someone outside of the self. Because of the greater cognitive complexity, this defense is more mature than denial. Identification is the most complex of the three defenses: The individual must be able to differentiate between self and others, to differentiate among others, to form inner representations of others, and to select some qualities of others and reject other qualities. Cognitively, identification is a complex defense and is thus considered more mature than denial or projection.

I reasoned that if these three defenses represent differing degrees of cognitive maturity, then they might be expected to be used by children of different ages—an immature defense would be used by young children, a mature defense by older children or adolescents. Reading the research literature, there was some evidence that denial *was* used more by younger than by older children, but there was little or no empirical research regarding the use of other defenses in relation to children's age.

With this general framework in mind, I proposed a theoretical model that would encompass both the idea that different defenses emerge at different points of development, and that each defense has its own developmental history (Cramer, 1991a). The model is illustrated in Figure 1.1. *Denial*, the simplest defense, was hypothesized to be most prominent among very young children but to decrease in use as they grew older. *Projection*, somewhat more complex, was hypothesized to increase and become predominant during later childhood and early adolescence. *Identification*, the most complex, was hypothesized to develop slowly from childhood on, becoming most important in late adolescence. Notice that, in this model, it is assumed that defenses *develop* during the child's life. Although one defense may predominate at a particular age, the other defenses are present, either in preliminary or residual form.

EARLY RESEARCH STUDYING CHILDREN AND DEFENSE MECHANISMS

The next task was to find evidence that would, or would not, support the model. A study of the existing literature found consistent evidence that the use of the defense of denial was more characteristic of young children than of older children or adolescents (Glasberg & Aboud, 1982; Goldschmid, 1968; Hill & Sarason, 1966; Smith & Danielsson, 1977; Smith & Rossman, 1986). The fact that these studies had used different measures to assess the use of denial gave credence to the conclusion that this was a real phenomenon, not dependent on a particular assessment method. In contrast to these studies of denial, there was little information about developmental differences in the use of projection or identification, but what did exist was consistent in showing that the use of these two defenses increased from childhood to adolescence.

Although research studies that related age to defense use, other than denial, were scarce, the developmental perspective on defense use was also supported by studies in which other indications of developmental level were related to defense use. Less mature defenses, such as denial, were found to be related to less mature levels of ego development (Bond, Gardner, Christian, & Sigal, 1983; Haan, Stroud, & Holstein, 1973; Jacobson, Beardslee, Hauser, Noam, & Powers, 1986; Vaillant & McCullough, 1987), lower levels of IQ (Feather, 1967; Miller & Swanson, 1960; Rump & Court, 1971) and less mature levels of psychosocial development (Vaillant & Drake, 1985).

There were also provocative findings showing that developmental differences existed in children's understanding of how defense mechanisms work. Not only were young children shown to have less understanding than older children, but there was an age-related pattern for the understanding of specific defenses found in several different studies. Specifically, denial was better understood by 8- and 11-year-olds than by 5- to 6-year-olds. Projection was better understood by 11-year-olds than by 8-year-olds, although many 11-year-olds did not understand projection, and none of the younger children understood this defense (Chandler, Paget, & Koch, 1978; Dollinger & McGuire, 1981; Whiteman, 1967).

The realization that there was a parallel between the age of understanding specific defenses and the age at which there was a decline in the use of those defenses raised the intriguing possibility that defense use and defense understanding might be linked. Could it be that, once a child understands how a defense works, she abandons the use of that defense because it no longer serves its function? Because the effectiveness of a defense depends on the user's ignorance of its disguise function, it is no longer an effective defense once an individual understands how the defense is disguising an unacceptable thought or feeling. This line of reasoning, if correct, would suggest that the use of a defense must precede its understanding because understanding it destroys its function. However, before this hypothesis could be tested, more definitive information on the development of defense mechanism use was needed.

THE USE OF NARRATIVE MATERIAL TO STUDY CHILDREN'S USE OF DEFENSES

From a preliminary study of 42 children ages 5–12 years, I devised a method for coding narrative material for the presence of the three defense mechanisms of denial, projection, and identification. (The specifics of this coding system are discussed in Chapter 15.) The criteria for the coding system were, first, that the coding categories for each defense were derived from theoretical descriptions of that defense, and second, that the coding system would demonstrate age differences in the use of the defenses. The final set of coding categories is presented in Table 2.1. An extensive Defense Mechanism Manual (DMM) was prepared, providing rules and examples for each of the coding categories. When this DMM was used to score the children's TAT stories for the use of the three defenses, the results were generally consistent with the theory of defense mechanism development. Dividing the children into three age groups, I found that denial, the least complex defense, was used more often by the youngest children and steadily decreased in use in the two older age groups. In contrast, identification, the most complex defense, was used least often by the youngest children and increased in use across the older age groups. The use of projection, of middling complexity, was used more than denial but less than identification in all three age groups.

The next step in looking for support for the theory of defense mechanism development was to apply this new method for assessing defenses to the narrative productions of a different, larger group of children. For this purpose, more than 300 children, ranging in age from 5 to 16 years, were studied. For each of four age groups (5 years, 9 years, 14 years, and 16 years), the use of denial, projection, and identification was determined by coding their TAT stories. As shown in Figure 2.1, denial was used most frequently by 5-year-olds. After that, its prevalence decreased, and it was used

TABLE 2.1. Defense Mechanism Manual Coding Categories:
Denial, Projection, Identification

Denial

1. Omission of major characters or objects
2. Misperception
3. Reversal
4. Statements of negation
5. Denial of reality
6. Overly maximizing the positive or minimizing the negative
7. Unexpected goodness, optimism, positiveness, or gentleness

Projection

1. Attribution of hostile feelings or intentions, or other normatively unusual feelings or intentions, to a character
2. Additions of ominous people, animals, objects, or qualities
3. Magical or autistic thinking
4. Concern for protection from external threat
5. Apprehensiveness of death, injury, or assault
6. Themes of pursuit, entrapment, and escape
7. Bizarre story or theme

Identification

1. Emulation of skills
2. Emulation of characteristics, qualities, or attitudes
3. Regulation of motives or behavior
4. Self-esteem through affiliation
5. Work; delay of gratification
6. Role differentiation
7. Moralism

infrequently by older children. Projection, in contrast, was used more frequently than denial by age 9 and into adolescence. By later adolescence (age 16), identification had become predominant, being used more frequently than either projection or denial (Cramer, 1987).

A critical test of theory and research is its replication by an independent researcher from a different laboratory. This critical test of the theory of defense mechanism development occurred 10 years later, when John Porcerelli and his colleagues used the DMM to code narrative stories of 150 children and adolescents from a different region of the United States (Porcerelli et al., 1998). The youngest children in this group were slightly older (7 years) than the youngest group in my study (age 5); Porcerelli also included college students in the investigation. As may be seen in Figure 2.2, the results from his independent study virtually replicated my earlier results. They show the same pattern of defense use—the sharp drop in the use

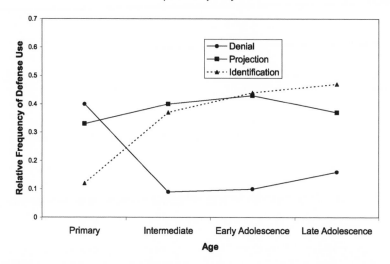

FIGURE 2.1. Defense use in four age groups. From Cramer (1991b); reprinted with permission from the *Journal of Personality.*

of denial after the early years, the greater use of projection during later childhood and adolescence, and the continuing increase in the use of identification until it becomes predominant in late adolescence. Not only was the pattern of results the same, but the relative magnitude of defense use across the two samples was very similar. That is, the points on the two graphs, when matched for age and placed one over the other, were nearly identical.

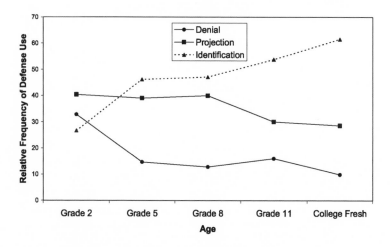

FIGURE 2.2. Defense use in five age groups: Replication.

A third independent study using the DMM to assess age differences also yielded results confirming the original study. Adolescents in the 11th grade were found to use more identification and less denial than students in the fifth grade (Raush, 1994). A similar decrease in the DMM assessment of the use of denial was found in a fourth study by Silverman (1999), and an increase in identification from grade 4 to grade 6 was found by Avery (1985). The latter study also found the use of identification to be positively related to Loevinger's (1966) ego level in the fourth, fifth, and sixth graders.

These studies are all consistent in demonstrating the hypothesized developmental pattern of defense use. A possible drawback, however, is that they were all cross-sectional studies. The findings for each age group came from different children who differed not only in age but possibly in other pertinent characteristics. Although these studies were conducted some 15 years apart and in different regions of the country, it is possible that cohort differences between the age groups, rather than true age differences, might somehow explain the age differences in defense use.

Although this seemed unlikely to me, the only real answer to this possibility was to carry out a longitudinal study, following the same children as they grew older. For this purpose, another research study was carried out, in which the same children were followed from age 6 to age 9; during this time, they were examined at three or four different ages for their use of defense mechanisms (Cramer, 1997b). The cross-sectional data had shown

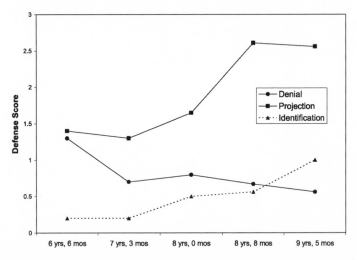

FIGURE 2.3. Longitudinal study of defense development: Ages 6 years, 6 months to 9 years, 5 months. From Cramer (1997b); reprinted with permission from the *Journal of Personality.*

that during this time frame, the use of denial decreases whereas projection increases. The longitudinal study provided an opportunity to see whether this pattern occurs in individual children.

The results of the study are shown in Figure 2.3. Between age 6 years, 6 months and 7 years, 3 months, there was a statistically significant decrease in the use of denial. Further, there was a statistically significant *increase* in the use of projection between ages 8 years, 0 months and 8 years, 8 months. Thus, within a single group of children, the same change in the use of defenses that was demonstrated in the cross-sectional studies was noted in the longitudinal study as well.

ARE DEFENSES BEING ASSESSED?: THE VALIDITY OF THE DMM

The results of these studies, as well as others discussed later (Cramer & Gaul, 1988; Cramer & Brilliant, 2001), clearly support the prediction that children of different ages use different defenses and that there is a developmental pattern in the predominance of the three defenses. Looked at from a different perspective, these results demonstrated that the DMM coding system is measuring developmental changes—that is, the coding system is assessing something that changes with age. But how do we know that we are really assessing defense mechanisms? In other words, how do we know that this defense coding system is *valid*?

Theory provides us with several postulates which, if supported by empirical research, give evidence of construct validity. First, once the function of a defense becomes conscious, it should be given up. Second, the use of defense mechanisms should increase under conditions of stress. Third, the use of defense mechanisms should protect the person from psychological upset. Finally, the use of defense mechanisms should be related to other facets of personality in ways that make sense psychologically.

The following section addresses the question of how the conscious understanding of a defense mechanism changes the use of that defense. Subsequent chapters demonstrate how stress influences defense use, which in turn reduces psychological upset, and how defense use is related to personality and personality change.

UNDERSTANDING A DEFENSE SHOULD PRECLUDE ITS USE

Defenses work—that is, reduce anxiety and protect self-esteem—because people are not aware of their function. The purpose of attributing one's

own anger or envy to others is to absolve oneself of the discomfort of harboring unacceptable thoughts or feelings. To realize that this negative perception of others is based on the attribution of one's own negative emotions
would be to acknowledge that one has such unacceptable emotions; such a
realization would be a cause for self-reproach and anxiety. To be aware of
the operation of the defense should thus render its disguise function ineffective.

Why should children shift away from using denial at 7 years of age? As
discussed below, it turns out that this is the age when children are able to
understand how denial works—its "disguise" function becomes clear to the
child. It seems likely that this new cognitive ability is part of the larger
change in cognitive development that is occurring around age 7. At about
the time that children shift from using denial to using projection, a more
general cognitive reorganization is occurring. As described by Piaget, it is at
this age that children move from the preoperational stage of cognitive development to the concrete operational stage. Their thinking becomes more
complex; they are able to consider more than one dimension at a time, and
they develop the capacity for perspective taking. Theoretically, these new
cognitive abilities should contribute to the "demystifying" of denial and its
subsequent replacement with projection.

A study of children provided confirmation for this theory. This study
was prompted by theory, but it also made use of two previous research
findings. First, as just discussed, it had been demonstrated that around age
7 children shifted from using denial as the primary defense to using projection. Second, as discussed, previous investigations had shown that few
children younger than 7 years understood the functioning of denial, and
practically none understood projection. In contrast, the large majority of
11-year-olds understood denial, but few were reported to understand projection. Thus there was a parallel to be seen between the developmental
sequence in the use of denial and projection and the developmental progression in the understanding of these defenses, with use preceding, in age,
understanding.

To investigate whether this pattern—defense use, followed by defense
understanding, followed by reduction in defense use—actually occurs,
more than 100 children from two age groups were examined (Cramer &
Brilliant, 2001). The younger group (mean age = 7 years) was chosen because this is the age at which many children shift from using denial as the
predominant defense to using projection. Presumably, this shift should be
related to their increased understanding of denial, so that those who understand denial should be less likely to use this defense. The older group (mean
age 10) was chosen because this is the age at which most children are using
projection as the predominant defense; those who are using this defense
should have little understanding of it. For the occasional child in this age

group who understands projection, his use of the defense should be minimal.

The children were assessed for their use of defense mechanisms and for their understanding of defenses on separate occasions. First, we had the children tell stories, which were then coded for defense use. In addition, we took a measure of their IQ using the well-standardized Peabody Picture Vocabulary Test. Two weeks later we presented the same children with short stories—vignettes—in which a child character displays the use of a defense. For example, one of the denial vignettes described a child who had been rejected by a playmate; the rejected child then says to his mother, "I don't care; I didn't really want to play with him."

Our child subject was read this vignette and then asked to explain *why* the boy said that. There were two vignettes illustrating the defense of denial and two illustrating projection, matched for gender with each subject. The explanations of the defense in the denial and projection vignettes were coded according to a system we had devised previously, summed over two vignettes. A score of 2 indicated "no understanding"; 4 = "minimal understanding"; 6 = "partial understanding"; and 8 = "full understanding" of each defense.

We determined each child's use of denial and projection and understanding of each defense. The results indicated that the younger children, as a group, used denial more often than the older children, as would be expected. The results also indicated that the younger children had less understanding of denial than did the older children. Most relevant, among the younger children there were differences in level of understanding (see Figure 2.4). To determine how defense understanding related to defense use, the 7-year-olds who had partial or complete understanding of denial (scores of 6 or 7) were compared with those who had minimal or no understanding (scores of 2–5), to determine if there were differences in the degree to which the two groups made *use* of denial. This comparison showed that those who had greater understanding of the defense used it significantly less often (see Figure 2.5).

Similar analyses of the use and understanding of the defense of projection were carried out with the older children. The older group showed more understanding of projection than did the younger group; however, among the older children there were also differences in level of understanding (see Figure 2.6). When defense use was related to defense understanding for this older group of children, there was a clear linear relation between the use of projection and the understanding of projection: Children who had no understanding made the greatest use of projection; those who had more understanding used the defense less (see Figure 2.7).

Taken together, the findings from the younger and older children support the hypothesis that (1) there is a developmental pattern in both the use

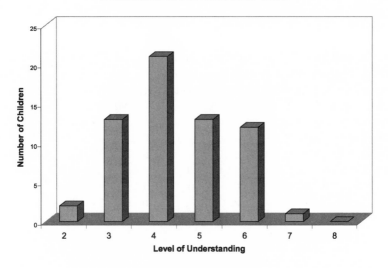

FIGURE 2.4. Understanding denial: Grades 1 and 2.

and understanding of defenses, (2) use and understanding are linked in the developmental progression, and (3) this linking is especially strong during the developmental period for which the defense is age appropriate. Use of a defense precedes its understanding; once it is understood, it is used less often and is gradually superseded by a more complex defense that is not yet understood.

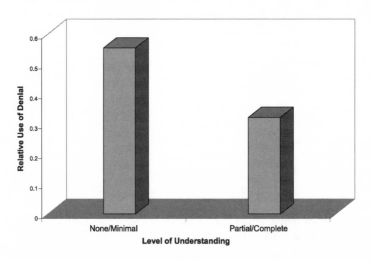

FIGURE 2.5. Use and understanding of denial: Grades 1 and 2.

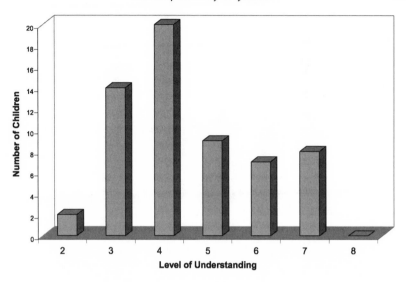

FIGURE 2.6. Understanding projection: Grades 4 and 5.

DEFENSE USE IN ADOLESCENCE

As discussed above, studies with the DMM indicated that the use of identification was found to be greater among late adolescents (mean age = 16 years) than early adolescents (mean age = 14 years, 6 months; Cramer, 1987). This finding was replicated by Porcerelli et al. (1998), who found, in addition, that the use of identification was even greater among college students as compared to the younger students.

In an early study using the DMI as the measure to assess defense use, a comparison of a younger adolescent group (mean age = 14 years) and an older group (mean age = 16 years) failed to show differences in defense choice (Cramer, 1979). Possible relations between adolescent developmental level and DMI defense choice was then approached in a different manner by Levit (1993), who reasoned that adolescent developmental differences in defense use might be easier to discover if the index of development were based on level of ego maturity rather than chronological age. Accordingly, the DMI scores of 66 adolescents, ages 14–19 years, were related to level of ego development, as assessed by Loevinger's Sentence Completion Test (Loevinger & Wessler, 1970). The results indicated that adolescent level of ego development was negatively correlated with the choice of turning against the object (TAO) and positively correlated with reversal (REV) and turning against the subject (TAS), the latter relation being due primarily to the girls in the sample. The results with projection and principal-

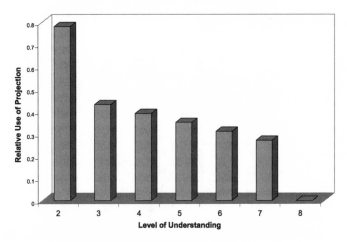

FIGURE 2.7. Use and understanding of projection: Grades 4 and 5. From Cramer and Brilliant (2001); reprinted with permission from the *Journal of Personality.*

ization (PRN; i.e., isolation, intellectualization, and rationalization) were not significant.

A conceptually similar study was carried out by Evans and Seaman (2000; discussed further in Chapter 6). Based on the DSQ-78, adolescents were divided into two groups: "mature" and "immature" defense users. The mature group showed greater ability to differentiate among various domains of their self-concept (e.g., parent relationships, peer acceptance, athletic and scholastic ability, romantic relationships, friendships, and physical appearance), suggesting a higher developmental level in the adolescents who used more mature defenses.

The immature group showed less differentiation among the various domains of the self-concept, suggesting a kind of developmental delay. Although the defense of identification is not part of the DSQ defense measure, the use of mature defenses by these adolescents was related to increased differentiation of the self-concept, or delineation of self-identity. The authors concluded that these findings support the theory of defense mechanism development.

Although these findings do demonstrate a relationship between defense choice and level of ego development, they do not address the issue of whether adolescent defense use changes with age. This question of change was investigated in a sample of 516 Finnish adolescents (Tuulio-Henriksson, Poikolainen, Aalto-Setala, & Lonnqvist, 1997). Using the DSQ-72, these young men and women were assessed for defense use at age 16 years and again at age 21 years. The results indicated an increase in scores on the mature scale and a decrease on both the immature and neurotic scales.

DEFENSE USE IN ADULTHOOD

The DMM has been used to study defense use in young adults and in early adulthood. Participants in the Block and Block (1980) longitudinal study were assessed for defense use at age 23 years on the basis of stories told in response to six TAT cards (Cramer, 1997a, 1999b; Cramer & Block, 1998). The results were consistent with the expectation that denial would be used less frequently than projection in this age group. However, as compared with samples of undergraduate college students, these young adults were relatively low on identification, using it less frequently than projection.

Similar findings come from a study of early adulthood (mean age = 34 years) from the intergenerational study carried out at the Institute of Human Development, University of California, Berkeley. DMM assessment of defense use indicated that projection was used more frequently than either denial or identification (Cramer, 2003b, 2004).

Both of these studies show that, with samples of individuals from young and early adulthood, the relative importance of the use of identification has decreased, as compared to its predominance in late adolescence (Cramer, 1987, 1995; Porcerelli et al., 1998). This difference may reflect the fact that the issue of identity development (and the related use of identification as a defense; see Chapter 5) is of primary importance for the late adolescent, but its salience decreases in adulthood. Evidence for this assumption comes from another longitudinal study of college students (Cramer, 1998b; see Chapter 7). On entry to college at age 18, identification was these students' predominant defense mechanism. However, by the time they became seniors, their use of this defense had significantly decreased ($p < .06$).

This idea of the declining salience of identification after late adolescence was also discussed by Hibbard et al. (2000) to explain their finding, using the DMM, that identification was related to attachment style in Asian women (who were 20 years old) but was not related in white women (who were 24 years old). Despite the cultural differences, the authors suggest that because identification is more typically a task of late adolescence, there may be different implications of using it at younger and older ages.

Little is known about *change* in defense use as adults grow older; more often, age differences have been studied. There are, however, several hypotheses about the kind of change that might be expected and the reasons for such change. The regression hypothesis (Gutmann, 1964) suggests that as people grow older, they may return (regress) to using defenses that were characteristic of an earlier period of development; thus older age would be associated with the use of immature defenses. An alternative point of view is represented in the growth hypothesis (Vaillant, 1977), which posits that older people use increasingly effective defenses that are less distorting of reality; thus older age would be associated with the use of mature defenses.[3] Yet a third viewpoint, the contextual hypothesis (McCrae, 1984), suggests that changes in defense use associated with age are due to the different types of stress that different age groups encounter, rather than to age-based developmental changes.

Most studies of *difference* in defense choice at different adult ages have relied on the DSQ. Andrews et al. (1993), using the DSQ-72 and DSQ-40, found that the use of "immature" defenses decreased in age groups from 18–25 to 35–50 to beyond 50 years. Age findings for the "neurotic" and "mature" defenses were not reported.

Another study using the DSQ-36 to investigate age differences created three age groups: adolescents (ages 17–23 years, mean = 19 years), middle age (40–47 years; mean = 43 years) and older age (63–70 years; mean = 66 years) (Whitty, 2003). A comparison of the 40 individuals in each age group indicated that the adolescents had higher scores on the Immature scale, whereas middle- and older-age individuals did not differ. Also adolescents had lower scores on the Mature defense scale, whereas the two adult groups did not differ. A further study of 354 women, ages 26–70 years, found that the DSQ-40 Mature scale was positively correlated with age (Romans, Martin, Morris, & Herbison, 1999).

In an additional study, a variation on the DSQ-78 was devised for assessing both adolescents and adults (Steiner et al., 2001). This questionnaire, termed the Response Evaluation Measure (REM-71), was completed by 1,487 adolescents ages 13–19 years (mean age = 16 years) from local suburban high schools and by adults found at a local airport (ages 20–39 years, $n = 192$; older than 39 years, $n = 196$). Based on a factor analysis of the 71 items designed to represent 21 defenses, two factors emerged, differing in defense maturity.[4] When the three age groups were compared, the less mature factor scale showed a significant decrease across the three ages. Also scores on each of the 14 defenses comprising this factor (e.g., Displacement, Projection, Undoing, Splitting, Dissociation) were significantly lower as age increased. This decrease occurred primarily between adolescence and early adulthood (ages 20–39 years). Scores on the more mature factor scale did not differ across age, due to the finding that some defense scores were higher (Intellectualization, Suppression, and Humor), some were lower (Altruism, Idealization) and some remained the same (Reaction Formation).

In another study of individuals ages 20–95 years, the relation between age and use of DSQ-88 defenses was determined (Costa, Zonderman, & McCrae, 1991). Age was found to be negatively correlated with the DSQ

Maladaptive Action factor and positively correlated with the DSQ Self-Sacrificing factor. However, as the authors pointed out, the magnitude of the correlations was relatively small (–.12 and .27), suggesting only a weak relation between age and defense use.

The findings of studies based on the DSQ are thus consistent in showing that the use of immature defenses is less frequent as age increases, and that the greatest decrease occurs between adolescence and middle age. They are inconsistent, however, on the question of age differences in mature defenses, possibly due to the different defenses used to comprise the Mature scale in the different studies.

One further study of age differences used the DMI to assess self-reported defense use in seven age groups, ranging from early adolescent (age 12 years) to older adulthood (age 70 years and above; Diehl, Coyle, & Labouvie-Vief, 1996). In contrast to the findings using the DSQ, this study found an increase in the immature defense of REV with age. The older groups were also more likely to report using PRN, whereas the younger age groups reported greater use of projection and TAO.

A problem with drawing developmental conclusions from these cross-sectional studies is that it is difficult to know the degree to which the findings reflect cohort differences. Cross-sectional studies involve individuals from different generations; age differences that are found may really represent different generational experiences (Costa et al., 1991). They may also reflect group differences in education, IQ, or current economic or social status, among other variables. After reviewing a large number of cross-sectional studies, Costa et al. (1991) concluded that, among adults, there is minimal evidence that defense use is related to age. They based this argument, in part, on findings that defense use in adults is related to personality characteristics.[5] Since they assumed that personality characteristics are stable in adulthood, not changing much after age 30, the implication is that defense use is also stable. However, more recent studies have demonstrated significant personality change in adulthood (Aldwin & Levenson, 1994; Cramer, 2003b, 2004; Haan, Millsap, & Hartka, 1986; Helson, Pals, & Solomon, 1997; Helson & Stewart, 1994; Helson & Wink, 1992; Helson, Kwan, John, & Jones, 2002; Roberts, 1997; Srivastava, John, Gosling, & Potter, 2003).

To avoid this problem of cohort differences, a time-consuming longitudinal study is required. Such a study has been carried out by Vaillant (1990, 1993), who followed college men into adulthood. Between the ages of 20 and 35+ years, Vaillant found a decrease in the use of immature defenses (although dissociation/neurotic denial occurred frequently in adulthood) and an increase in mature defenses. This study is discussed further in Chapter 10.

CONCLUDING REMARKS

In this chapter we have reviewed the theory of defense mechanism development. Defense mechanisms are seen to develop out of biologically given
motor reflexes, which then come under conscious control and continue as
volitional behavior. The schema for these behaviors are eventually internalized and represented ideationally, creating the foundation from which mental mechanisms of defense emerge.

The developmental theory of defense mechanisms includes two main
premises: (1) different defense mechanisms become predominant at different periods of development and thus are related to chronological age; and
(2) each defense has its own developmental history. Following from my interest in the developmental pattern of defense formation, I chose to study
three defenses that represent increasing complexity and maturity: denial,
projection, and identification. This research required the creation of a
method to study defense use in children.

A coding scheme was developed to use in conjunction with narrative
material (TAT stories) provided by children of different ages. As hypothesized, it was found that the use of denial was characteristic of young children, projection predominated in late childhood and early adolescence,
and identification was most characteristics of late adolescence. These developmental findings have been substantiated in four further cross-sectional investigations from independent laboratories, as well as from further studies of my own. They have also been confirmed by longitudinal
study.

In our work with children we also provided evidence for the validity of
the DMM as a method to assess defense mechanisms. Given that defenses
are theorized to be successful because they function outside of awareness, it
follows, theoretically, that once a person becomes aware of the defense and
its function, it would no longer be useful. A controlled study of children
demonstrated that the change in the use of defenses with age is related to
the child developing an understanding of the functioning of individual defenses, and that, once the nature of the defense is understood, it is used less
often.

Developmental studies using a different measure of defense mechanisms (the DSQ) also demonstrated that immature defenses are used less
frequently by adults than by adolescents, who use them less frequently than
children. On the other hand, the use of mature defenses is more prevalent
in adulthood than in adolescence. Within the adult years, it appears that
the use of immature defenses is less frequent among older adults, whereas
the use of mature defenses does not differ across adult ages; however, there
are some exceptions to these general findings. Of some interest is the finding that the use of identification, as assessed by the DMM, decreases in

prevalence by early adulthood, as compared to late adolescence. It seems likely that this finding is related to the decreasing salience of the issue of identity/identity development that characterizes the late adolescent period. Considered from a different perspective, this finding suggests that a continuing reliance on identification as a defense after late adolescence may have important implications for psychological functioning.

PART II

A Closer Look at Three Defenses

In the next three chapters we take a closer look at the defenses of denial (Chapter 3), projection (Chapter 4), and identification (Chapter 5). As discussed in Chapter 2, these three defenses are chosen for study because they represent three different points in defense development during childhood and adolescence. Here I focus on a theoretical and clinical understanding of these defenses. In each case I trace the ontogenetic line of the defense development and the various forms the defense may take. The chapters include a discussion of how each defense may occur as part of normal development, as well as illustrations of the defenses in connection with psychological disturbance. The universality of these defenses is illustrated through a consideration of several myths and fairytales.

An understanding of the nature of these defenses—both their development and their components—is critical to recognizing their occurrence in narrative material. A careful reading of these chapters is therefore essential to become proficient in the use of the DMM. More important, reading these chapters should increase one's general understanding of how defenses develop, how they function, how they have informed cultural myth, and how they appear in clinical material.

CHAPTER 3

Denial

Though knowing the truth, he may act as if it did not exist.
—FENICHEL (1945, p. 145)

Denial functions through the disavowal of whole percepts
and the substitution of a wish-fulfilling fantasy. . . .
—LICHTENBERG AND SLAP (1972, p. 781)

The first defense mechanism to be discussed in detail, denial, is also one of the earliest defenses available to the child. Along with primary repression, denial is available to serve a defensive function during the earliest months of life. Whereas primary repression protects the child from being overwhelmed by instinctual demands, denial functions to ward off upsetting perceptions of the external world (Freud, 1940).[1]

To understand the nature of this defense mechanism, I begin by discussing the various components of denial—the mental processes involved in its operation and the ways in which it may be manifest. This discussion is followed by a recounting of several well-known folktales in which significant aspects of the stories rely on the mechanism of denial. The question of the development of two different forms of denial and their developmental course is considered next. The results of laboratory studies showing the early use of perceptual denial illustrate one form of denial, and a literary study of *Candide,* which exemplifies denial through the imposition of a personal fantasy onto reality, illustrates the second form. The intertwining of these two forms of denial is illustrated by yet another folktale. The functioning of denial is then considered in several clinical cases. Finally, the ways in which denial may be manifest in projective storytelling are illustrated.

43

COMPONENTS OF DENIAL

The defense mechanism of denial, in its simplest form, is easy to conceptualize. In popular lore, it is seen in the advice "Just ignore it, and it will go away." Theoretically, denial in this form refers to a mental operation in which attention is withdrawn from external stimuli that, if recognized, would cause psychological pain or upset. The focus here is on a defense mechanism that functions to ward off external reality. It was this external focus that characterized the early descriptions of denial (e.g., Freud, 1911, 1923, 1924).

In subsequent writings, however, the concept of denial was expanded to include a warding off of certain internal stimuli, accompanied by a covering over, or a "screen," which substituted for the painful thought (e.g., Freud, 1925; Fenichel, 1945; Jacobson, 1957). This conception created some difficulties in distinguishing denial from repression. Theoretically, denial was seen as directed against memories that were preconscious (i.e., potentially available to awareness), as distinguished from repression, which was directed against unconscious memories (i.e., unavailable to consciousness under ordinary circumstances; cf. Jacobson, 1957; Moore & Rubinfine, 1969; Sjoback, 1973). In either case, the means by which the "warding off" or "disavowal" of events occurs in denial has been expanded to include not only the withdrawal of attention but also a variety of other mental operations. A consideration of the components of denial, as these have been discussed in the literature, indicates that this defense, as it occurs in adults, is more complex than what would be involved in a simple ignoring of reality.

A most primitive component of denial is the failure to see what exists in reality. To not see or not hear what is "really" there, when it occurs in an adult, indicates a severe breakdown of reality testing that we associate with a psychotic condition. Theoretically, this "not seeing" can occur through the total withdrawal of attention from the event, or through a "negative hallucination."

Denial may also be manifest in a less extreme form through a physical or psychological withdrawal from the painful situation; reality may be ignored. Denial in this form is less absolute, for it allows the possibility to bring the denied event back into focus through, for example, sensitive questioning on the part of a therapist. Another component of denial, related to ignoring reality, involves making mistakes in reality testing (misperception) or misinterpreting the meaning of events.

These components of denial, with the possible exception of the last mentioned, are all closely tied to the functioning of the perceptual system. It is this system that provides our first bridge to the outside world as well as our only means for protection against it. It is for this reason that a defense based on the malfunctioning of the perceptual system is considered so primitive.

Denial, however, occurs in other forms. An event may be perceived but only accepted in a negated form, as in "It didn't happen that way."[2] Less extreme than outright negation, but serving the same purpose of avoiding painful anxiety, is the operation of minimizing the anxiety-arousing event or ridiculing its importance. A related mental operation is that of overexaggeration to such proportions that the existence in reality of the described event must ultimately be denied. Reversal—changing the experience of the event into its opposite—may also be grouped with these manifestations of denial. Although we think of negation, minimization, exaggeration, and reversal as occurring primarily in the verbal domain, such distortions are clearly possible on a perceptual level. In any case, this method of dealing with an upsetting experience by changing its psychological "size" can be understood as a derivative of the perceptual distortion that forms the base of this defense.

Denial is also expressed through "enacted daydreams," the satisfactions of which may replace the disappointments of reality (A. Freud, 1936). Although these are common enough in the make-believe play of children, they are less likely to be acted out by adults. Instead, these daydreams remain as internal fantasies but may continue to function as part of denial.

Such fantasies serve denial in several ways. If the unreal can be made to appear true, then the real may be delegated to the realm of the untrue. In this case the fantasies, unaffected by external events, acquire a salience that rivals external reality. Eventually these fantasies come to exist as an alternative reality. The denial function of this personally constructed alternative reality is manifest when it is imposed on the external world. Real events are then recognized only insofar as they conform to the fantasy. The occurrence of unfounded optimism and elation in the face of objective failure is a manifestation of this component of denial and may be understood as a result of the substitution of a personal fantasy for objective reality.

These various components of denial can be subsumed under two broad categories. First, some operations are closely tied to the perceptual system; they ward off reality through not seeing, through avoiding, or through distorting what is perceived. At the basis of these operations is an interference with the registration of perceptual experience.

A second form of denial occurs more on the cognitive level and involves the construction of a personal fantasy. The individual's involvement in this fantasy rivals the perception of reality and replaces it in significant portions of her experience. These fantasies may also be imposed on reality with an insistence that other people agree with the fantasy and ignore reality. The perceptual system may continue to function, but it takes second place to the much preferred personalized fantasy.

The remaining components of the defense of denial—negation, minimizing, maximizing, ridicule, and reversal—may occur in conjunction with either of these two forms of denial and provide the link between them. They may be used to ward off reality by changing perception in such a way that reality is no longer threatening, or they may be used to modify the internal meaning of a perception so that it agrees with the personal fantasy construction.

DENIAL AS SEEN IN FOLKTALES

It is interesting to note the ways in which denial appears in well-known folktales. Sometimes the entire plot is based on the main character's use of this defense, which provides the tale with either a comical note or a heightened dramatic quality. In these stories, denial occurs on a perceptual level. Examples of such tales are "The Emperor's New Clothes" and "Little Red Riding Hood." In other instances denial appears in the form of a personal fantasy imposed onto a situation that is otherwise bleak and ugly. Examples of this type of tale are "Cinderella" and "Snow White."

Perceptual Denial

In "The Emperor's New Clothes,"[3] two rogues come to town with a promise to weave a most beautiful cloth, so fine that it can be seen only by a very wise man. The emperor, who is very vain and especially fond of clothes, requests a suit to be made of this extraordinary material and pays the two rogues handsomely. He recounts the anticipated beauty of this cloth and the personal qualities necessary to see it to his courtiers. As time passes, the courtiers are sent to report on the weaving, and eventually the emperor himself goes to see the new suit of clothes.

As we are aware, no cloth was being woven. Nevertheless, after each visit by the royal court, the beauty of the cloth was praised; that is, the nonexistence of the cloth was denied. Each viewer attributed his difficulty in seeing the cloth to his own stupidity, believing that if he were smarter, he would be able to see the (nonexistent) cloth. The denial is carried to an extreme when the emperor rides through the town in a grand procession, wearing the new suit. The townspeople praise the beauty of the new clothes. The end of the story turns on the pronouncement of a little child, who looks at the emperor and cries aloud, "But he hasn't got anything on!"

The theme of this tale is based on the most primitive component of denial—failure to perceive what is there or, in this case, what is *not* there. The tale makes it clear to the reader that, in reality, there is no cloth and no suit. Yet we are asked to believe that the wise men of the town behave otherwise. It is noteworthy that to convince readers that this collective misperception is believable, the author must provide some sort of explanation as to how such a primitive operation as perceptual denial could come about in men who are not psychotic. This explanation is carried out by the introduction of the fantasy that only wise men can see the cloth. In this way the author draws in the component of a self-serving personal fantasy—that each man believes he is not stupid—to bolster the plausibility that perceptual denial could occur in a group of adults. The author is also intuitively correct when he places the use of denial in the context of vanity and narcissism. It is the wish of these men to see themselves as smart that facilitates the disavowal of reality.[4]

The literary conceit of the tale comes when a child unfrocks the defense. The defense of denial, quite inappropriate for grown men, is exposed by a youngster who, under ordinary circumstances, might be expected to participate in the defense. It is this juxtaposition of the old being fooled by the primitive, while the young sees clearly past his years, that highlights the folly of the tale.

Tales of pure perceptual denial are hard to find, perhaps because they are so difficult to present. For to describe this mechanism, the reader must first be apprised of reality, and then a character who misperceives this reality must be introduced. Inevitably, some sort of explanation for this character's perceptual errors must be given. In the case of the emperor, the explanation is the personal fantasy. In the case of the comic strip character Mr. Magoo, the explanation stays on the perceptual level: Mr. Magoo is extremely nearsighted.

One well-known fairytale that does make use of the schema of presenting reality and then portraying reality as denied is Little Red Riding Hood.[5] In the early part of the tale the reader and Red Riding Hood encounter a wolf. Red Riding Hood has a short conversation with him, presumably giving her an opportunity to see what he looks like. Yet, even at this early point in the story, the denial of reality is stated explicitly: "Red Riding Hood did not know what a wicked animal he was, so she was not a bit afraid of him."

While the girl gathers flowers, the wolf runs ahead to grandmother's house. After disposing of the old woman, the wolf puts on her clothes and climbs into her bed. Eventually, Red Riding Hood arrives; "She felt quite frightened but she did not know why." Systematically, she examines the body in the bed and denies the significance of what she sees. She comments on the big ears, the big eyes, the big hands, and the big teeth of the wolf, but the meaning of these perceptions—that the wolf is in bed, not grandmother—does not register.

In the end, of course, such massive denial breaks down; reality overwhelms and the wolf consumes her. Then, perhaps out of consideration for his reader, the author provides one more denial to reduce anxiety: The wolf's stomach is cut open, and the little girl springs out, whole and hearty.

The dramatic high point in this tale is carried out through the repetitive noting of specific perceptual details—the various parts of the wolf's body—in conjunction with a continuing failure to recognize what is seen. That Red Riding Hood has had the opportunity to know, in reality, that this is a wolf and not her grandmother is assured by her prior experience with both. And although she did not know to be afraid on her first encounter with the wolf, she does experience fear on the second meeting. So it is neither lack of reality experience nor lack of fear that explains Red Riding Hood's failure to recognize the dangerous situation she is in. Rather, her failure in reality testing and her denial of the meaning of her perceptions can be understood as a defensive maneuver: If the wolf can be denied, so can her fear.

The Imposition of a Personal Fantasy

The second type of denial, in which an emotionally pleasant, self-sustaining fantasy is imposed on an otherwise bleak and unfulfilling reality, is a common motif in fairytales. For example, Cinderella, who lives in dirt and ashes as a servant in the home of her cruel stepfamily, is transformed into a beautiful maiden who marries the prince. Snow White, cast out to die by a wicked stepmother, is rescued by a life-giving prince.[6]

It is interesting, however, to see how this type of denial is played out in the lesser characters and to note its inevitable failure. In "Cinderella," the attempt to enact a personal fantasy that is at odds with reality forms the basis for the characters of the stepsisters. In reality ugly, mean, and coarse, they appear at the ball dressed in finery, acting the part of potential sweethearts to the prince, seemingly oblivious to the discrepancy between their fantasized view of themselves and the unattractive picture that others perceive. The discrepancy between their personal fantasy and reality comes into dramatic focus when they attempt, despite the obvious elephantine dimensions of their feet, to squeeze them into a noticeably tiny glass slipper.[7] In this grotesque attempt we see the continuing belief that they are dainty, petite, and glamorous take precedence over the glaring reality of a big foot confronted with a petite shoe.

Another example of the insistent imposition of a personal fantasy onto reality occurs in the character of Snow White's wicked stepmother. Like Cinderella's stepsisters, she is quite vain. Although probably attractive in reality, the magnitude of her beauty is of continual concern to her. Indeed, her character is driven by the personal fantasy that she must be the *most* beautiful, and it is this fantasy that she puts to the test and imposes, time after time, in her query: "Mirror, mirror, on the wall, who is fairest of us all?"

In this repetitive insistence that her fantasy be verified by another, we encounter one of the frequent accompaniments of this type of denial: the insistence that someone else agree with, or mirror, the person's own (fantasy) view of herself and the world. When this need for mirroring, which is a normal part of the child's early life, occurs in an adult in conjunction with denial of the sort described here, it has a peremptory aspect. Others must agree with the queen's personal fantasy. If they do not, as came to pass with the mirror ("Queen, thou art the fairest in this hall, But Snow White's fairer than us all"), then a furious rage may be unleashed. In the case of the queen, this fury was directed toward Snow White, who must be eliminated because she challenged the queen's fantasy. Another possible outcome would have been to shatter the mirror—to destroy the one who does not reflect, or validate, the personal fantasy.

Denial and Pathology

In these fairytales there is something ludicrous about the insistence of the sisters and the queen in imposing their personal myth on reality: in the case of the sisters, because of the obvious discrepancy between their personal fantasy and reality, and in the case of the queen, because of her repeated need for validation. But there are other occasions when this type of denial evokes feelings of pathos or can be accepted as "in the service of the need to survive" (Geleerd, 1965, p. 123).

A poignant example of this type of denial is given by Anna Freud (1973) in her description of an English child during World War II. As was true for many wartime children, 3-year-old Billie had been removed to a shelter in the country, which was physically safer than his home in the big city, but separated him absolutely from his mother. In an attempt to deny this devastating reality, he focused instead on a personal fantasy that his mother would come and claim him, and he imposed this fantasy on those around him. He would repeat, over and over, that Mother would come, and he listed, monotonously, the various garments she would put on him before he left in a fantasized departure with her. A request to stop this litany lowered its volume to sotto voce, but he continued to enact the fantasy in his movements, putting on various articles of imagined clothing.

The pathetic quality of this attempt to make reality conform to his personal myth is striking. Although, objectively, his behavior is no less silly than that of the stepsisters, the emotions evoked are different. For we understand that this is a child struggling for survival in a situation he is largely helpless to modify. The world events that necessitated removal from his mother are gigantic and too devastating to accept, and his inner capacities to effect change are extremely limited. In the face of imminent destruction, which he is powerless to influence, the alternatives are to give up (psychological annihilation) or to believe that things are different from what they are.

The frantic enactment of the denial fantasy in this little boy is a good example of Geleerd's "denial in the service of the need to survive" (Geleerd, 1965, p. 123). As she points out, the real world is indeed filled with many horrors and potential catastrophes: illnesses, wars, accidents, hurricanes, tornadoes, earthquakes, and floods. Yet we continue to live our lives as if those realities did not exist—that is, they do not form part of our personal worldview. The imposition by terminally ill patients and their families of the fantasy of health and recovery is well known.[8] Although we know the statistics regarding airplane crashes, we believe we are exempt from those probabilities and we continue to fly. Although we have seen our own country blow up entire cities in atomic warfare, we continue our lives without concern that we might be destroyed on a moment's notice. Even though we have seen our own skyscrapers demolished into flaming death traps, we continue to live and work in similar buildings. In these and many other instances, a personal fantasy of survival is imposed on a reality that indicates otherwise. Geleerd speaks of this type of denial as both normal and instinctive, with its origin in the wish to live. By and large, these denial fantasies do not interfere with human relationships and are not linked to unresolved unconscious conflicts. As with Billie, we must believe that we will survive in order to do so.

The implications of these situations are that, under certain conditions, the use of the defense of denial is normal and nonpathological: when (1) the external reality is overwhelming and immutable, or (2) the person, due to chronological immaturity, has no capacity to change or make an impact on reality. Denial of self-destruction related to wars, floods, and accidents is of the first type. The denial seen in Billie is of the second type: He had neither physical nor psychological capacity to effect a reunion with his mother.

The use of denial becomes pathological when neither of the above conditions is present, although frequently the individual may believe them to exist. For example, beneath the denial fantasy of superiority and elitism may be the warded-off view that the world will always be critical and rejecting, and one will always be alone. This distorted view of reality carries the same sense of absolute immutability as does the reality of life-destroying natural events, and the associated pain is handled in the same way—it is denied through the imposition of an alternative reality. Through this fantasy, what is felt to be immutable is avoided.

Pathological denial may also occur in adults who feel they have no capacity to affect reality, a condition that occurs when ego development is arrested. Their experience is like Billie's: They feel unable to act, to think, and to hold their own feelings. They do not believe that there is anything they can do to change the unhappy situation. Their interpersonal problems frequently center on the insistent search for someone else to think and act for them and to take care of their feelings. The helpless, and hopeless, passivity of these patients is pervasive. Their experience of inadequate ego resources, which is normal and age appropriate in young children, reflects a pathological lack of ego development when it occurs in adults. In such circumstances, feeling oneself to be powerless and without internal resources, denial is an available solution.[9]

THE DEVELOPMENT OF TWO FORMS OF DENIAL

In this section I propose that the components of denial emerge in a somewhat orderly fashion: that some appear not long after birth, whereas others depend on the development of the cognitive capacity for an elaborate internalized fantasy representation. I would like to begin with two extremes as starting points. In one case, I start at the beginning of life—the baby during the first year. In the second case, I begin with the young adult. In both cases, to make a clearer illustration, I rely on examples in which denial is used to a pathological extreme because it is easier to see in this exaggerated form. However, I argue that this is but an amplification of the normal course of events. In the first case I trace the development of the components of perceptual denial from birth forward. In the second case I trace the components of denial through fantasy retrospectively, from the idealization fantasy of the young adult back through its earlier manifestations in childhood and infancy.[10]

Perceptual Denial

Theoretically, the prototype for denial is to look and not to see. In the absence of physical incapacity, we understand this "not seeing" to be the result of withdrawing psychological attention from the external world. Looking and not seeing, as it occurs in infants, is the most primitive and earliest form of denial, in which the perceptual system simply shuts down. Although other components of denial involve some change or modification of reality, this most basic component functions by ignoring reality altogether. What is not there cannot produce any pain.

The failure of the infant to respond to stimuli that are clearly present may be the result of the withdrawal of attention from the external world, or may be due to the functioning of the "stimulus barrier," or some combination of these two. The stimulus barrier concept, as defined by Freud (1920), refers to an innate protective mechanism, present in most infants, that prevents the baby from being overwhelmed by excessive external stimulation. As such, it can be understood as an early component of denial.[11] The functioning of the stimulus barrier appears to alternate with periods of alert inactivity, in which the baby pays attention to what is going on in the external world. Moreover, there appear to be innate differences among infants both in the presence of periods of innate activity and in the presence–absence of the stimulus barrier (Wolff, 1959; Bergman & Escalona, 1949). These differences suggest the possibility of biological differences in the propensity to use denial.

Primitive as this component is, it is possible to point to an even earlier predecessor of this shutting off of perception. From the beginning, the infant comes with what Spitz called "the prototype of all defense" (1957, p. 76)—namely, the capacity to fall asleep when overwhelmed with excessive stimulation. The near-total withdrawal of attention from the outside world that occurs in sleep is, then, the earliest manifestation of perceptual denial.[12]

The capacity of the infant to effect a similar kind of attention withdrawal, while awake, is the next step in the development of perceptual denial. It represents a maturational shift in which that which was a physiological response is now carried out through a psychological mechanism.

The ability to look at, yet not see, has been strikingly documented in René Spitz's moving films of institutionalized infants raised under conditions of severe emotional deprivation.[13] In these profoundly disturbing recordings, we see babies who sit with wide open eyes, but their eyes are vacant of images; reality does not register. Sudden lights produce no blink; sudden noises, no startle. These infants, for whom the world has offered only pain, do not appear to perceive anything.

The same phenomenon has been documented by Selma Fraiberg (1982). From an intensive study of 50 deprived infants, Fraiberg reported on 12 babies who showed the greatest psychological impairment in emotional development. Under normal circumstances, when infants experience discomfort and are separated from mother, they search out the environment to locate her, as a source of comfort. These infants, neglected or abused by their mothers, might understandably be expected to find mother a source of pain. Lengthy videotapes, showing the reactions of these infants when they were physically separated from their mothers for a brief period of time, indicated that they failed to see mother, even though she stood directly in their line of vision. Moreover, they showed no reaction to her clearly spoken voice. Fraiberg describes this chilling phenomenon as follows:

> The baby is scanning the room, his eyes resting briefly on the stranger, the cameraman, or an object in the room, and in the scanning he passes over his mother's face without a sign of registration or recognition. There is not a pause in scanning or a flicker on his face that speaks for registration. In situ-

ations where gaze exchange or a gesture is nearly unavoidable because of the line of vision or the proximity of baby and mother, we see the patterns again and again. It is as if perception has selectively edited the picture of the mother from the pictures in the visual survey. (1982, pp. 619–620)

If [mother] is for the moment outside the baby's visual field and she speaks to the baby or calls to him, there is no automatic turning in the direction of her voice, and there is no alerting or signs of attention. The editing process has taken place again. (1982, p. 620)

Fraiberg discusses this failure to see (i.e., to register) as a defense behavior against perceiving the mother, who, for these infants, has been the source of negative experiences. She also discusses the failure to see as a defense that may "belong to the biological repertoire and is activated to ward off registration and, conceivably, a painful affect. When the visual and aural registration of this percept is closed off or the registration is muted, the associated affective experience remains dormant, that is, not called up by perception" (Fraiberg, 1982, p. 620).

In terms of the basic characteristic of perceptual denial—the warding off or blotting out of the perception of external reality—the defense described by Fraiberg fits the theory perfectly: An external object is clearly present and in such a position and form that the infant would normally be expected to perceive it, but the object is not seen. Further, there is a clear emotional explanation for this not seeing: The object, mother, has been a source of deprivation and abuse to the infant. These findings also fit very well with our theoretical understanding of the mother's role in facilitating the child's capacity for reality perception. As we understand it, the capacity of the infant to perceive reality is closely related to the same capacity in the mother, as it pertains to the infant. I refer here to the mother's capacity to perceive her infant realistically, and her capacity to reflect this perception back to the infant—to mirror, to help him perceive himself as he is.

In Fraiberg's study this defense was observed as early as 3 months of age and continued to be seen throughout the first 3 years of life in these children (the time span of the study). Although Fraiberg's infants were part of a severely pathological group, a similar defense has been observed under conditions of stress in a "normal" population of 12-month-old babies (e.g., Ainsworth & Wittig, 1969; Ainsworth & Bell, 1970; Ainsworth, Blehar, Waters, & Wall, 1978), in which the mother–child relationship was strained; the continued use of this primitive defensive response at 1 year of age likely reflected the conflicted relationship.

This kind of defensive denial of reality through active physical avoidance has been documented through numerous empirical studies. For example, in an investigation of separation anxiety in infants, Tennes and Lampl (1969) constructed a situation in which mothers and their infants, who enjoyed a good relationship, played together in an observation room. After a time, mothers were instructed to leave the room, while the infants remained with an unknown caretaker. The most usual reaction of these normal infants, ages 9–13 months, was to cry. When they were picked up by caretakers and held in a position that did not require them to look at their caretakers, there was a noticeable relaxation, and the crying stopped. However, if the caretakers positioned the infants so that they were in the infants' line of vision, the babies would turn their heads so as *not to see* the caretakers. If this attempt to avoid perception was not successful, they resumed crying.

Here again we see the defensive component of avoiding the perception of reality during the first year of life. In reality, the mother was absent. To perceive the face of the caretaker would be to perceive mother's absence and the pain associated with that. To avoid perceiving the caretaker's face is to avoid the pain. That the perception of reality is painful because it confirms the mother's absence is seen in the infants' crying when required to look at the caretaker, even though the caretaker herself has never been a direct source of pain for the infants. However, when the babies were held so that they need not see the caretaker, they stopped crying and assumed a relaxed, limp, and somewhat "heavy" posture characteristic of younger babies sprawling on their mother's shoulder or lap; this tempts one to think the position allowed them to imagine (hallucinate) that they were sprawled on mother—a fantasy they could continue as long as the perception of reality could be avoided. But this moves us into denial through fantasy.

Further research using this method involving mother, infant, and unknown caretaker, known as the "strange situation" (Ainsworth et al., 1971), has demonstrated that some infants consistently avoid looking at their mother after the mother has left them for a brief period of time and then returns. This type of "avoidant" behavior on the part of the infant is related to the mother's behavior: Observations in the home revealed that the mothers of these avoidant infants are likely to be rejecting and emotionally unresponsive. As described by Main (1981), this type of avoidance likely serves a defensive function of disrupting the normal attachment pattern, which, if activated, would lead to rejection by the mother and thus to anger and/or anxiety in the infant. The defensive avoidance protects the child from this negative experience (Cassidy & Kobak, 1988; Main, 1995, 2000).

Equally striking behavior that fits the criterion of denial has been observed in an experimental study of normal, nonstressed infants, ages 4–6 months (LaBarbera, Izard, Vietze, & Parisi, 1976). In this study the investigators first demonstrated that the babies could discriminate between faces that portrayed joy and those that portrayed anger. Subsequently, they found that the babies avoided looking at the angry faces in favor of the joyful faces. They concluded that the avoidance of the angry faces comes about in these young infants because they possess no other coping responses to handle the implicit threat of the anger. Within the present framework, we can understand this perceptual avoidance as a manifestation of the defense of denial.[14]

The empirical data from these investigations provide good evidence for the early functioning of denial. The descriptions of the infant looking at, but not seeing, fit very well with the hypothesis of the withdrawal of attention and with the concept of "negative hallucination" in which what exists is hallucinated to not exist; that is, through hallucination, the object is removed from existence.

To look but not to see is a defense the infant can use before any capacity for voluntary motor activity exists. Lying flat on his back, the baby shuts out whatever configuration of physical stimuli fall on his open eyes. However, once the infant has developed the capacity to voluntarily move his head, he may change position so that the noxious stimulus no longer is in his line of vision. This capacity to look past the object provides the beginning of another component of denial: the component of avoiding or "overlooking" reality. Reality is not totally blotted out, but the infant's perception is adjusted so that it is *as if* that reality does not exist.

The two components discussed thus far—attention withdrawal and avoidance—occur on a perceptual level. Denial occurs either by not seeing or by avoiding seeing. The components of denial that emerge subsequent to these early months involve, in some way, the child's attempt to *change* the perception so that it becomes less painful. These subsequent components— misperception, reversal, and negation—are closely tied to perception but their operation requires some additional *cognitive* input from the child.

In misperception, the perception of an object is changed into something other than what is present in reality. Whereas previously a disturbing perception was blotted out or avoided, the normally developing ego makes such an extreme denial of reality less possible. Instead, the disturbing perception is now acknowledged but is changed into something that is less painful. The result is a misperception, generally of a benign sort, which functions to alleviate anxiety by changing (i.e., apparently changing) external reality. This process is in contrast to the malevolent misperceptions that occur in projection, in which anxiety is alleviated by changing internal reality—the internal frightening impulse is placed outside the self. Examples of this developmental shift from avoiding a disturbing stimulus to changing the stimulus into something less disturbing are found in the experimental work of Smith and Danielsson (1982); young children, when tachistoscopically presented with a frightening image, changed it into something more benign.

In a closely related component of denial, reversal, a disturbing perception is changed into its opposite. Reversal may occur in several spheres of functioning. Affective reversal is a common phenomenon in toddlers, whose tears of frustration are transformed, sometimes with help from adults, into trickles of laughter. In the studies of Fraiberg, affective reversal, as a defense, has been documented as early as 9 months and was regularly observed to emerge during the age range of 9–16 months. For example, a 9-month-old infant who experienced starvation in his early months is described while being subjected to his mother's "game," in which she repeatedly takes away his bottle and pretends to drink it herself. Rather than cry or protest, he laughs excitedly (Fraiberg, 1982).

If we can assume that deprivation of food produces pain in a hungry infant, then the laughter indicates that pain has been transformed into pleasure, and that the affective meaning for the infant of the mother's behavior has been reversed. This defense behavior, occurring at 9 months of age, is an example of affective reversal, a component of denial. Reversal may also occur through changed cognition—the animal that was first thought to be huge and ferocious is now labeled a little puppy. On the perceptual level the experience of shifts in figure and ground seems to involve the same kind of mechanism, in which the opposing image replaces the initial perception. Experimental studies of figure–ground reversal, using ambiguous figures, have suggested that the capacity to make such a reversal increases with age.[15]

Another component of denial that allows reality to be both perceived and rejected at the same time is negation. In this case, disturbing perceptions, thoughts, and feelings register but are rapidly transformed by the addition of the negative sign, the "not." Thus, the big dog is "not big," the wish to inflict injury on the frustrating object is changed into "I don't want to hit her," and the subjective experience of terror is changed into "I'm not afraid." The perception, which can no longer be totally avoided, is acknowledged only through negating its meaning.

A poignant example of this kind of denial comes from a 4-year-old boy who had spent some time playing alone at the fringe of a group of children. As they played, he watched them with interest, even longing, but when they glanced at him he would look away, avoiding any contact. This approach–avoidance behavior continued for a while, until it culminated in his spontaneous statement: "I don't need anyone to play with me" (Kristen Kemple, personal communication, February 16, 1990).

The concept of the "no," or the negative, is one that appears in the child's cognitive capacity around the age of 2 years. This is an important development because it allows the child to deny the existence of reality by making a negative judgment about it.

Negation may function hand-in-hand with reversal; if reality is not what it appears to be, then there is a greater possibility that a reversal—the opposite of reality—may be true. Consider the functioning of these two components in the statement of the little boy who says, "I'm not a small boy—I'm bigger than anybody I know." First there is the negation of reality— "I'm not small." Here the boy's perception of his own smallness is counter-manded by the attachment of the negative sign, which permits the percep-tion by negating it. Once *small* is negated, it is then logically more possible to change the perception to *bigger,* for although a boy cannot logically be both small and big at the same time, a boy who is "not small" can logically be big. Thus, given the initial negation, the reversal becomes logically possi-ble.

The playing out of such negations and reversals in the form of stock characters has fascinated children for years. The near-sighted, wimpy re-porter Clark Kent is transformed into Superman; the lame newspaper boy becomes Captain Marvel Jr.; David Bruce Banner, quiet-spoken research scientist, is changed into the Incredible Hulk. These, and the host of other reversible characters in pop literature, graphically portray the functioning of negation and reversal. Using these components of denial, the characters become "not weak" and assume qualities of strength and moral power be-yond anything known to mortals.

At the same time, the portrayal of these negations and reversals in the media are often troubling to young children. As they struggle to grasp real-ity and to distinguish between the real and the unreal, the manifestation of the components of a defense mechanism as though they were actually hap-pening in reality may create considerable confusion and anxiety. Fantasy creations by adults that co-opt the child's arduous attempts to come to terms with reality are unnecessarily disturbing to the child.

The introduction of these components of denial depends greatly on the acquisition of language and on grasping concepts of continuous dimen-sions. Their functioning is now largely removed from the perceptual realm, although the mechanisms involved in figure–ground reversal may be a per-ceptual analogue. But the disturbing experience is changed primarily on the cognitive level, and the change *appears* to be under the conscious control of the individual. Such individuals are known to their friends as being "prone to exaggerate." Children, less charitable with each other, may refer to such an individual as a "liar." What is not recognized in such statements is that, to the extent that the exaggeration is part of the defense of denial, it is not under the conscious control of the individual. The defensive exaggerator believes in his distortions of reality as if they were true; to not do so would be too painful. Yet the denial is eventually seen through by others, for the discrepancy between what is and what is said about it is too great.

These, then, are the components of perceptual denial as they emerge in the developing child. Those most closely tied to the perceptual system largely disappear by adulthood, but there are certainly many instances in which an adult "fails to see" or "doesn't hear" something that, if recognized, would cause pain. More frequently, to the extent that denial is a defense used by adults, it is the components of minimization-maximization that are manifest. Misfortunes are downplayed and successes are expounded upon and expanded.

Denial through Fantasy

To understand the components of the second type of denial, we take the reverse journey: from adulthood back to infancy. The essence of this type of denial involves the imposition onto reality of a personal fantasy that has a positive emotional tone and serves a self-sustaining purpose. In its most elaborate and developed form, this kind of denial occurs as an idealization: Experiences are assigned highly personalized interpretations; aspects of reality are given unusual significance or value in such a way that they conform with a preconceived fantasy, the purpose of which is to sustain the self and protect the individual from pain.

One of the clearest examples in literature of the imposition of an idealized fantasy onto reality occurs in the tale of *Candide*.[16] As in many cases of idealization, Candide's need to see the world as the best of all possible worlds derives from a significant early figure in his life. This mentor, Pangloss, is for Candide, "the greatest philosopher of the province, and, therefore, of the whole world." Like Pangloss, Candide sees the events of life as being evidence for this world being "the best of all possible worlds." As he moves through life, Candide experiences flogging, starvation, being forced into service, and having a chamber-pot dumped on him. At the same time, Pangloss contracts syphilis, which results in his losing the end of his nose, his eye, and his ear. The two travelers witness the devastation of Lisbon as the result of an earthquake. Yet they continue to impose onto these massive misfortunes the belief that "everything is for the best."

Significantly, when Pangloss is hanged, there is a slight weakening in Candide's fantasy system; in the absence of Pangloss, the fantasy is more difficult to maintain. However, the myth is soon shifted to a new object: "It is certainly the new world which is the best of all possible worlds" (p. 28). When, after more calamities, he finally reaches El Dorado, Candide is again ready to impose the fantasy; not knowing what he might find, he decides "Probably it is the country where everything is for the best; for there must be one country of that sort."

The tenacity with which this fantasy is clung to, despite overwhelming evidence to the contrary, forms the ironic motif of the tale. Yet there is evidence, too, that Candide has perceived something of reality; halfway through his adventures he recounts that "in spite of what Dr. Pangloss said, I often noticed that everything went very ill in Westphalia" (p. 55). And there is a suggestion that he has some insight into his defense of denial when he refers to his optimism as "the mania of maintaining that everything is well when we are wretched" (p. 63).

Nevertheless, Candide continues in the attempt to make reality conform to his myth. He meets another learned man and immediately attempts to impose his belief system on that individual to create a new idealized object to take the place of the departed Pangloss. Candide says to the learned Martin: "Sir, no doubt you think that all is for the best in the physical world and in the moral, and that nothing could be otherwise than as it is" (p. 79). The reply, however, does not confirm the idealization, for Martin, who has his own belief system says "Sir, . . . I do not think anything of the sort."

Candide's need to continue the idealization is great; if part of his myth is too flatly and directly contradicted, he still maintains the idealization of the genius companion. This defensive maneuver occurs again when he meets Pococuranta, a man who is dissatisfied with everything, who says, in essence, that nothing is for the best. Candide overlooks the discrepancy with his fantasy belief system and instead imposes the "great man" fantasy: "Oh! What a superior man. . . . What a great genius this Pococurante is! Nothing can please him" (p. 95).

But giving up the "all is for the best" myth is not without consequence. On the occasions when this fantasy fails, Candide sinks into a deep depression. When the belief in the idealized other dissolves, he is left to experience the feelings of insignificance, abandonment, and fragmentation against which the defense protected him. The clear connection between failure of defense and experience of painful depression is made in the juxtaposition of Candide's statements: "How right you are, my dear Martin! Everything is illusion and calamity!" followed by "He fell into a black melancholy and took no part in the . . . amusements. . . . Martin was not consoling. Candide's melancholy increased" (p. 86). Yet a part of the defense was maintained (and no doubt maintained him), for Candide continues to believe that, although it is inaccessible, there is, in the country of El Dorado, a place in which everything is for the best.

It is interesting how Voltaire helps Candide move out of this infantile approach to the world. What is lacking in Candide is the capacity for reality testing, an ego function. In the immature ego, the processes of assimilation and accommodation do not occur; reality is not taken in, and structures are not modified on the basis of experience. Change, or development, in the ego does not occur.

Voltaire's solution to this state of stagnation, of ego arrest, is to propose that *work* is the key to getting on with life. Thus Martin says, "Let us work without theorizing . . . 'tis the only way to make life endurable" (p. 114). Psychologically, we may understand this as a call to mobilize the ego functions—the capacities for perception, reasoning, judgment, action;

that is, the capacities for individual initiative—and to abandon the passively fixed ideas in the idealizations, fantasies, and philosophies.

This kind of misinterpretation of reality in terms of an idealized fantasy may be seen as the most highly developed, mature form of denial; it occurs among adults who are overly optimistic, overly positive, overly contented. It is one aspect of what is known clinically as "Pollyannish denial." The denial occurs not in terms of a failure to perceive what is there, but rather in an imposition of a highly personalized interpretation of what the perceived events mean. The meaning is distorted to make it more pleasant and more self-enhancing.

Starting with this component of denial as the most mature, let us move backward on the developmental continuum and identify earlier components. One fantasy commonly imposed onto reality by adolescents is known to clinicians as the "family romance" fantasy. In this imagined reality the adolescent imagines that his parents are not his real parents, who, if known, would be quite different from the parents with whom he lives. In a variation of this fantasy, it is only one of his parents who is a false parent.[17] The use of the idealization component of denial occurs most often in the evaluation of persons. The tendency to exaggerate or maximize the positive characteristics of an individual while underplaying or minimizing his or her shortcomings forms a familiar part of hero worship in the adolescent years. Such maximization or minimization of the qualities of the individual bring about a concordance between the internal myth of the idealized object and the experience of the object in reality.

Another component of this aspect of denial that emerges in adolescence or earlier occurs in the form of a daydream: The adolescent or child drifts out of reality into a daydream, a fantasy, in which an interesting alternative experience to reality occurs. In this realm, the impossible becomes possible, failure becomes victory, weakness becomes strength. Such fantasies may rely on some of the components of perceptual denial, such as reversal, but they are used on a conceptual, rather than perceptual, level.

Daydreams or fantasies of this sort are similar to the idealization component of denial in that they provide an alternative set of experiences that are more pleasant than those that occur in reality. However, they are also different in that the daydreamer generally recognizes the unreal nature of the fantasy and can acknowledge that it was only a daydream. Yet, in an interesting way, the possibility of attributing experience to the realm of the unreal (i.e., the daydream) in itself can provide the possibility for a further defense; other "real" experiences may be treated as though they, too, were unreal, were only daydreams, and did not really happen. Thus, the capacity to have daydreams provides both an alternative reality and a way to disavow the events of external reality on a conceptual basis.[18]

The predecessor of daydreaming can be seen clearly in the "enacted daydreams" of childhood. Through dramatic play, children act out their wishes, hopes, and preferences for the way they would like the world to be. The dramatic world of play takes precedence, for a time, over the world of reality, and the self-enhancing pleasures of success, beauty, and power are experienced to a degree not possible in the real world of childhood. Here, too, is the imposition of a personal fantasy onto reality for a period of time. While involved in such play, it is often extremely difficult for the child to shift back to the adult's reality. For the time being, the enacted fantasy is the preferred reality, and objective reality is rejected.

Fantasy play, most characteristic of the beginning school years, has its origins as early as 2 years of age, when the capacity for symbolic play emerges. At about this age the toddler may be observed using objects in quite novel ways (Kavanaugh, Eizenman, & Harris, 1997). The meaning of objects is no longer restricted to their primary function; a cup is no longer only something to drink out of, but may become a boat to carry a minia-ture toy mouse across the pond. At mealtime the unwanted vegetable may be transformed, at the child's request and with the aid of an adult, into a buzzing airplane that circles the airport before landing in the child's mouth. This kind of play may or may not be defensive, depending on the purpose it serves. But in either case, it illustrates an early occurrence of the process of imposing a personal, idiosyncratic interpretation onto reality.

Thus, as early as 2 years of age, we may see a component of denial through fantasy—of the imposition onto the world of an alternative, per-sonal reality that is more pleasant, and satisfying. Is it possible to find an even earlier component of this type of denial? It seems to me that it is, at least in terms of psychoanalytic theory. According to theory, when the in-fant experiences hunger, he cries, and the painful sensations disappear with the experience of being fed. Through association, the cessation of pain is linked with the appearance of the source of food: the breast or bottle. Gradually, a mental representation of pain comes to evoke a mental repre-sentation of the food source. When it does not appear in reality, the mental image is maintained and perhaps intensified, for the purpose of diminish-ing pain. This phenomenon, known in the theory as "hallucinatory wish-fulfillment," involves the same general process as do the other components of denial through fantasy. There is an experience of psychological pain, in response to which the mental apparatus constructs an alternative reality (the imaged or hallucinated food source) that is more satisfying than objec-tive reality. This, I suggest, is the earliest component of denial through fan-tasy. However, at this early stage of life, the fantasy is manifest through the perceptual system in an hallucination.[19, 20]

When physical or psychological needs are consistently not gratified in reality, the infant must find some way to feel good. By turning away from reality, the child may begin to construct a fantasy in which the experience of pain and helplessness prompts ideas of omnipotence. In this fantasy, the child believes she has some magical power to control the caretaker. Such a fantasy involves a denial of reality as well as certain aspects of projection. As described by Novick and Novick (1998, 2002), when the caretaker continually fails to meet the infant's needs, feelings of intense, helpless rage are defended against by the creation of omnipotent beliefs that she is able to control or destroy the other. This delusion of omnipotence becomes a safeguard and a source of self-regulation (Novick & Novick, 1998, 2002). It should be understood that this kind of omnipotent fantasy signals pathological development and a hostile defensive reaction to failures of reality (Novick & Novick, 1998).[21]

In this section, I have traced the development of two forms of denial. Beginning with infancy, we have followed the course of perceptual denial from its origin in the physiological "shutting down" of the perceptual system in sleep, through perceptual avoidance and then perceptual distortions, evolving into the conceptual counterparts of these misperceptions (e.g., reversal, maximization, minimization). Taking the reverse course, we have traced the developmental history of denial through fantasy from its full-blown conceptual form in the adult, as seen in the imposition of a personal fantasy onto life's events, back through the use of idealization and daydreams in adolescence, to the dramatic play of childhood, and returning finally to infancy and the wish-fulfilling hallucination—a perceptual phenomenon. By considering both the perceptual and conceptual components of denial, I have illustrated how, over the course of development, "Denial functions through the disavowal of whole percepts and the substitution of a wish-fulfilling fantasy" (Lichtenberg & Slap, 1972, p. 781).

ANOTHER FOLKTALE

Again we turn to the realm of fairytales to illustrate how the two forms of denial intertwine to produce an arrested character structure. In "The Snow Queen,"[22] Kaj and Gerda are dear childhood playmates. One day an evil magic mirror shatters, and slivers of glass are blown into Kaj's eyes and into his heart. It is the nature of this mirror, even its fragments, that it distorts people's perception. The good is minimized, and the bad is magnified. And this is what happened to Kaj. With the glass is his eyes, he overlooked the beautiful blossoms of the rose bush and noticed only their irregularities and imperfections. He was solely interested in looking at snowflakes. In addition, the fragment of mirror in Kaj's heart turned it into a lump of ice. As a result, his former fondness for Gerda was replaced with cruel teasing.

Soon after, Kaj is kidnapped by the Snow Queen and taken to her palace, which is made of ice, snow, and biting winds. "Little Kaj was blue with cold—nay, almost black—but he did not know it" (p. 142). "He went about dragging some sharp flat pieces of ice which he placed in all sorts of patterns. . . . In his eyes they were excellent and of the greatest importance: this was because of the grain of glass still in his eye" (pp. 142–143).

Meanwhile, Gerda worries about him and goes in search. After a very long journey she locates him in the queen's palace. Delighted, she approaches him, but he does not recognize her. "He sat still, rigid, and cold" (p. 143). But she flung her arms around him, and her hot tears "fell upon his breast and penetrated to his heart" where they "thawed the lump of ice and melted the little bit of the mirror which was in it" (p. 144).

Kaj was then able to cry, and his tears washed the glass out of his eye, so that he was able to perceive Gerda. "He knew her and shouted with joy" (p. 144).

The possibility for parallels between this tale and the arrested development that is associated with the use of the two forms of denial is intriguing. Kaj's problem begins with the "bad mirror" experience, parts of which he incorporates.[23] This experience with the bad mirror affects Kaj in two ways. First, his center is frozen; his emotional development is stunted. This psychological arrest is further reinforced by the second result of the bad mirror experience: his inability to perceive reality. Through the components of minimization and reversal, his perception of reality is distorted; he does not see that which does not fit with his cold heart. Initially, the nature of the distortion in the fairytale is in the opposite direction to that usually found in denial. Kaj's distortion changes positive into negative, in keeping with the coldness of his heart. But once he reaches the queen's palace, his denial functions in its more usual manner, whereby the negative is ignored or replaced with an acceptable fantasy. Kaj does not know (i.e., fails to perceive) that he is frozen with cold. And he imposes his inner fantasy that he is doing something important onto his essentially random behavior with the pieces of ice. His disavowal of reality reaches a climax when he fails to recognize Gerda.

Through design or happy fortune, Gerda brings about a successful therapy. She focuses on the frozen heart. Her warmth and holding manage to "unstick" that arrested center of development and to allow Kaj to discard the frozen view of life. Once this fantasy is dissolved, Kaj is able to cry and thereby correct his distorted perception.

CLINICAL EXAMPLES

Let us turn now to examples of the manifestation of the two forms of denial in several young adults seeking psychotherapy.

An unusually attractive young woman, stylishly dressed in the mode of her peers, entered my office for the first time. Despite her "together" appearance, she was clearly distressed: Her hands shook, her lips quivered, and she was struggling with losing control. Within minutes, she was sobbing uncontrollably, the cause of which upset I had not yet had the opportunity to discover. What was striking (and has remained fixed in my memory) was her reaction to the flow of tears and the heavy sobs. As the tears continued, she said to me, "I'm a very happy person." I looked at her, somewhat questioningly, and she repeated, "But I really am a very happy person."

In this mini-example there is a striking demonstration of both forms of denial. In the external observable reality of the situation she was crying heavily; in reality, such sobs are not associated with happiness. Yet in her opening comments, she makes no reference to these sobs and ignores their implication. At the same time we see the imposition of a personal myth on the situation. For reasons at this point unknown, she imposes the fantasy that she is a very happy person, and when it is not mirrored, she insists on its truth. The wish for the myth to be true is stronger than the perception of reality.

Another young woman, who had been through a stormy relationship with a man slightly older than herself, was finally able to say that the affair was over. The ending of the relationship had been exceedingly painful for her; the more he withdrew, the more desperately she clung to him. Work circumstances necessitated a geographical distance between them, which helped ensure a physical separation.

It was because of the upset associated with the breakup of this relationship that Dee entered therapy. Many of the early sessions were spent in recounting the last few months of the affair, with a gradual shift of focus from how awful she felt to how she was sure there was something else that she could have done to change this man's feelings toward her. She then described her attempts, repetitively, to get him to see things her way, to get him to understand her. This need to have others see the world as she did (i.e., to have her inner representation mirrored) became a recurring one in the therapy.

However, the initial expression of this need appeared in a repeated request that I tell her what to do about the young man, because she felt helpless to figure it out on her own. As she had also solicited advice from a number of her friends, and from her family, I asked why she needed my direction as well. Although her initial response was that I was an "expert" and so could give better advice, she added that she had not liked the advice given by others. Exploration of this helped her realize that what she really wanted from me was not advice but that I, unlike her friends, would agree with her own plan of action—that is, that I would validate her perception of the situation. The real focus here was not so much on denying reality as on an insistent attempt to create a situation in reality that matched her internal, anxiety-reducing fantasy. On a limited scope, this could be seen in the attempt to have me validate her belief that it would be a good idea to send him a long, explanatory letter, which would then repair the relationship. On a broader scope, it was seen in her persisting fantasy that the relationship with the young man still existed and would be resumed after the current hiatus.

The difficulty in these cases comes when the internal, alternative view of "reality" (i.e., the fantasy) cannot be matched in the external world. The angry frustration with this failure is not infrequently followed by an expression of hopelessness regarding the external world—"there is nothing there for me"—meaning, there is nothing there that matches my inner view. This hopelessness about the external world, it should be pointed out, occurs when denial breaks down; it is not a product of denial. It is not so much, then, that external reality is totally denied, for my patient could give reasonably accurate descriptions of the events surrounding her concerns, as that an alternative fantasy reality is preferred. As another young woman told me, "I know it's not true, but I want to think of it this way."

During the first several months of treatment, Dee continued to contact the young man by letters and phone calls, with the idea that, given another chance, she could explain herself well enough that he would have to accept her view. It was in the reporting of these and other similar ventures in months to come that a second aspect of denial became apparent. In the course of these communications, Dee repeatedly made direct or indirect requests to see him, often in the context of a thinly disguised rationalization around mutual interests or common friends. Characteristically, he responded with a polite refusal, offering as reasons, for example, that he was busy at work but that he might be less busy 5 months hence, or that relatives had invited him out at the time of her proposed visit but he might be visiting friends in her town later in the year. On occasion, when his social graces failed him, he would give a vague response of being "unsure, but I'll let you know."

Inevitably Dee, who was quite bright, would miss the implication of these remarks. She interpreted his remark about being busy at work to mean that he really wanted to see her and would invite her as soon as possible. She understood his loyalty to his relatives and looked forward to his promised visit to her in the spring. She heard "I'll let you know" as an offer of a meeting, the time and place to be arranged later.

Though these are but a few examples, they were repeated many times with this man and in subsequent relationships with other men. Dee failed to recognize not the objective reality of what was said, but rather the implications, the import. Because of the associated pain, Dee denied the meaning of these experiences: that she was being rejected. It is the meaning of the event, rather than the event itself, that is changed in such a way as to avoid psychological pain.

I close this section with two rather extreme examples of denial through fantasy—extreme because the personal myth is so basic to the patient's self-concept and yet so obviously false in the face of incontrovertible reality. At the basis of both myths was the feeling in the individual of absolute uniqueness.

A college student I had been seeing for some time was facing the usual anxieties surrounding graduation and entry into the outside world. Despite several interviews and inquiries from prospective employers, he had not yet landed a job for the upcoming year; a number of his friends were in the same unemployed position, although others had secured a position. Understandably distressed, he began writing letters to organizations whose focus included his area of interests. One of these businesses invited him for an interview, which he accepted with excitement. On his return, there was something unreal in the way he spoke about the meeting, which prompted me to ask how many other people he thought might be applying for the job. To my surprise, he responded that no one else would apply for this job, for no one else had his combination of interests. Somewhat incredulously, and perhaps insensitively, I asked him whether, of the thousands and thousands of young people graduating from college at this time and looking for a job, there might not be some who had interests similar to his own. He replied, with irritation, that he didn't know any and then became enraged that I would ask such a question.

A second example comes from a successfully employed professional woman who had grown up in a Jewish family in Brooklyn. Well into the therapy, we were discussing the extreme aloneness she had felt as a child. This emotional aloneness—in part, due to her mother's illness and her father's absence—was, during her early life, experienced primarily on the physical level, in the absence of people and things (e.g., toys) from her life. It was in explaining to me why no people inhabited her early world that the denial fantasy emerged. She told me that her parents wanted the family to associate only with Jews, and since there were no other Jews in Brooklyn, there was no one with whom to associate. When I questioned this myth, she maintained it steadfastly, despite my reminders that she had told me about the people across the hall celebrating Passover and her memories of her Jewish cousins living nearby. That this myth continued unaltered was revealed when, visiting Brooklyn several months later, she looked in the phone book and was surprised to find other listings with her own Jewish name.

At the heart of both these fantasies was the personal myth of uniqueness—a myth that both "explained" the loneliness and isolation felt by these two individuals and at the same time bolstered their self-regard. The personal fantasy helped both individuals deny painful aspects of their life—that they might not be chosen for a position, that they might have lived in a situation of emotional and social deprivation. But the unreal way of "seeing" the world, when revealed, indicated a significant failure in reality testing. The continued use of the defense of denial beyond its developmentally appropriate time had produced distortions in thinking.

THE USE OF DENIAL IN PROJECTIVE STORIES

We discussed earlier how denial can be used by accomplished authors for dramatic purposes, as in "The Emperor's New Clothes" and "Little Red Riding Hood." It is also possible to identify the use of denial in the productions of unsophisticated storytellers. In this section two children's stories, both told in response to a TAT picture, are reproduced and then analyzed for the occurrence of denial in the story. In both cases the child was responding to TAT Card 17BM, which depicts a bare-chested man clinging to a rope. The following tape-recorded story was told by a 10-year-old girl.

> *He looks like he's in the circus and those people climb the things that get on the rings. And he looks like he's gonna f . . . fall. So he's holding on very tightly. And he's going up the rope. And when he gets there, he's gonna do something. And he might fall. He doesn't wanna fall because there's no net down at the bottom, so—it looks like it's daylight out and he has tights on and—I don't know if he has something else on, I don't know that. And he has short blond hair, and he's climbing the rope, and when he gets up there he, he might slip and fall down, down, down, and hurt himself from a rope burn, but I don't think he'll do that, and at the end he'll fall and bump his head— (laughs)—he will fall and bump his head, and then he felt like crying but he didn't. So they took him to the hospital and he didn—he lost his memory because he hit his head on the rock, because this was during practice and then he's okay after a while.*

This story provides a good illustration of the use of denial to ward off anxious feelings. Anxiety around the possibility of injury appears early on, when the storyteller falters on the word "fall," followed by the coping response of "holding on tightly." But the concern about falling continues ("And he might fall"), and the danger is amplified ("no net down at the bottom"). The storyteller attempts to move away from the dangerous situation by focusing on a description of the picture ("It looks like it's daylight out") and of the man. But this latter maneuver immediately gets her into trouble again over the anxiety aroused by looking at the possibly naked man, who she then hurries to clothe ("he has tights on"). But even this denial of his nakedness is not sufficient to quell her anxiety, and two blatant statements of denial immediately follow: "I don't know if he has something else on," "I don't know that." Her attention is then focused on the uppermost extremity (i.e., least anxiety-provoking part) of his body ("he has short blond hair"), and from there she slides back into the first anxiety-arousing theme of falling. Now the possibility of getting hurt is stated overtly for the first time, and the first blatant use of denial in connection with the theme of falling appears ("but I don't think he'll do that"). The defense is not successful, however, and the anxiety theme of falling and bumping his head continues. The denial then is shifted to the reactions of the fallen man, who "felt like crying but he didn't." Another attempt at denial is made around the visit to the hospital but is aborted ("he didn . . . "). The story returns to the issue of injury but concludes with a blanket denial ("he's okay after a while"). Interestingly, the choice of type of injury—to not remember ("he lost his memory")—is itself congruent with the predominant defense mechanism of denial employed in this story.

In this story denial is accomplished primarily through the use of verbal negation, although there is a touch of denial on the perceptual level around the man's nakedness. In the second example, from a 5½-year-old girl, we see denial on a more primitive level. Denial creates a perceptual distortion and a disruption in reality testing. Again, the story was tape-recorded as the child looked at TAT Card 17BM.

This is a statue, climbing down a rope. [What happens?] He falls and then breaks. And then somebody builds him back up, and he does the same thing over again.

Although nearly all children, regardless of age, see the figure clinging to the rope as a live man, this little girl turns the figure into a statue. Given the subsequent course of the story, it appears that she is concerned about the possibility of the figure falling. To quell her anxiety about injury or death, she denies that the figure is alive; if it is not alive, it cannot be hurt and cannot die. This denial is carried out through a misperception; the human being is misperceived as a statue. However, this denial is not completely successful. It leads to a disruption in reality testing, in which the statue exhibits animate behavior by "climbing down a rope." When the concern about falling and its consequences is expressed ("He falls and then breaks"), we see how the perceptual denial allows the child to avoid and undo the anxiety-laden fear of death: Because it is a statue, the pieces can be put back together again, and so there is no harm, nothing to be feared.

But the issue is not put to rest completely, for the whole process is then repeated.

CONCLUDING REMARKS

We have seen that denial develops out of a prototypic physiological response in which the infant rids himself of disturbing external stimulation by withdrawal into sleep. This means of avoiding unpleasant perceptions continues through mental operations in which attention is withdrawn from external stimuli, so that they are avoided or "not seen."

As memory traces are laid down and the capacity for cognition develops, additional means for dealing with upsetting perceptions of reality become available. In addition to simply blotting out the disturbing percept, the child may misperceive it—that is, change the percept into something it is not, but something that is less threatening. Or, as language and the capacity for applying the negative develop, the percept is acknowledged through its negation. Similarly, the development of the mental operation of reversal makes it possible to change the percept, or its qualities, into the opposite. Further along, denial may occur by means of the related mental operations of minimization, maximization, or exaggeration, or in an attitude of nonchalance or indifference in the face of threat or danger.

Along with this disavowal of what is present in reality, denial may occur through the substitution of an alternative fantasized reality. Early in life, this wish-fulfilling fantasy may occur perceptually, as in a dream or an hallucination. Later, it may occur in playacting, and still later, in daydreams in which unsatisfactory reality situations are replaced with gratifying fantasies and unfounded optimism.

Thus the two forms of denial develop and, at least later in life, often intermingle. The resulting character style and its attendant difficulties have been illustrated through the presentation of folktales and clinical case studies.

CHAPTER 4

Projection

> The first judgment of the ego distinguishes between edible
> and nonedible objects: the first acceptance is swallowing,
> the first rejection is spitting out.
>
> —FENICHEL (1945, p. 146)

The second defense mechanism to be discussed in detail, projection, has its beginnings in the earliest years of the child's life but does not become predominant until late childhood and early adolescence. In the broadest sense projection protects the child from disruptive anxiety by attributing unacceptable feelings, wishes, and impulses to someone else; the disturbing thoughts are placed outside of the self—"ejected" into the external world and attached to some other object.

Like the chapter on denial, this chapter begins with a discussion of the components of projection—the mental processes involved and their manifestation in behavior. Several folktales are then considered to illustrate the different components of projection. The next section traces the development of projection from its earliest form in infancy to its mature form in preadolescence. Another folktale, which contains several forms of projection, is then presented. The chapter continues with an illustration of the use of projection in a clinical case and concludes with a demonstration of how projection is manifest in projective storytelling.

COMPONENTS OF PROJECTION

The defense mechanism of projection is more complex than denial, both logically and psychologically. It involves the capacity to differentiate between inside and outside, between self and other. It requires the ability to make judgments—pleasure–pain, good–bad, acceptable–unacceptable. Projection is carried out by breaking the connection between the conscious ego and certain thoughts or impulses and then attributing the origin of these thoughts elsewhere. In this way the individual remains unaware of their personal origin.

In denial a whole percept or mental representation is disavowed and may be replaced by a wish-fulfilling fantasy. In projection, however, the representation is split, with the positive segment allocated to the inside (the self, the ego) and the negative segment to the outside (the other). Schafer (1954) defines projection as "a process by which an objectionable internal tendency . . . [either an] id impulse or superego attitude . . . is unrealistically attributed to another person or to other objects in the environment instead of being recognized as part of one's self" (p. 179). The phenomenon of "splitting" is basic to the mechanism of projection.[1]

In its broadest sense the term *projection* has been used to encompass any process in which inner phenomena are allocated to the external world. It has been suggested that some of these processes are better referred to as *externalization,* because they lack certain critical features of projection proper—for example, there may be an awareness of the personal origin of the thought or feeling (Novick & Kelly, 1970; Novick & Novick, 1996b). However, because these processes are generally accepted as precursors of projection proper, and hence form a necessary part of a developmental theory of projection, they are included in this discussion of the components of projection. In the normal course of events, we have no difficulty distinguishing between a perception and an idea. A perception is a mental event, the origin of which we attribute to the external world. An idea, on the other hand, is a mental event, the origin of which we attribute to our internal, psychological world. Perceptions refer to something "out there," whereas ideas reside within.

There are, however, exceptions to this general rule. On occasion an internal memory-image can be confused with a perception and falsely assumed to have the same external origin as the perception. We refer to this phenomenon as a hallucination, which is perhaps the clearest manifestation of projection. Colloquially, this component amounts to "seeing something that isn't there." It may be contrasted with one of the components of denial, which involves not seeing what *is* there.

The experience of the projected hallucination is not confusion between memory-image and percept. Rather, the hallucination is assumed to exist in the external world in the same way that the source of a percept exists in that world. Indeed, both hallucination and perception involve the projection of a mental image onto the external world; thus the mechanism of projection has a normal perceptual process as its base. The difference between the two lies in the true source of the image.

Although the projection of a full-blown visual image onto the external world occurs infrequently, projection of other mental representations such as wishes, feelings, and impulses is a more common phenomenon. This component of projection—the assumption that one's own feelings, thoughts, or wishes exist in others—takes two forms. In the first case, the individual assumes that the other shares his own thoughts, beliefs, or feelings—that the two of them "think alike." This tendency to generalize one's own internal state to account for the behavior of others may involve both negative and positive feelings, and the individual may be aware that he is making such a generalization. This process clearly involves the attribution of an internal tendency to an external object, but it may or may not be defensive, depending on whether its purpose is to prevent the individual from experiencing painful anxiety. Animistic thinking, in which human motives, feelings, and thoughts are attributed to animals or inanimate objects, is a special example of generalization (Novick & Novick, 1996b). Again, such animism may involve the attribution of negative or positive characteristics to the object, and the individual who engages in this type of thinking may be aware of the attribution. The central feature that justifies including generalization and animism as components of projection is that an internal tendency is attributed to an external object and is used to explain that object's behavior.

Though animistic thinking is associated with primitive or early levels of individual and cultural development, this form of projection occurs in contemporary adult society in the phenomenon of projective identification—experiencing oneself in another by attributing one's own feelings and thoughts to that other.[2]

This attribution of one's own mental representations to others brings about a further component of projection—namely, the alteration of reality. Projection alters the perceived character of the outside object (Knight, 1940); it alters what is perceived, what is intended, and the interpretation of what occurs. When projection is used as a defense, this alteration or misperception makes the experience of events more negative, or more ominous, than they are in objective reality.

Another component of projection may occur in connection with this ominous alteration of reality. As the world becomes more frightening, the individual may attempt to develop an "explanation" for the disturbing happenings. In some cases the explanation takes on a logically consistent form, with conclusions following closely from premises. Here projection contributes to the formation of a delusion in which circumstantial reasoning and ideas of reference contribute to the further alteration reality. The delusion may be relatively benign, as in an unfounded belief that one is being looked at or talked about, or it may take a more bizarre form involving a more extreme alteration of reality.

The belief that the world is a frightening, ominous place contributes to the creation of still more components of projection. On the one hand, the belief in threatening external forces leads to the attempt to protect oneself from the imagined danger. This may take the form of physical escape, the creation of protective barriers against attack, or attempts to disguise oneself. The felt need for protection may also result in a kind of wariness that includes a hyperalertness to being tricked or misled. On the other hand, the belief that one is endangered may result in attempts to disarm, capture, or destroy the dangerous other, the imagined assailant.

Each of the components of projection discussed here is based on placing one's own inner mental representations onto objects in the external world. In yet another component of projection, the mental representation is not put outside the self; rather, the *origin* of the representation is made external. Here the cause or responsibility for the thought is attributed to the external world. The individual is aware of having unacceptable thoughts, feelings, or impulses, but he or she attributes the source of these ideas to someone else. Thus, to relieve the anxiety of disclosing a discomforting thought in psychotherapy, it is not uncommon for certain patients to add, "You wanted me to say that." In more pathological cases the individual may experience his actions and thoughts as being under the control of another, with delusions involving magical or supernatural forces that influence behavior.

These various components of projection can be grouped into three broad categories.[3] The first group includes operations in which the individual, although projecting his own thoughts or feelings onto external objects, is at the same time aware of possessing those feelings himself. These operations have been referred to as the *generalization* of one's own thoughts, feelings, or self-image onto others. At the base of these operations is a cognitive weakness, namely, the failure to differentiate between self and other, between animate and inanimate.

The second form of projection involves a clearer separation between self and other. Although the individual in some cases recognizes the existence of the unacceptable characteristics as his own, he attributes the responsibility for these characteristics to someone else. In other cases he may be unaware of these characteristics in himself. Either way, because of the attribution of responsibility, he is not "at fault" for his thoughts, feelings, or actions.

The third form of projection is based on the individual's attribution to others of thoughts, feelings, wishes, or impulses that exist within herself but of which she is quite unaware. This is projection in its most classical form. The projected thoughts or feelings are generally ones that are unacceptable to the individual.

PROJECTION AS SEEN IN FOLKTALES

The three categories of projection just discussed are found in various folktales. Often the projection is carried out in these tales through the use of two related characters—twins or brothers, master and servant—with the unexpressed thoughts or feelings of one character being overtly expressed by the other.

The first category of projection—the generalization of psychological attributes—is illustrated in two tales: "The Castle of No Return" and "The Giant Who Had No Heart in His Body." The second category—attribution of responsibility—is illustrated in "Little Claus and Big Claus" and "The Tale of Lord Peter." The third category—projection proper—is discussed in connection with the Homeric "Hymn to Demeter" and "The Tale of Anpu and Bata."

The Generalization of Psychological Attributes

In some folktales attributes or characteristics of the central character are generalized to a second person or to an object, and the tale revolves around the sharing of these attributes by the two characters. The story of "The Castle of No Return"[4] involves twin brothers, one of whom is about to leave home while the other remains behind. So that the homebound brother can know the fate of his twin, a bottle of water is left at home. The exploring brother explains: "If the water stays clear that means I am doing well, but if the water becomes troubled it means that things are going badly." When the water subsequently becomes "troubled," the second brother sets out to rescue the first. It is the sharing of the troubled state between the man and the water that prompts the rescue.

The assumption that one character's attributes can be found in another object has been used in fairy tales to bring about the character's punishment. For example, in "The Giant Who Had No Heart in His Body,"[5] six sons of the king are turned into stone by a giant who has no heart. A seventh son, named Boots, sets out to rescue his brothers and discovers that to kill the giant, he must find the giant's heart and then destroy it. With the help of a princess, Boots learns that the giant's heart is located in a duck's egg. After a search, he finally locates the egg and squeezes it. "As soon as ever he squeezed it the giant screamed out." When Boots squeezed it again, "the giant screamed still more piteously and begged and prayed so prettily to be spared, saying he would do all that the prince wished if he would only not squeeze his heart in two." Thus the giant is made to restore the six brothers to life. As soon as this is done, "Boots squeezed the egg to pieces, and the giant burst at once." Thus revenge on the giant is carried out by attacking the part of him that is located in the duck. This tale provides a good example of generalization (i.e., placing of parts of oneself within another), demonstrated when the attack on the duck results in pain to the giant.

Attribution of Responsibility

Although the tale of "The Giant Who Had No Heart" best illustrates the mechanism of generalization, it also contains a variant on the mechanism of splitting, with the "bad" qualities attributed to one character while the "good" qualities reside in another. In this tale the bad qualities reside in the giant, whereas the good "heart" is placed in the duck's egg, although the splitting is not complete—the giant feels pain when the egg is squeezed.

This form of projection is portrayed in a number of folktales. Often it occurs in a tale of two main characters, one of whom is good, simple, and honest whereas the other is more clever, devious, and manipulative. What the former would never do, the latter carries out with abandon. The components of projection exemplified in these tales include splitting, followed by externalization of part of the main character's self-representation, and an attribution of responsibility for unacceptable actions to this externalized "other."

Three examples of tales of this sort follow. The first two, "The Maiden in the Tower"[6] and "Little Claus and Big Claus,"[7] illustrate the type of tale in which the connection between the wishes of the first character and the actions of the second is explicit. In the first tale the heroine tells us that a parrot speaks for her. In the second story Little Claus consciously pretends that his bag, which actually contains some horse hides, is covering a "magician" who speaks Little Claus's thoughts. Both the reader and Little Claus are aware of the transfer of responsibility for these thoughts from Little Claus to the "magician."

In a second type of tale in which responsibility is attributed to another, the connection between the wishes and actions of the two characters is less explicit. This type is illustrated in the story of "Lord Peter,"[8] in which a cat carries out the guileful manipulations that elevate poor Peter's status, while Peter remains naive and somewhat bumbling. There is no suggestion that Peter is in any way responsible for the cat's devious behavior. Only the reader is aware that the cat is acting to fulfill Peter's need to rise out of poverty and become a wealthy man. In this way the defensive function of the attribution of responsibility is made more apparent.

"The Maiden in the Tower" provides one of the best folktale illustrations of projection in which the shift of responsibility from the main character to another is clearly spelled out for all to see. In this story a godmother confines a young girl with beautiful golden hair to a tower for safekeeping, with her pet parrot, so that no man can carry her off. However, a prince gains entry to the tower. The girl is frightened and wishes to escape from him but does not know how. The prince eventually gets her to agree to leave with him, but she delays him until the next day. This delay allows for the return of the godmother. The prince is hidden behind a curtain, but the parrot repeats, over and over, the statement, "Godmother, lover hidden there." When the godmother asks the girl what the parrot is saying, the maid replies, "Oh Godmother, he only says what I teach him to say," thus clearly explaining the mechanism of projection. As a result of the explanation, the godmother discovers the prince and rescues the maid from her abduction. In this way the maid, who is unable to speak out against the prince, in fact accomplishes the deed through the words of the parrot. As a result of this attribution of responsibility, the prince cannot punish her. However, the maid's reply to her godmother makes it clear that she is, in fact, responsible for all of the parrot's words.

In "The Tale of Little Claus and Big Claus," Little Claus is a needy, small-time farmer whose worldly possessions are inferior to those of Big Claus. Little Claus is also greedy and vain; when Big Claus loans him the use of his horses, Little Claus boasts to passersby that he owns the animals. As a result of his direct expression of covetous greediness, Little Claus is roundly punished; his only horse is killed. He then sets off on a journey, intent on selling his horse's hide.

At nightfall he requests lodging at a farmhouse but is refused by the farmer's wife with the explanation that her husband is away. Consequently, Little Claus climbs on top of a shed to find a place to sleep for the night. From this vantage point he is able to see over the closed shutters into the house, where he spies the farmer's wife entertaining the village sexton, whom the farmer dislikes intensely. The wife has set out an elaborate meal, with meat and fish and wine and cake. Little Claus longs for some of this food and peers ever more intently at the feast.

At this point the farmer returns home unexpectedly. The wife, fearing her husband's wrath, hides the food in the oven and the sexton in a chest. When the farmer sees Little Claus, he invites him into the house to eat and to sleep. For a meal, the wife sets out a dish of coarse groats, which the farmer eats eagerly. Little Claus, however, yearns for the lavish fare he knows to be hidden in the oven. But, perhaps remembering his previous punishment for the open expression of his greed, he does not personally take the responsibility for obtaining this food. Instead he steps on the bag containing the horse's hide, causing it to squeak. When the farmer asks about the noise, Little Claus says he has a magician in the bag, and that the magician tells him there is a meal of meat, fish, wine, and cake in the oven. The food is then discovered, brought to the table, and consumed.

By having this imaginary character speak for him, Little Claus is absolved both of his greed and of the responsibility for his previous voyeurism. He then repeats the "magician" trick to disclose the whereabouts of the sexton. In this way he satisfies his wish for revenge on the wife who refused to give him shelter, while again attributing the responsibility for this action to another.

The connection between Little Claus and the magician is obvious to all, but in "The Tale of Lord Peter" there is no conscious link between the character of Peter and his cat. Although the attribution of responsibility for unacceptable actions occurs in both cases, in the tale of "Lord Peter" it occurs in a way that more closely parallels the function of a defense—that is, Peter is unaware of attributing his wishes to another.

Peter, the youngest of three brothers, has no money or way to survive after his parents die. His brothers take what few possessions the family owned and set out to try their luck in the world. Peter is left with nothing but the family cat; clearly, he is "in need." Whereas Peter is portrayed as a simple, honest fellow who is incapable of lying or presenting himself falsely, the cat is shown as a clever manipulator who engages in a series of outright lies to help Peter. Further, the cat is responsible for bribing others to lie about the status of his master, whom he calls "Lord Peter." The cat designs a series of deceits in which he instructs Peter to pretend to the king that he is a man of wealth and station. These subterfuges, cleverly maneuvered by the cat, involve the successive commandeering of game, sheep, cattle, horses, and, finally, a grand palace. In each case the cat is made responsible for the king being misled into thinking that all this bounty belongs to "Lord" Peter.

Throughout, Peter maintains a kind of naive innocence, simply following the commands of the cat: Peter does as he is told. The frequent repetitions of the cat's manipulations and bribes make it clear that Peter is in no way responsible for the deception. In the end, the king acknowledges Peter's superior status, Peter's needs are met, and his conscience is clear.

Projection Proper

In the previous two tales it is clear how splitting (i.e., the creation of two characters, one honest and one devious) is used to allow the main character to externalize unacceptable aspects of himself and to attribute the responsibility for unacceptable actions to another. It is also possible to find illustrations in folktales of the type of projection we have referred to as "projection proper," as in the Homeric "Hymn to Demeter" and "The Tale of

Anpu and Bata." In these cases the unacceptable wish is depicted as clearly residing in the character to whom it truly belongs, and the attempt of this character to project the wish onto another is laid bare for all to see.

One of the earliest literary examples of this form of projection occurs in the Homeric "Hymn to Demeter."[9] This hymn, written before 650 B.C. by followers of Homer, recounts the tale of Persephone, daughter of Demeter, being snatched into the underworld by Hades. Demeter is enraged by this abduction. To appease her anger, Zeus sends Hermes to Hades to ask for the release of Persephone. Hades does not want to disobey Zeus; he allows Persephone to see her mother, but he reminds the daughter that he, too, is a god, and while she lives with him she will reign as a queen and will receive all the privileges and gifts that belong to a queen. Hearing this, "Persephone rejoiced and jumped up quickly with joy. But secretly he slipped her a pomegranate seed, a sweet one, to eat, a precaution so that she would not stay everyday up there with the venerable Demeter. . . . "

This passage is all that is said about the eating of the pomegranate seed—an act that ensures Persephone's return to the underworld and her status as queen. However, when her mother chastises her for having eaten the seed, Persephone changes the story. She relates: "But secretly he slipped me a pomegranate seed with a sweet taste, *and forced me, unwillingly, violently, to eat it*" (p. 127; emphasis added).

Clearly, Persephone shifts the responsibility for the forbidden act to Hades through her addition of the elements of force and violence. In this sense the tale illustrates the second form of projection—attribution of responsibility to another. But the implication of Persephone's remarks goes beyond this meaning, in her intimation that Hades has sexually seduced her. It is this aspect of the story that led one psychologist (McClelland, 1963) to suggest that the third form of projection we have characterized—namely, the projection of an unacceptable impulse onto another, with a lack of awareness of this impulse existing in oneself—is also illustrated in the "Hymn." Although Persephone is characterized as "prudent" and "good," she displays some ambivalence about her lover, and being his queen is not without its rewards for her. McClelland has argued that, despite Persephone's protest that Hades seduced her, the reported seduction stemmed largely from Persephone's own unacknowledged attraction to her lover.

The functioning of projection proper is shown even more clearly in the ancient Egyptian tale of "Anpu and Bata."[10] Anpu, his wife, and his handsome younger brother Bata all live together. Bata cares for the cattle, plows the field, and is described as hardworking, obedient, and steadfast. The story revolves around a scene in which Anpu's wife invitingly lets down her hair and attempts to entice Bata. But he becomes enraged at her suggested crime, pointing out that she and Anpu are "as parents" to him. The wife becomes afraid of what she has said and done, but Bata promises not to reveal her evilness. Nevertheless, Anpu's wife, fearful of being found out, devises a scheme to absolve herself of any wrongdoing and to dispose of Bata at the same time. When Anpu returns from the field, his wife presents herself as disheveled. She accuses Bata of having tried to seduce her, vows that she refused him, and claims that he had beaten her in an attempt to prevent her from telling of his misdeed. Anpu then sets out to kill Bata, who flees.

The wife's projection of her sexual wishes onto Bata, to absolve herself from the guilt connected with her unacceptable wish, is clearly laid out for the reader. Her claim that he made sexual advances to her is a projection of the sexual advances she makes to him. Although Anpu is taken in by this defense, the reader is not.

As the story is told, Bata is honest and moral in the extreme. His virtuousness, however, is so absolute as to be almost unbelievable. One wonders whether, when he encounters Anpu's wife letting down her hair, he might not have been just a bit tempted. This raises the possibility of a double projection in this tale—one explicitly stated for the reader, the other implicit and not openly disclosed. One analyst (Bettelheim, 1976) pointed out that, inasmuch as the tale is told from the viewpoint of the younger brother, it is possible that Bata, in the context of the wife's hairdressing, had projected onto her the sexual desires that he did not dare to acknowledge in himself. Thus the wife's attribution of desire to Bata may have had some slight basis in reality. This possibility raises the interesting point that projections often have a grain of truth. Impulses or thoughts tend not to be projected randomly. Rather, the object of the projection may actually harbor a slight tendency to feel or think in accord with the projected feeling or thought.

THE DEVELOPMENT OF PROJECTION

As in the chapter on denial, I propose that some of the components of projection appear relatively early in life, whereas others depend on the emergence of more complex cognitive capacities. As with denial, we find that the prototype for projection lies in a physiological response present shortly after birth. Further precursors for projection are hypothesized to be present during the early months of the infant's life. However, I argue that projection cannot occur[11] until the child has developed internal standards for good–bad and acceptable–unacceptable.

"Projection may be defined as a method . . . whereby the subject attributes his own unacceptable unconscious tendencies to an object and then perceives them as tendencies possessed by the object" (Knight, 1940, p. 335).

The cognitive requirements for this mechanism to be carried out include at least the following:

- A differentiation between inside and outside.
- A differentiation between self and other (object).
- A differentiation between acceptable and unacceptable as determined by social mores.
- A differentiation between conscious and unconscious mental representations.

These requirements necessitate that the defense mechanism of projection develops later in the life of the child than the mechanism of denial.

However, before these cognitive abilities are developed, the early prototype for projection occurs in a physiological response that is present in the infant shortly after birth. When the young baby finds something in his mouth that is disagreeable or "bad," he spits it out. The baby gets rid of the unpleasant sensation by expelling the object into the external world. Unlike projection proper, the unpleasant feeling is not attached to any other person or thing—an operation that would require the recognition of objects separate from the self.

This possibility of ridding himself of a painful sensation also exists at the other end of the baby's alimentary canal. As the bowel or bladder fills and distends, discomfort increases but is relieved by expelling the feces and urine into the outside world.[12] Popular sayings sometimes convey this idea of defecation as a way of ridding the body of pain: Thus an adult man recalls his mother instructing him, many years earlier, that when he went to the bathroom it was to "put a *pain* in the pot."

The capacity to separate the pleasurable from the unpleasurable soon becomes possible on a psychological level with the laying down of memory traces. As with denial, this new capacity represents a developmental shift: What was a physiological response can now be carried out through a psychological mechanism. During the early months of life, the infant is repeatedly forming memory traces of his experience, many of which occur in connection with his mother. It is believed (e.g., Spitz, 1965) that these memory traces are laid down along affective lines. Thus some memories represent the "good" mother—the one who satisfies the infant's needs—whereas other traces represent the "bad" mother—the one who fails to satisfy the infant adequately. Representations of the "good mother" are stored separately from representations of the "bad mother," a situation that sets the stage for the infant to retain the "good" representations as his own and to expel the "bad" representations into the outer world.

For this precursor of projection to occur, two cognitive capacities must have developed. First, there must be some beginning development of the ego capacity for memory and for the development of memory structures organized according to affective dimensions. Second, the capacity to differentiate between internal and external, or between the "I" and the "non-I"—a capacity that Spitz (1966) places at the fifth or sixth month of life—must have developed. Once these are in place, mental representations that are associated with pleasure are incorporated into existing memory structures, whereas representations that cause unpleasure are projected into the external world. As Novick and Kelly (1970) discussed, this precursor of projection helps create the "purified pleasure ego" (Freud, 1915, p. 136), which in turn contributes to the development of the self.

Although the initial determination of the pleasure–unpleasure quality of a mental representation may be based on the gratification or nongratification of physiological needs, psychological factors soon become important determiners of the affective quality of an experience. Those experiences of the self and mother that are associated with mother's closeness, approval, and positive regard form the basis for a pleasurable/good/rewarding memory structure, which is kept "inside." Experiences of self and mother that are associated with mother's withdrawal, disapproval, and anger form the basis for a painful/bad/punishing memory structure, which is relegated to the "outside." The organization of memory traces along these lines allows the phenomenon of "splitting" to occur. With the establishment of such splitting, the psychological mechanism that is subsequently to be used for projection is in place.[13]

At the same time, the early closeness of mother and infant serves as a precursor for the defense of projection, forming a basis for generalization and the belief that the other thinks and feels the same as oneself (projective identification), or even that the other has put thoughts into one's head (Stolorow & Lachmann, 1978).

Not until the end of the second year does the infant normally begin to fuse the memories of the "good mother" with those of the "bad mother," eventually forming a more realistic image of mother as a distinct, integrated individual who is associated with both pleasurable and unpleasurable feelings. At the same time, the dual representation of the "good self" and the "bad self" are fused to form a single self-representation.[14] Further, the source of the *self*-representation is allocated to the inside, whereas the source of the *object*-representation (i.e., mother) is allocated to the outside.[15] This increased differentiation between self and object provides the opportunity for the next precursor of projection to develop.

As the child becomes more aware of a world separate from himself, he begins to try to understand it. These early attempts to understand natural phenomena are partly determined by what the child has come to know about himself. He "understands" what he sees around him in terms of what he consciously knows and feels about himself. In the young child, this is a normal mode of thinking (i.e., nondefensive). Examples of such animistic thinking abound in Piaget's discussion of early preoperational thought. For example, a young child observes a string attached to a box unwind after it was wound up and remarks that the string "wants" to be unwound because it "knows" that it is twisted. Another child states that the clouds move because the sun pushes them with its rays (Piaget, 1929). This type of thinking, in which other people and objects in the world are assumed to be like oneself and are understood by fitting them into one's own pattern, is, in Piaget's theory, an example of the principle of assimilation. Novick and Novick (1996b), in their discussion of projection, refer to this primitive system of thought as generalization, whereby conscious inner experiences are generalized to, and assumed to be shared with, other persons and things.

At the same time, although the child attributes his own feelings, wishes, and intentions to others outside of himself, he consciously perceives these characteristics as part of himself. Unlike the situation in projection proper, the child is aware of having the same feelings that he attributes to others, and these feelings may be either positive or negative.

Although such generalization, or animistic thinking, is natural in the young child's attempt to understand what goes on around him, it may serve a defensive function at times. When the assumption that others are like oneself is exaggerated—when the sharing of attributes is too extreme—the self and the other become as one—that is, a fantasy fusion of self and other occurs. This merging protects the young child from the painful feelings associated with separation and loss of the other. In this fusion of self and other through the assumption of shared characteristics, we also see an early form of projective identification.

As the child continues to develop, he becomes more aware of cause-and-effect relationships. In human relationships the issue of cause and effect is translated into the question of responsibility—that is, who, or what, is responsible for what has happened. In the young child's life, it is very often the parents who are responsible for what happens. The baby cannot move himself from place to place; he is moved by the parents. The toddler does not arrange to go to nursery school; he is placed there by an adult. This long period of dependence on the parents contributes greatly to the child's attribution of responsibility to others—responsibility not only for his physical situation and his emotional well-being, but also for his more specific thoughts, actions, and feeling states.

This attribution of responsibility becomes defensive when it is used to protect the individual from feelings of shame or guilt. Thus the boy who reveals to his therapist that he would like to see his mother undressed quickly adds, "You wanted me to say that," and so relieves his anxiety. Clearly involved in this process is the development of some internal standard by which the child begins to evaluate his own behavior as acceptable or unacceptable— a standard which, if broken, causes anxiety. To acknowledge oneself as the person responsible for the unacceptable behavior would be too painful. Consequently, although the child remains conscious of the behavior, the cause or responsibility for the feelings, thoughts, or actions is placed elsewhere.

In recent years academic psychologists have investigated the attribution of responsibility in children under the topic of "locus of control." Using questionnaires and other interview methods, they have found that as children grow older, the locus of control for their behavior shifts from being predominantly external to being predominantly internal (e.g., Connell, 1985; Crandall, Katkovsky, & Crandall, 1965). Thus the child moves from assuming that others are responsible for his behavior to internalizing the responsibility.[16]

But this process does not occur in all individuals. The sociopathic individual is one in whom the internalization of responsibility fails to occur. Listening to such a person recount a multitude of encounters with the legal system, the continual and overwhelming attribution of responsibility to others is striking; for example, "If he hadn't have come into the bar, I wouldn't have hit him"; "People shouldn't leave their valuable property lying around, tempting one to take it."

In clinical practice it is not uncommon to learn that patients believe their feelings are being determined by others to a significant degree. They are convinced, even obsessed with the idea, that only the presence of a specific individual can "make" them feel good, just as, in their earlier life, they felt that mother was able to "take away the bad feelings" and to provide good feelings. It is quite foreign to them to think that the source of feelings is internal and may be related to intrapsychic conflict. They attribute the responsibility for their feeling state entirely to the "other" and engage in a relentless pursuit of that person.

The attribution of cause to the external world was the first type of projection that Freud identified (e.g., 1895). This type of attribution implies the development of an internal standard of judgment regarding acceptable and unacceptable behavior, and it stems from the child's long period of dependence on others. Unlike projection proper, the unacceptable thought or feeling remains in conscious awareness, internal to the individual; it is only the responsibility for the thought that is projected outward, onto another.

As the child continues to develop, he ordinarily finds it more and more difficult to accommodate these unacceptable thoughts or impulses as being part of himself. Further, the reaction of significant others reinforces the child's difficulty in integrating these discordant aspects into the self. To recognize these devalued characteristics in oneself is to suffer the feeling of a devalued self. One way to avoid such feelings of humiliation is to project the unacceptable characteristic onto another. Thus the 4-year-old who is struggling to learn to tie his shoes points an accusing finger at an older child and exclaims, "*He* can't tie his shoe." By ridding himself of these unacceptable aspects of his self-representation, he protects himself from disruptive anxiety and provides time for the remaining self-representations to integrate. In normal development, once the self-image has stabilized, the child can begin to reintegrate those aspects of himself that are less acceptable.

However, it is not uncommon to meet adults who continue to maintain a positive self-image by projecting onto others aspects of their self-representation they consciously find unacceptable. For example, a newly married woman found herself puzzled when neighbors, about whom her husband had ambivalent feelings, expressed their regrets that a prior commitment had kept her from joining them for cocktails. Because she had no knowledge of either the commitment or the cocktail party, she spoke to her husband. He explained to her that *he* had made a prior arrangement, and he assumed that she must also be busy; thus his refusal of the neighbor's invitation. Some time later the couple attended a social gathering but left early at the husband's request. Subsequently, he queried his wife about her reaction to a particular woman. Having fallen prey, on previous occasions, to his projections, she withheld comment, only to endure his explosion, "It was obvious you didn't like her and wanted to leave early!" Among his neighbors and colleagues, this man was known for his warmth and friendliness—a self-image that he fostered. When the couple built an addition to their house, the inevitable delays as well as incompetent workmen frustrated both husband and wife. However, the husband referred to these frustrations as residing only in the wife: *She* was upset, *she* was angry. While he encouraged her to deal with the contractor and to insist on completion of work promised, and suggested that *she* convey *her* feelings of frustration and anger, he maintained cheerful relations with the builders. At the completion of the house, he was still the "nice guy," while she had become the shrew.

In this example it is assumed that the man was unaware of his externalization of unacceptable aspects of himself. In other cases, however, one individual may knowingly attribute some characteristic to a second person, in order to use that individual for his or her own gain. These are clear instances of manipulation. However, the dividing line between a calculated shifting of blame and externalization of a part of the self-representation to avoid humiliation can be fuzzy. Thus, while one individual may be used (manipulated) as the receptacle for unacceptable parts of the other's self-representation, the latter individual may be unaware of this process and thus unconscious of the manipulation.

The final stage in the development of projection in the child requires the emergence of several other cognitive capacities. In projection proper, an unacceptable thought, feeling, wish, or impulse of which the individual is unaware is projected onto another. This impulse is manifest in the form of a fantasy; thus the child must have reached a level of cognitive development in which fantasy is possible. Cognitively, the individual toward whom the impulse was once directed (i.e., the object of the impulse) now becomes the agent of the impulse, whereas the original agent becomes the object. It is this latter characteristic that clearly differentiates projection proper from its other forms. In all the other forms the relief from anxiety comes from placing something that is internal onto the external world; the inside is rid of something objectionable or is defensively merged with the external.[17] In projection proper, not only is the unacceptable internal impulse made external but, because of the change of object, this impulse is now directed back at the self: "I hate him" becomes "He hates me."

It is this last characteristic—the direction of the unacceptable impulse toward the self—that renders this defense relatively ineffective for the avoidance of anxiety. To become the object of one's own unacceptable fantasies is clearly maladaptive, although it does allow one a (false) sense of control if one believes that one can escape from the presumed external source of danger.

However, to the extent that individuals—children or adults—externalize parts of themselves or project representations of their own unacceptable impulses onto others in whom those characteristics do not exist, they are altering reality—or rather their perception of reality. To see something that is not there—and, in the case of projection, this something is almost always negative, punishing, and unacceptable—is to distort reality, to suffer a breakdown in reality testing. This distortion of reality forms the basis for the unwarranted suspicion and hyperalertness that accompany the use of projection over extended periods of time; it also creates the felt need for protection from threat and sometimes for a "reactive" aggressive stance.

ANOTHER FOLKTALE

An old folktale embodies many of these forms of projection. In the Grimms' story of "The Goose Girl,"[18] a princess and her servant set off on a journey to a foreign land where the princess is to marry a prince. As a parting gift, the princess's mother gives her a handkerchief containing three drops of her (the mother's) blood.

The servant is portrayed as a mean, bad person who haughtily refuses to help the princess and, indeed, steals her belongings during the journey. The good princess, on the other hand, does nothing in retaliation. She remains "humble" and forgets about the servant's rudeness. The only protests that are heard occur through the mother's handkerchief, which cries out, "If my mother knew it, it would break her heart."

As the trip continues, the servant forces the princess to exchange clothes and horses with her and to swear, on pain of death, that she will tell no one of the exchange. When they arrive at the prince's castle, the servant is dressed in the grand robes whereas the princess appears in unattractive, "mean" apparel. The princess says nothing about the trickery.

The false princess, however, fears that the princess's talking horse, Falada, will reveal what she has done. She then accuses Falada of having upset her on the trip by his wrongdoing, and the prince unwittingly has Falada's head cut off. But the true princess arranges to have the head mounted on the town gateway. Each day, as she passes beneath the gate on her way to her new job of tending geese, she calls out "Alas! dear Falada, there thou hangest!" The horse's head, which has retained the ability to speak, replies, "Alas! Queen's daughter, there thou gangest. If thy mother knew thy fate, her heart would break with grief so great."

When she arrives in the fields with the geese, the princess lets down her hair to comb and curl it. The young boy who accompanies her would like to pluck out some of the golden strands of hair, but the princess calls upon the wind to blow his cap away. While the boy chases his cap, she finishes her coiffure, and he is prevented from annoying her.

The boy finally informs the king of these strange happenings. The king observes them himself and then questions the "goose girl" as to their meaning. She refuses to answer him, explaining that, under pain of death, she has given her oath not to tell. Finally, he convinces her to give the explanation to a cooking stove. She concludes her revelation to the stove by again saying, "If my mother knew it, it would break her heart." The king listens through the stove pipe and discovers the deceit.

A banquet is arranged at which the king, the prince, the false princess, and the true princess are present. The king puts a "riddle" to the false princess, in which he asks what should be done to a person who deceives his master. The king then tells a story of a servant who has usurped his master and again asks what the punishment should be for such a person. The false princess decries that the person should be dragged through the streets in a barrel full of sharp nails. The truth is then revealed, the would-be princess/servant receives her own punishment, and the prince marries his true bride.

The tale is replete with examples of the various forms of projection. In the beginning of the story there is the clear splitting between the "good" princess, who appears to harbor no feelings of malice, revenge, or even anger, and the "bad" servant, who becomes increasingly malicious as the tale develops. Then, on top of this straightforward division of good and bad between the two characters, a second form of splitting occurs through the device of exchanging clothes. Through this conceit, a splitting of good and bad now occurs *within* each character as well as between the two characters. The princess now appears "bad" and "mean" on the outside, remaining "good" on the inside, whereas the reverse is true for the servant.

An additional form of projection occurs through the recitations of the handkerchief. Although the princess says nothing, her protest is spoken by the handkerchief; the princess's thoughts are projected onto this magical cloth. Interestingly, the projection is carried even further, for the handkerchief laments that it is the *mother* who would be upset; there is no suggestion that the princess herself might be disturbed.

Yet another form of projection occurs in the servant's generalization of her own hostile feelings to the horse Falada. Inasmuch as she has done wrong to another woman, the servant assumes Falada will do wrong to her. A further projection is manifest when the servant accuses Falada of wrongdoing during the trip, whereas the wrongdoing was clearly carried out by the servant.

The use of projection occurs yet again in the declarations of the horse's head. Whereas the princess keeps to her oath of silence, the horse reveals her identity ("Alas, Queen's daughter"). Again there is the projection that it is the queen, not the princess, who would be distraught about the situation.

The inability of the princess to take even the slightest assertive action on her own part and the need to project responsibility for such assertion onto some other object occurs again in the fields with the young boy. Clearly, the princess does not want him to fool with her hair, but the responsibility for shooing him off is projected onto the wind, which causes him to run after his cap. The princess remains, as ever, blameless.

When the trickery is finally revealed, the princess does not tell her story directly. By speaking to an inanimate stove, she does not violate her oath not to tell "any human creature"; the story is projected into the stove pipe, which in turn relays the tale to the king. The princess remains "honorable."

Even the final punishment of the bad servant occurs through a form of projection. The king "projects" the deceitful characteristics of the servant onto another character and then invites the servant to determine the punishment for that "other." The misdoings and the punishment are then returned to the servant, their rightful owner.

CLINICAL EXAMPLE

In the following clinical example, we see the function of projection and note its greater complexity to denial.

Elaine, a patient in late adolescence whose inability to function at college had led her to return home and begin therapy, experienced considerable difficulty in forming relationships outside her immediate family. The few merged attachments she had experienced in her life were characterized by mutual exploitation—physical and material exploitation on the part of the other, emotional exploitation on her own part. Not surprisingly, she had eventually become disillusioned about each of these relationships.

After some time in treatment she was able to strike up a friendship with a young man whom she had known during childhood. From her description of him, he seemed noticeably different from her earlier choices. However, his unwillingness to allow merging and his failure to exploit left Elaine feeling confused and rejected. Although in her previous relationships Elaine had repeatedly telephoned the person or "dropped in" unexpectedly, in this newly developing friendship she steadfastly refused to call the young man, insisting that he would have to call her. Some time elapsed during which he did not call, about which she felt both hurt and angry. Nevertheless, she refused to contact him, even when she learned from a mutual friend that he was hoping she would call. Much of the time, however, she was out of touch with her feelings of anxiety and anger that he did not call, tending instead to dismiss him as "boring."

One early summer evening, accompanied by her sister, she drove past the young man's house, thinking she might have a "chance" encounter. He was, in fact, out on the lawn and waved to her; she stopped and began to chat with him. She described this conversation as friendly and pleasant and was surprised to find him so cordial. He invited Elaine and her sister to a small party to be held at a friend's studio later that evening, asking her to come around 9:00 P.M.

Elaine and her sister returned home to prepare for the party. However, they delayed their departure and when they arrived at the studio at 10:30, the windows were dark and no one was to be seen. Understandably, Elaine was upset by this disappointment. Her subsequent reaction well illustrates the use of projection.

When she came to see me the next day, she related these events and then added her "explanation" of why all of this had happened. She believed the young man had purposely pretended to her that there was going to be a party to trick her and make her feel foolish. Further, his reason for doing this was to get revenge on her, because *he was angry that she had not called him* in the previous weeks.

Although Elaine agreed that he had never played any mean jokes on her before, nor on anyone else that she knew of, she held to her explanation, which was based on the projection of *her* anger that he had not called.

The issue of her late arrival and the possibility that the party might have closed down or moved to another location by that time were dismissed by Elaine on the basis of an angry phone call she had made to the young man the next morning. The purpose of this call—"to catch him in a lie"—was carried out by Elaine herself telling a lie about the time she

rrived at the party, implying that it was shortly after nine. When he apolo-
ized about the party not getting off the ground, adding that a few people
ad come later (i.e., after Elaine had presumably come and left), she had
er "proof" that he had lied. With this "evidence" of his dishonesty, she
vas able to express her anger at him directly. This "justified" anger was
naintained until a few days later when she learned from an acquaintance
hat the party had, in fact, been held, but that only a few people had come
nd it had closed down around 10:00.

In this clinical example we can trace the functioning of projection in a
airly straightforward way. Elaine's initial feeling of anger during the week
efore the party because he did not call was too painful for her to experi-
nce, for to do so would put her in touch with her great disappointment
nd her feelings of being rejected—a rejection she felt resulted from her
ndesirability and unworthiness. Through delaying her arrival at the party,
he helped create a situation in which it was possible for her to project both
he anger and the reason for the anger onto the young man—*he was angry
because she did not call*. At the same time, the projected explanation of his
"malicious" behavior provided her with an external justification for ex-
ressing her anger toward him. The issue of rejection remains, but through
rojection, the rejection is now clearly seen as due to his maliciousness. The
ainful possibility that the initial "rejection" was due to her own (felt)
ndesirability or unworthiness is now well out of the picture: The anger
an be expressed without Elaine's experiencing a narcissistic wound.

THE USE OF PROJECTION IN PROJECTIVE STORIES

To say that we can find evidence of projection in projective storytelling may
eem self-evident because the assumption is that the entire story is based on
he projection of the thoughts, feelings, concerns, and values of the story-
eller. Yet the kinds of thoughts and feelings and the manner in which they
re expressed may differ widely across individuals. In looking for evidence
f defensive projection in stories, we note the occurrence of themes that
vould be unacceptable if enacted by the storyteller in real life. We also note
he expression of thought patterns that take the same form as that of the
lefense mechanism (e.g., one character attributing his thoughts to a second
:haracter or to inanimate objects).[19]

This section presents and analyzes stories told in response to TAT Card
17BM (a man clinging to a rope) for the occurrence of projection. The storytellers are three boys, ranging in age from 7 to 15 years old.

The following tape-recorded story was told by an 11-year-old boy:

*Once there was a story about a man and he was building a house and
then some warriors came along and broke down the house and were*

trying to kill him. Luckily he escaped and went away on his horse. Trying to get into the government building, he climbed up a rope and got in and killed the emperor.

This story, although short, is striking in its demonstration of the use of projection both by the storyteller and by the main character in the story. Although the TAT picture depicts a single man clinging to a rope, the storyteller adds a band of murderous warriors, an escape horse, and a murdered emperor. There is nothing in the picture to suggest these characters; they are clearly derived from the storyteller's own aggressive fantasies, projected onto the benign stimulus card. However, beyond the storyteller's projections we see within the story itself the use of projection by the hero. The story begins with someone else trying to do something to the hero—that is, trying to kill him—which the hero then ends up doing to someone else. In the beginning, a man, apparently minding his own business, is benignly building a house. Along come some men described as "warriors," to whom are attributed both the intention of destroying the man's work and the wish to kill him. The story concludes, however, with the hero himself carrying out the intentions that had previously been attributed to the warriors— namely, killing someone.

As another example of the use of projection in a TAT story, the following was written by a 15-year-old boy:

The person is John Freen—Ace secret agent. He is trying to escape from the Castle of Death! He had already killed the evil Calipso and plans to blow up the foundation! He is climbing down the rope on the side of the castle. He must work fast—for in 10 minutes the castle will be blown sky high!—Freen is feeling nervous tension, fear of death. He feels the moon and the cold darkness are against him!

This story portrays many aspects of projection. There is, first of all, the idea of someone secretly carrying out dangerous acts, hidden from others. At the same time, this individual is in danger of being trapped by others. Although he has killed, he fears being killed. There is a continual interplay between his aggression toward others and his fear of aggression from them. This fear of attack from others reaches its high point when the hero, who has himself planted a bomb that is about to blow him up, now feels that "the moon and the cold darkness are against him."

From another vantage point the several ominous additions to this story—the evil Calipso, the death castle, and the bomb—are all reflections of the way in which the storyteller reacts when placed in a stressful situation. Aggressive feelings of the storyteller are projected onto objects and people in the environment, which then become ominous, just as happens within the story when the hero displays animistic thinking in his attribution of aggressive feelings to the moon.

In a developmentally earlier form, the same theme of being caught, trying to escape, and the projection of anger connected with this frustrating situation and resulting in the addition of ominous people and objects to the story, is seen in the following story by a 7-year-old boy told about the same picture:

> *That man is on the rope. Because he is trying to get away. Because he doesn't want to get hurt, by the guards. The guards are bad. The guards have long, sharp things, and he is trying to get away from them. He is going to get pulled down and get eaten up.*

One way of understanding this highly aggressive story is as a statement of the child's experience with the examiner. The examiner asks him to tell story; he feels a demand made on him, from which he would like to get away. But he is not supposed to leave; the adult authority has told him to stay. The rise in his own anger about this situation is projected onto the authority, who he then fears may hurt him. According to this illogic, because the guards are perceived as angry and potentially hurtful, they are bad. The hostile feelings are, in addition, attached to concrete objects ("long, sharp things"), perhaps linking up with fears of phallic reprisal, which reinforces the need to get away. This increasingly anxious situation continues with a regression to an earlier form of aggressive fantasy—namely, the projection of the wish to destroy through devouring.

CONCLUDING REMARKS

We have seen that projection develops out of a prototypic physiological response in which the infant rids himself of a disagreeable sensation by ejecting it out into the environment. This expulsion of the unpleasant subsequently proceeds along psychological lines through the mechanism of splitting, in which "good" memory representations are felt to be internal whereas "bad" memory representations are experienced as external. For these early stages of projection to be possible, the following cognitive capacities must have developed:

- The capacity to differentiate between inside and outside and between self and other.
- The capacity to form memory structures organized according to the dimensions of pleasure and unpleasure.

Splitting is subsequently followed by generalization and animism, processes whereby the child assumes that his own thoughts and feelings are present in, and shared by, others. In neither of these early forms of projection is the child unaware of his own feelings.

With the beginning of early childhood, the emergence of several cognitive capacities makes possible the development of further forms of projection. These cognitive capacities include:

- The development of internal evaluative standards.
- The separation of conscious and unconscious thought processes.
- The capacity for representing an impulse in fantasy.
- The capacity for understanding cause and effect and separating the causative agent from the object affected.

In conjunction with these cognitive developments, projection in the form of attribution of responsibility appears next. While the unacceptable impulse remains inside and conscious, the cause of the impulse is projected outward, onto another. This is followed by the projection of unacceptable aspects of the self-representation onto others, to maintain a valued self-image. Finally, projection proper develops in which an unacceptable unconscious impulse is projected onto another, and a reversal of subject (agent) and object occurs.

Although the precursors of projection can be found in infancy and toddlerhood, the greater complexity of cognitive capacities required for the functioning of projection, compared with denial, suggests that the relative importance of projection increases in the early school years at the same time that the use of denial is declining. Moreover, it is at this time that the child develops clearer internal standards of good and bad, acceptable and unacceptable, superego formation, and a shift in moral judgment from consequences to intentions—critical elements in the functioning of projection. Moreover, because projection in a mild form does not seriously distort reality, and may even serve a positive function for the individual by making him more empathic and thus "understanding" of others, the use of projection may decline only slightly throughout the periods of childhood and adolescence. Certainly we can see extensive use of projection as a means of ensuring group cohesiveness through the formation of adolescent cliques and in the functioning of their "in groups" and "out groups."

CHAPTER 5

Identification

Identification refers to modifying the subjective self or behavior, or both, in order to increase one's resemblance to an object taken as a model.
—SCHAFER (1968, p. 16)

Identification represents a process of modifying the self-schema on the basis of a present or past perception of an object which is taken as a model.
—SANDLER (1960, p. 150)

Identification used as a defense replaces "a real object relationship by making good a loss through the internalization of the lost object."
—MENAKER (1979, p. 215)

Identification is also "a necessary, normal, positive developmental aspect of ego growth . . . it is that mechanism without which human relatedness would be impossible."
—MENAKER (1979, p. 215)

The hungry infant's longing for oral gratification is the origin of the first, primitive type of identification. . . .
—JACOBSON (1954, p. 99)

We are what we eat.

The mechanism of identification is considerably more complex than those of denial and projection. As with projection, identification requires the capacity to differentiate between self and other. However, identification further involves a differentiation and modification within the ego; new ego structures—including the superego and the ego ideal—develop as an integral part of the process of identification. As with the other two defenses,

93

the beginnings of identification may be seen early in life. Different from denial and projection, identification continues to develop through adolescence.

The literature shows a considerable inconsistency and some confusion in the use of the term *identification*. In one review, 8 different definitions of identification were discussed (Sanford, 1955); in another, 10 further definitions were considered (White, 1961). Clearly, the concept has come to embrace a large variety of phenomena.

Beyond these multiple definitions of identification, a second source of confusion has contributed to the lack of clarity surrounding the concept. It is characteristic of the literature in this area that the terms *identification, introjection,* and *incorporation* are often used interchangeably (cf. Bronfenbrenner, 1960; Compton, 1985; Knight, 1940).[1] This situation leads not only to semantic confusion; it also creates considerable confusion when the defenses are seen from a developmental perspective, because incorporation is a primitive mechanism based on the physiological prototype of "taking in" food, whereas identification is developmentally advanced, requiring structural modifications in the ego based on experience. I differentiate among these three mechanisms in this chapter.

From the multitude of definitions offered, it is possible to summarize the main features of identification:

- A change that occurs in the ego (i.e., the personality, behavior, or motives of the individual).
- The change is in the direction of becoming *like* some other individual, group, or cause.
- The change serves the purpose of maintaining an affective relationship with a significant other.
- The change is related to the development and maintenance of self-esteem.

A comprehensive definition of identification has been offered by Schafer (1968):

> In its fullest sense, the process of identifying with an object is unconscious, though it may also have prominent and significant preconscious and conscious components; in this process the subject modifies his motives and behavior patterns, and the self representations corresponding to them, in such a way as to experience being like, the same as, and merged with one or more representations of that object; through identification, the subject both represents as his own one or more regulatory influences or characteristics of the object that have become important to him and continues his tie to the object; the subject may wish to bring about this change for various reasons. . . . (p. 140)

The idea that identification may occur "for various reasons" points up yet another complexity—and possible source of confusion—regarding this mechanism. On the one hand, there is a *defensive* identification that occurs as a way of avoiding anxiety and maintaining self-esteem. With this mechanism the anxiety caused by the loss, or anticipated loss, of a significant other is attenuated by recreating that other internally. Defensive identification may also include a modification of the ego to include the parents' standards and prohibitions, so as to maintain their approval and to control unacceptable impulses.

On the other hand, there is a *developmental* identification in which the child modifies his ego, on the basis of experience, to become increasingly independent, individuated, and autonomous from significant others. This kind of identification is a necessary part of normal psychological development that contributes to the formation of conscience, of the ego-ideal, and finally of "identity." In contrast to defensive identification, developmental identification leads to a structural change in the self-representation (Horner, 1983).

A final source of confusion in the use of the concept of identification stems from the fact that the term refers to both a *process* and an *end state*. As a result of the process of identification, modifications in the ego occur. These new ego structures represent the end state of identification. Some of these identifications may continue throughout life; others will change with experience (they may be modified or abandoned); and new identifications will be developed during latency and adolescence.

Thus the process of identification takes experiences with the outside world and places them inside to create new ego structures. Projection, on the other hand, takes internal mental representations and places them outside to rid the ego of sources of anxiety. Identification, in that it serves to modify the ego in accordance with experience, shares some features with Piaget's concept of accommodation.

COMPONENTS OF IDENTIFICATION

Let us look now at three main components of identification—incorporation, introjection, and identification proper (Meissner, 1974). With incorporation, the motive is to possess, to have, to become merged with the object. There is little or no distinction between the subject and the object; the boundaries are fluid and ambiguous. A very primitive, primary process type of mentation allows this process to function; the subject takes all of, or part of, another person (or thing) into herself, and this incorporation causes positive or negative changes in her feelings and experience. Although this type of primitive thinking is generally restricted to either infancy or conditions of psychosis, it can be seen in both fairytales and the fantasies of young children. An example is given later in this chapter: A 4-year-old boy told a TAT story in which a young boy eats the muscles of a giant to become a giant himself.

With introjection, there is a somewhat clearer distinction between the self and the object, although the boundaries are still somewhat fluid. Some theorists (e.g., Meissner, 1974) describe the motive of introjection as the desire to be the *same* as the model—that is, to achieve identity with the object. Others (e.g., Schafer, 1968) stress that the aim is to continue a relationship with the object by displacing this relationship from the outer to the inner world. In either case, representations of important others are established internally via introjection. These may include multiple representations of the same person, each carrying with it the valence of the emotional relationship existing at the time of introjection. Thus there is the representation of the loving mother, the angry mother, the depriving mother, the supporting mother, and so on. Introjection may also occur in the internalization of the parents' code of prohibitions; however, in contrast to identification and the development of the superego, these introjects stand apart from the ego (i.e., they do not effect a change in the ego). Satisfying or violating them is based on the child's concern for her parents' reaction, not on a sense of meeting her own internal standards. Prohibitions based on introjection are relatively weak (i.e., easily disobeyed or circumvented), compared with those based on the superego. As with incorporation, introjection may be influenced by primary process thinking. It is accompanied by poor reality testing and may involve magical thinking.

In contrast with incorporation and introjection, identification requires that the other person be recognized as separate. The motive of identification is to be *like* the model; this requires that there be both a cognitive and affective differentiation between the self and other, for to be like another, one must recognize that the other is different from the self. Identification aims to transform the ego along the lines of the other; it involves the internalization of both the regulations and the characteristics of others in the environment. Regulations include the demands, control, guidance, prohibitions, punishments, and gratifications of the significant other, as well as the rebellion against, or surrender to, these. Characteristics include the behavior patterns, motives, defenses, skills, and attitudes of the significant others. In all of these ways identification functions as a defensive or as a developmental mechanism. In all cases the mechanism of identification serves either to protect or enhance self-esteem.

Once regulations are internalized through the process of identification, they can be projected back onto the environment (e.g., onto an authority figure), without losing their basically internal position. The attribution of demand or (nonmagical) control to others is therefore at base a reflection of identification (Fenichel, 1945). Also the newly developing aspects of the self formed through identification can be externalized onto others and vicariously "tried out" in this way to see how they fare in reality (Novick & Kelly, 1970).

In addition to these three identification processes, two other components are related to the development of identification: imitation and learning. These parallel components interact with the identification processes and facilitate the development of identification (Gaddini, 1969; Meissner, 1974). Imitation of the parents' behavior serves, in the beginning, to maintain the relationship with the nurturing other; subsequently, it facilitates the development of skills that allow the child to function separately from the parent. Whereas imitation may be lasting or momentary, *learning* refers to a relatively lasting change in behavior as a result of experience. Learning comes about through the selective reinforcement of certain imitative behaviors.

Through imitation and learning, children become functionally more like their parents; this increasing similarity paves the way for identification with the parents to occur. Once children have added the behaviors and understandings to their repertory that allow them to act a little bit like the parents, they can, through identification, *become* like the parents. In other words, the behaviors must exist before children can use them as a means for identification; it is through imitation and learning that the behaviors are established. In this sense both imitation and learning are components of identification.

The way in which identification takes place and the types of identification that are formed depend on a variety of factors (cf. Schafer, 1968, pp. 171–179). The occurrence of identification in any one child depends on constitutional differences such as temperament or activity type, on stage of development, and on the multiple appeals of the identification—the variety of wishes it will fulfill and the array of problems it will solve. In addition, it depends on the character of the individuals who serve as models, the parents' and significant others' reactions to the developing identifications, and the nature of the child's other experiences, especially as these further the integration or disruption of the identification process.

IDENTIFICATION AS SEEN IN FOLKTALES

The legends of many cultures present the idea that humans can acquire various characteristics through the incorporation or introjection of other beings, or parts of other beings, who possess the desired characteristic. Thus, in Greek mythology, Zeus swallows his pregnant wife, Metis, and shortly after he is able to give birth to Pallas Athene. In addition to acquiring his wife's capacity for childbearing, he also acquires her command over wisdom and knowledge; for Zeus claims, after swallowing her, that "she gave him counsel from inside his belly."[2] Zeus acquires other powers by incorporating his second wife, Themis, who controlled the cycle of the seasons and was known for her righteousness, justice, and equity.[3]

The acquisition of wisdom through incorporation also appears in Celtic myths. In one tale Fionn accidentally eats the burned flesh of a sacred animal and, as a result, he obtains supernatural wisdom.[4] In another, the goddess Cerridwen wishes to compensate her unfortunate, repulsive son by giving him knowledge. She prepares "a cauldron of inspiration and science." As she goes to gather "herbs of virtue," she leaves her clansman Gwion to stir the pot. Accidentally, three drops of liquid from the pot fall on Gwion's finger, which he puts in his mouth. Then, "he found himself [the] master of knowledge." The acquisition of knowledge through incorporation does not stop at this point, however. Cerridwen, enraged at Gwion's acquired knowledge, subsequently engages in shape-shifting; she transforms herself into a hen and Gwion into a piece of grain. Cerridwen then swallows him and thus takes the knowledge into herself. Subsequently, she gives birth to a son, Taliesen, who possesses this knowledge.[5]

Another example of incorporation occurs in the Bulgarian folktale "The Language of Animals."[6] In this story a shepherd saves a serpent from a fire. In return, the serpent takes the shepherd to his father, who is king of all the serpents. The king offers the shepherd a reward for having saved his son. The shepherd requests that he be given the ability to understand the language of animals. The king fulfills this request by spitting into the mouth of the shepherd three times; from then on the shepherd can understand all animals.

It is not only knowledge that is acquired through incorporation. In Norse legends, the timid youth, Ingiuld, became very bold after he ate the heart of a wolf, and Hialto became strong and courageous after eating the heart of a bear and drinking its blood. Among the North American Indians it was believed that men who ate venison became swifter and wiser than those who ate the clumsy bear, and the great chieftains refused to eat the meat of any animal that was slow-moving or dull-witted.[7] Such ideas also appear in Icelandic, African, Korean, and Australian myths, among others.

Eating the organs of someone envied also occurs in a tale more familiar in Western European culture. In the story of Snow White, the wicked queen, consumed with jealousy and envy of Snow White, orders her killed and eats up what she believes to be Snow White's lungs and liver[8] or her heart.[9] Although it is not stated, it is perhaps implicitly understood that the queen hopes to acquire Snow White's beauty by incorporating into herself the girl's most vital organs.

Although many of the incorporation myths focus on the hero acquiring *positive* characteristics, a variant on this theme occurs in an American Indian legend. The Assiniboine tribe of the northern Rockies have a tale in which a reckless, wasteful brother assumes the grotesque physical characteristics of a monster he has wrongly eaten. After roasting the monster alive, he eats his flesh and then, day after day, his body becomes as that of the monster. He is covered with long black hair, and horns grow from his head; fish scales appear on his legs, which then become a tail. In the end, the bad brother loses his humanity altogether.[10]

Identification through imitation and social learning can be seen in the story of the "Three Bears," which tells of the little girl Goldilocks and three bears: a Great Big Bear, a Middle-Sized Bear, and a Wee Little Bear.[11] Goldilocks, while out playing, comes upon the bears' empty house, and, being curious, goes in. This entrance into a new environment gives Goldilocks the opportunity to try out different roles and to discover that only the role of the Wee Little Bear—the one most like her—fits comfortably. The porridge of the Great Big Bear is too hot, his chair is too hard, and his bed has a headboard that is too high. The porridge of the Middle-Sized Bear is too cold, her chair is too soft, and her footboard is too high. But the porridge, the chair, and the bed of the Wee Little Bear are just right, and Goldilocks appropriates each for herself. Without much reflection, she takes them over as her own, whole cloth.

The return of the bears is marked by a succession of imitations. The Great Big Bear says "Somebody has been tasting my porridge," which is then echoed by the Middle-Sized Bear and by the Wee Little Bear, who adds "and has eaten it all up." The Great Big Bear begins again, "Somebody has been sitting in my chair," which is echoed by the Middle-Sized Bear and by the Wee Little Bear, who adds, "and has broken it all to pieces." Once more the Great Big Bear announces, "Somebody has been lying in my bed," which is again echoed by the Middle-Sized Bear and by the Wee Little Bear, who adds, "and here she is!"

Part of the pleasure young child experience on hearing this story comes from the description of early aspects of identification—of Goldilocks trying out the role of bear, and of the little bear imitating the bigger bears. But the Wee Little Bear, it should be noted, does not simply imitate the big bears. There are additions made to the Wee Bear's refrains that differentiate him from the older bears. Significantly, this differentiation has been brought about through the introduction of a peer into his life. As the child's social world expands to include peers, there are more possibilities for developing skills, attitudes, and even changes in identification. The tale thus illustrates several of the early components of identification: appropriating the characteristics of others, imitation, and learning through experience with peers.

One other way in which an early form of identification occurs in folktales is seen in the child who inherits the qualities of the parent. In these stories the explanation for the child becoming like the parent is kept on the biological level; the process is automatic, without the conscious participation of the child. For example, in Irish myths[12] there are tales in which the magical powers of the parent are inherited by the child. That the child's acquisition of the parents' qualities is automatic (i.e., not due to experience or development) is made especially clear in an Irish myth in which the ambitions of the father are transferred to the child at the moment of conception.

THE DEVELOPMENT OF IDENTIFICATION

In discussing the components of identification, we examined the different processes of incorporation, introjection, identification, and imitation, noting that these terms have often been used interchangeably, leading to some confusion (cf. Knight, 1940). In this section on the development of identification, I propose the point of view that incorporation and introjection are precursors to identification, but they do not lie on a straight-line continuum with it. Rather, they are conceptualized as discontinuous processes, and each is prominent at a different phase of development.

Because this section on the development of identification is long and complex, it may be helpful to summarize it at the beginning. Incorporation—the process of taking in—is present shortly after birth and continues to function until the middle of the first year, when it becomes less prominent and is largely replaced by introjection. Introjection—the process of internalizing and establishing as separate mental representations the positive and negative relationships with the mother and emotionally significant others—predominates from that time until the end of the second year, at which time the process of primary identification takes its place. Coexisting with these three processes of incorporation, introjection, and identification, imitation functions throughout the first 3 years of life to help prepare the way for identification to occur.

The process of primary identification is followed, 2 years later, by the development of secondary identification, which occurs in conjunction with the formation of the superego. Then, in adolescence, the ego undergoes further reorganization, during which ties to the old (primary and secondary) identifications are loosened and new identifications are formed. From these consciously selected identifications, the ego ideal is gradually formed. The completion of this last process of identification marks the end of adolescence.

From this brief summary, it is apparent that the development of identification is considerably more complex than that of either denial or projection. In the first place, identification involves several different processes: imitation, incorporation, introjection, and identification proper. These identification processes, although they emerge at different points in development, do not form a psychological continuum; they are best understood as parallel lines of development that may interact to produce further mechanisms of identification. In addition to these processes, identification also refers to an end state, as seen in the concepts of primary and secondary identification. Primary identifications, formed during the first 3 years of life, serve as a defense against anxiety associated with loss of the mother and other dangers to the self. Secondary identifications, formed during the fourth and fifth years of life in conjunction with the development of the superego, serve as a defense against the uncontrolled expression of impulses. The identifications that contribute to the formation of the ego ideal occur during later childhood and adolescence.

Insofar as identification involves a modification of the self, the development of identification implies the existence of a self, however rudimentary. Consequently, to discuss the development of identification we must also discuss the development of the self and the differentiation of the self from the (m)other. The discussion of the development of the self during the early years of life is based on the study of separation–individuation by Mahler, Pine, and Bergman (1975), and on Spitz's (1957, 1965) analysis of the development of the self and the ego. Although aspects of Mahler's work—especially the idea of a symbiotic union of the infant with mother—have been called into question more recently (e.g., Silverman, 2003, 2005; Stern, 2000), there are significant points of agreement regarding early development between this theory and that of both Spitz and Piaget (1929, 1952). Although findings from current infant research conflict with the idea that the infant lacks differentiation from the mother, there is considerable agreement among these investigators, working from different theoretical perspectives, about the milestones relevant to the process of separation–individuation and to the development of the concepts of self and other. The discussion of the further development of the self during adolescence is based on the work of Blos (1962, 1979).

THE DEVELOPMENT OF PRIMARY IDENTIFICATIONS

The development of primary identifications at the end of the third year of life is preceded by the earlier processes of incorporation, introjection, and imitation. In the following discussion these identification processes are coordinated with the developmental models suggested by Mahler, Spitz, and Piaget. The implications of research on infant perception for the development of self (cf. Harter, 1982) are also considered.

Before birth, the infant-to-be is entirely merged with the mother. The embryo resides within the mother, surrounded by her. At the same time, the mother's life-giving supports of nutrients and oxygen flow into the embryo, and the residual waste flows back into the mother. The two organisms are biologically merged, having existed in the state of oneness for the better part of a year. It is not surprising that this sense of closeness should continue in the infant for a period of time after birth. The infant continues her existence by taking in the food that mother provides and depending on mother to keep her warm, comfortable, and protected.

At this stage of life the baby's primary mode of relating to the environment is "taking in"—primarily food but also other kinds of external stimulation. As with denial and projection, this physiological response provides the prototype for a subsequent defense. The response of "taking in" is the prototype for the psychological defense process of incorporation. In the first months of life the physical and psychological growth of the baby depends on incorporation of what mother provides; these incorporations relieve physiological/psychological tensions. In turn, the mechanism of incorporation provides the beginning of the identification process.[13]

During the early part of this stage, the infant begins to demonstrate the capacity to distinguish something in the environment beyond what he feels; that is, he shows an awareness of the "non-I" (Spitz, 1965). This development is seen behaviorally in the emergence of the smiling response to a visual stimulus representing a human face. Importantly, this response occurs as readily to a schematic representation of a face as to a living human face, suggesting that the response does not indicate the recognition of another person but rather the existence of something else out there. During this time, the infant also begins to imitate the facial configurations that he sees (Meltzoff & Moore, 1977, 1983; Spitz, 1958). It seems possible that the imitative processes interact with the incorporative processes to foster a psychological connection with the mother. In this way the baby's imitations may well serve a defensive function by preserving the attachment with the mother (Meissner, 1974, p. 522).

Although the baby is able to discriminate mother's face, voice, and smell from the same qualities of other women, and is able to discriminate among faces of unknown people (Bushnell, Sai, & Mullen, 1989; DeCasper & Fifer, 1980; Porter, Makin, Davis, & Christensen, 1992), there is as yet no capacity for object permanence (Piaget, 1952)—that is, no understanding that an object or person who disappears from sight continues to exist. Because mother is more clearly recognized as a distinct entity, the infant is exposed to the possibility that she may disappear, and the lack of object permanence creates the further possibility that when mother disappears, she is gone forever. Now a defense against the anxiety associated with the possible loss of mother is needed. It is suggested that the defensive process of introjection begins at this time.

During the second half of the first year of life, there is further evidence for the differentiation of the mother from other adults. Around 8 months of age the baby no longer smiles at all human faces; that response is reserved for mother or mother-substitute, and the presence of other adults may elicit reactions of discomfort (stranger anxiety). It is assumed that this differential response to mother versus others reflects the infant's association of mother with gratifying experiences; thus the mother's presence elicits a good feeling in the infant. This association of mother with a positive emotional feeling creates in the infant a mental representation that may be characterized as "good mother." At the same time there are occasions when mother is not able to provide immediate gratification. If the infant is assumed to form a "good-mother" representation following on experiences of gratification, then experiences of nongratification and frustration will lead to a "bad-mother" representation. In normal circumstances the good-mother representations are much stronger than the bad-mother representations at this stage of life, and hence the physical presence of the mother evokes a positive response from the baby.

A second important cognitive development is the beginning of the capacity for object permanence. Now the infant searches for an object that is hidden under a screen, whereas previously she behaved as though the hidden object had ceased to exist. This capacity is important in the continuing differentiation of the self, for it indicates that things and people outside of the infant continue to exist apart from the infant and her perception of them—an understanding that facilitates the differentiation of the infant from the mother.

As the baby is differentiating mother from others and beginning to develop an understanding that mother and others continue to exist separate from the baby, there is also evidence that awareness of the self is beginning to develop. In fact, there is evidence that babies at this age begin to show some self-recognition on a proprioceptive level. In a series of cleverly designed tasks using a mirror and various amusing attachments to the infant's body, Bertenthal and Fischer (1978) were able to show that 8-month-old infants had the capacity for proprioceptive self-recognition. Harter (1982) has termed this process awareness of a bodily self.

During this period, the infant shows increasing evidence of imitating the parent's gestures. In the interactions between the infant and the adult, there is often an immediate mirroring of the adult's gestures, frequently to the delight of the parent. This selective response on the part of the parent to the infant's imitative behavior reinforces those aspects of the baby's behavior. Insofar as these behaviors are like the parent's, the process of imitation contributes to the eventual identification of the child with the parent.

The differentiation during this period of mother and baby as separate beings allows for the development of emotional ties between them. In turn, the baby internalizes those emotional relationships. With this internalization, the defense of introjection begins. The inner representations of the good mother become one introjection or set of introjects; the representations of the bad mother become another. Once these relationships can be activated internally, introjection serves as a defense against the growing awareness that mother is separate and could leave. Introjection makes it possible to continue the relationship with mother intrapsychically, even if mother is not physically present.

As the child moves into the second year of life, the new capacities of the preceding period continue to develop, and there is an increased understanding of object permanence. This is also a period of increasing use of imitation. During this period, imitation includes copying the parents' gestures, tone of voice, emotions, and behavior; it is a time of pleasure in imitative games such as peek-a-boo and pat-a-cake. These imitative behaviors ordinarily occur only in the presence of the adult who serves as the model for the baby to imitate (McDevitt, 1979). Thus a 14-month-old infant, whose loving nanny took particular delight in singing Bach's vocal music during their daily walks, was heard to vocalize the "Gloria" aria from her stroller, quite on key. (At 5 years of age, this young girl's teacher said she had perfect pitch.)

Whereas imitation initially served to maintain a connection with the mother, it now helps the child gain skills needed for mastery and for functioning independently from the parent. The capacity to act like grownups eventually gives the child a sense of autonomy and the ability to act on his own in the absence of the parent (Meissner, 1974, p. 522). Imitation at this period can also serve a defensive function against anxiety associated with separation from, or loss of, the mother (Meissner, 1974, p. 521). As in the preceding period, introjection also serves this defensive function.

Toward the end of the second year of life, the first clear differentiation of a psychological self can be observed. This differentiation comes about, in significant part, as an outcome of the joint processes of imitation and introjection, which together produce a new defense: identification with the aggressor (explained below).

By 15 months of age the child is beginning to show deferred imitation— that is, the ability to imitate an adult's behavior and emotions even when the adult is not present—indicating that the child retains mental representations of the (m)other's behavior patterns. This kind of imitation is also seen in the role-playing games of this period—feeding and diapering the doll, putting it to bed, brushing its hair; all behaviors the adult has performed at some other time. This deferred imitation serves at least two functions in the development of self. In taking over some of the functions the mother had performed, whether on a play level with a doll or on a reality level as in feeding himself, the child further facilitates the differentiation of self from other. At the same time, the deferred imitation permits a continuing relationship with the mother in her absence.

The capacity for imitation serves a further role in the differentiation of self through the acquisition of the concept of "no." As the child becomes capable of independent action, he also becomes subject to the mother's prohibitions, often expressed by her saying "*No.*" In the child's experience, "no" becomes associated with a sense of frustration and ensuing anger. Through imitation the child learns to pronounce "no"; through introjection, the child becomes able to use "no" to express his angry feelings. However, by acting the same as mother acts, the child expresses these feelings without running the risk of losing his connection with mother. In the use of "no" to oppose the mother, the child is imitating the mother's verbal behavior and is acting the same as the introjected frustrating mother. Insofar as he is the same as the introject, the child maintains contact with mother and defends himself against anxiety over possible loss. This particular constellation of imitation plus introjection to produce the oppositional "no" is known, in theory, as identification with the aggressor, or, as Spitz prefers, identification with the frustrator (Spitz, 1957).

Not only is this occurrence a precursor to true identification in the sense that the ego is modified (with the development of the concept "no"), it also facilitates an objectification of the self and the mother. The will of the child is put into direct opposition to that of the mother, and thus the difference between the two individuals is brought into clearer focus.

Evidence for the increased awareness of the self at this time also comes from the experimental studies of infant perception. By 18 months of age, many infants recognize themselves in a mirror and recognize when the external self has been modified, as, for example, when a dot of red rouge has been applied to the infant's nose. This capacity for self-recognition is present in nearly all infants by 20 months of age. By 24 months of age, most toddlers are, in addition, able to apply their own name to their mirror image (Amsterdam, 1972; Bertenthal & Fischer, 1978; Lewis & Brooks, 1975). Longitudinal study of infants from 15 to 21 months of age has shown that the capacity for self-recognition occurs in conjunction with the use of personal pronouns (Lewis & Ramsay, 2004). Also, related to the clearer conception of the mother as a being with a separate, continuing existence of her own are the findings that object permanence, in Piaget's sense, becomes fully developed during this time.

Toward the end of this period a "crisis" occurs. The child who has been eager to share all his experiences with mother now begins to alternate between two contradictory modes of relating to her. Part of the time the child clings to mother, desiring great closeness and protection. At other times, the child angrily rejects mother's presence and offerings of help. This conflict between "clinging and cleaving" (Spitz, 1957, p. 124) may continue for the last 6 months of this phase, ending at the conclusion of the second year of life.

A number of theoreticians (e.g., McDevitt, 1979) have suggested that the resolution of this crisis depends on the functioning of identification. In this conceptualization, selective identification with parents helps resolve the alternating feelings of helplessness and ensuing clinging versus ambivalent autonomy and ensuing fighting that characterize the period. [14]

It is at this point in the child's development, then, that identification as a defense emerges: "[The child] now resolves his actual and intrapsychic conflicts between his own wishes and his parents' prohibitions, as well as his feelings of helplessness and his wish to please his parents, by selectively identifying with them" (McDevitt, 1979, p. 333). Imitative behavior patterns previously learned by the child help make him more like the adult model and thus facilitate the development of identification. Beyond this reliance on imitation, however, identification also requires the integration of introjections (Meissner, 1974).[15]

Around the end of the second year of life the use of introjection as a defense against anxiety associated with the loss of mother declines. In its place, the development of primary identification begins. Unlike the situation with incorporation or introjection, in which attributes of the "other" are either merged with the nascent self or held as internal representations distinct from it, identification involves a modification of the ego. To use Piaget's concepts, incorporation involves the process of assimilation, whereas identification involves the process of accommodation. In the latter case, internal psychological structures (the ego) change as a result of experiences with external reality (the other).

Over the next 12 months the consolidation of individuality progresses. The process of identification continues, the ego is modified accordingly, and the child's observation of her own self contributes to the sense of individuality, of difference from others. Thus a 3-year-old would often proclaim to her family, "I want to do what *I* want to do!"

During this time, object constancy is attained (in ordinary circumstances) with a further consolidation of the good-mother/bad-mother representations. This consolidation also results in giving a relinquishment of splitting as a defense. Possessing a consolidated internal image of the mother allows the child to identify with her—an identification that becomes psychologically available to the child for the same love, comfort, and sustenance the actual mother once provided. Many of the care-taking functions that mother contributed and that served to enhance the infant's developing self can now be dispensed by the child's internalized identifications with the mother. This enrichment of the self, in turn, enhances feelings of confidence, security, and self-esteem (Horner, 1983).

The process of identification contains a certain paradox. This process, in which attributes of the mother are taken over and become part of the child's own ego, not only results in the *differentiation* of the self from the (m)other, but also *preserves* the (m)other, both emotionally and cognitively, within the self. Thus identification allows the child to give up the mother and move toward autonomy while serving as an ego defense against anxiety or other dangers to the ego.

THE DEVELOPMENT OF SECONDARY IDENTIFICATIONS

The integration of primary identifications, in conjunction with the attainment of object constancy, completes the separation–individuation process in the child. These primary identifications are lasting parts of the ego, and they further the development of the self-representation. It is these identifications that make it possible for the individual to develop mature relationships with others (Horner, 1983; Menaker, 1979); through identification with the loving, caring mother, the child develops the capacity to become a loving, caring individual. In addition, primary identifications serve as a defense against anxiety over loss of the identified-with others.

Around the fifth year of life secondary identification begins. According to classical psychoanalytic theory, this process occurs in conjunction with, and as an outcome of, the Oedipal conflict. As the child gradually gives up his or her now sexualized attachment to the parent of the opposite sex, this loss is filled through an identification with one or both parents. In the usual case, the boy identifies with his father and the girl with her mother, but the opposite may occur; in any case, there is generally an identification with both parents, the relative strength of each identification being determined partly by the relative strength of biologically given masculine or feminine dispositions and partly by the social configuration of the family. Freud (1923) considered that all children are bisexual and that the presence of both masculine and feminine dispositions in the child allows him or her to identify with both father and mother.[16]

Although the resolution of the Oedipal conflict requires a giving up of the parent-as-partner, the modification of the ego by means of identification allows the relationship with the abandoned partner to be maintained. This process comes about through a special type of modification of the ego—namely, through the structuralization of the superego. Just as the same-sex parent was once perceived as the obstacle to the child's realization of his wishes to be his other parent's partner, through the process of identification the child now creates the same obstacle within himself. That part of the ego that is modified to carry out this function develops into the superego. With the development of the superego, the child maintains within himself the parents' prohibitions and threats as well as their protection and reassuring love.

Self-esteem can now come from doing the right thing, rather than solely from the approval or disapproval of some external person. Meeting the demands of the superego can now bring the sense of security and pleasure that was once derived from the attitude of the parent toward the child. Similarly, not meeting the demands of the superego can produce guilt and the sense of being unworthy or unlovable.

According to classical theory, the superego, through the process of identification, functions as a defense against the expression of libidinal impulses toward the opposite-sex parent and aggressive impulses toward the same-sex parent. However, an alternative explanation for the development of secondary identification, which does not invoke the hypothesis of the Oedipal conflict, is possible. From early on, as part of normal development, the child tries to do things like his parents. The ensuing development of ego skills facilitates mastery and autonomy, creates competencies, and may also serve a defensive function against loss of the parent's support. With the establishment of object constancy and primary identification, the child aims to do what his parents do; he identifies with their activities, and this identification is facilitated by his previous imitation of their behavior. A good part of what parents do is determined by their standards and ideals. To identify with the parents, the child also identifies with their standards and ideals, which includes accepting the prohibitions connected with them.[17] Out of the initial aim of identifying with the parents' activities comes the eventual identification with their prohibitions (Fenichel, 1945, pp. 102–103). This process can be seen as an alternative route to the development of the superego and secondary identifications.

Once the secondary identifications are established, they coexist with the earlier primary identifications that formed a considerable part of the ego's structure. The two processes of identification are parallel; they interact and facilitate one another (Horner, 1983) and, throughout the elementary school years, play a part in the child's acquiring skills, learning about the academic and social world, and developing ways to control his emotional reactions. There is even evidence that identification with the parents' defenses is important in the child's selective development of his own defense mechanisms (Thelen, 1965).

With the onset of adolescence, the identification with the parents— which had provided both structure and organization for the child's ego and superego—now begins to be disrupted. The emotional ties with the parents of childhood that came about through the processes of primary and secondary identification are loosened, and a second individuation process begins (Blos, 1962, 1979). Whereas the first individuation process, concluded by age 3 years, occurred as the child established internal ego identifications with the mother, the second individuation has a reverse purpose; the process now requires a disengagement from the internal identifications to allow the young person to become independent from the family, to develop extrafamilial relationships, and to choose her own individual identity.

One of the results of the loosening of ties with former identifications is a certain degree of instability and reorganization in the adolescent ego,[18] accompanied by a kind of ego weakness, experienced as a sense of loss, of emptiness or insufficiency, aptly expressed in the question, "Who am I?" In an effort to protect the ego organization, various maneuvers may be tried, including the formation of new identifications. These identifications may be formed with the heroes or heroines from the world of sports, entertainment, or fiction; they may be formed with an individual chum or with a group. Identification with these new objects may provide the kind of security and self-esteem that was previously derived from identification with the parents, thereby facilitating the adolescent's separation from the emotional ties to the parents of childhood. Moreover, identification with a group—the members of which are, to varying degrees, involved in the same process, helps to relieve guilt feelings connected with the disengagement and bolsters the tenuous self-esteem of the adolescent adrift.

Some of these young people, threatened with the sense of ego impoverishment and depression stemming from the loss of childhood identifications, seek to restore the good feeling by merging with political, philosophical, aesthetic, or religious ideologies or with available social movements. Others may adopt the mechanism of *negative identification* in which a "new" identification is based on an unconscious wish to become the *opposite* of the parental identifications (Erikson, 1968). Yet others, also wishing not to be like the parents, will use the process of *counteridentification* (Menaker, 1979) to consciously strive to create a self that is new and *different* from the parental mode. Shifting among these various possibilities for identification helps create the changing and turbulent personality of the adolescent. Still others, defending against the ties to parental identification but having no replacements, experience a sense of alienation (Berman, 1970).

The loosening of emotional ties to the parental identifications and the increasing identification with others have two further important implications that contribute to the late adolescent's "identity": first, the weakening of the power of the superego and, second, the development of the ego ideal.

At the beginning of latency, the superego, which developed from parental identifications, helped maintain the child's sense of security and self-esteem through the internalization of the emotional tie to the parents. The partial relinquishing of this tie at adolescence means, in turn, that the basis of the superego is weakened. The superego loses some of its rigidity and power, while the ego and the ego ideal take over some of the superego's functions.

The ego ideal may be viewed as an aspect of the superego; both share a common function of regulating behavior and attitudes toward the self. Violation of the superego's edicts results in feelings of guilt, and a discrepancy between the ego ideal and the self-representation creates a feeling of lowered self-esteem or shame. Although both the superego and ego ideal begin in early childhood, they do not evolve from the same origins or at the same point in development.

It is beyond the scope of the present work to provide a detailed discussion of the origin of the ego ideal, but it is important to note that this aspect of the ego has as its origin a kind of primitive self-love (primary narcissism) that sustains the helpless infant and older child through the many, inevitable defeats he will experience. Later, as adolescence begins, this self-love is manifest in narcissistic identifications and attachments. At the end of early adolescence, the phase of narcissistic object choice ends with a process of internalization that gives rise to a new institution within the ego: namely, the ego ideal. This process parallels an earlier internalization, the identification with the parents, that gave rise to another new part of the ego: the superego.[19]

The ego ideal takes over some of the functions that had previously been part of the superego. New, often temporary, identifications with extrafamilial others as well as with the contemporary (i.e., not infantile) parents influence the content and direction of the ego ideal. In turn, the ego ideal comes to reflect the individual's identity. The self-love, first associated with primary narcissism, now takes the form of self-esteem based on striving to match the ego ideal. Whereas in childhood this sense of self-esteem was based on an identification with the parents and their expectations, with the emergence of the ego ideal the sense of self-esteem is less dependent on external sources; rather, it depends only on those sources with whom the individual has chosen to identify and has internalized as part of his ego ideal.

The development of the ego ideal, based on new identifications and emotional experiences outside the family, continues throughout adolescence. It becomes "most urgent" at the end of adolescence. In fact, the end of adolescence is defined by the completion of the ego ideal. The superego continues as an agency of prohibition, whereas the ego ideal is an agency of aspiration. Although superego demands can be met, ego ideal strivings are never fully satisfied. These strivings involve delay and a state of anticipation; there is a continuous pursuit of achievements that are never fully attained: It is the persistent striving that sustains the feelings of well-being (Blos, 1979, p. 323).

The ego ideal gives men and women their sense of identity. It is the constant, unrelenting influence that determines the adult's striving. It makes it possible to ignore the risk of mortality, allowing humans to accomplish great feats of heroism, sacrifice, and creativity. "One dies for one's ego ideal rather than let it die" (Blos, 1979, p. 369).[20]

This final stage in identification, then, involves a sifting, discarding, and consolidation of earlier identifications. It also involves the creation of an unobtainable ideal, the seeking after which, with the attendant delay of gratification and sustained effort, is a source of self-esteem. It was undoubtedly about this experience that Robert Browning wrote, "Ah, but a man's reach should exceed his grasp, Or what's a heaven for?"[21]

EXAMPLES OF IDENTIFICATION IN LITERATURE

An intensive search of children's literature for stories exemplifying issues of identification yielded an interesting result: It was very difficult to find children's stories that revolve around this developmentally more advanced process. However, two excellent works from adult literature take the issue of identification as a central theme. The first of these—*Henry IV, Parts 1 and 2*—portrays the process of identification in an adolescent prince, whose struggles are taken seriously. In contrast is the tale of *Don Quijote*, in which the identification of a middle-age Spanish gentleman with heroic knights of old provides a pathetic farce.

Henry IV

An excellent example of an adolescent's struggle with identification is found in Shakespeare's play *Henry IV.*[22] In this historical drama King Henry assumes the throne by murdering his predecessor, while his son, Harry, carouses with his buffoon pal, Falstaff. More important than the political intrigue, the plot continually revolves around the question of conflicting identifications. In the beginning of the play, Prince Harry has identified himself with Falstaff, a glutton devoted to instinctual gratification and lacking in conscience. Throughout the play, this identification is signified by use of the prince's nickname "Hal." In choosing to identify with a character so opposite from his father, the king, Prince Harry provides us with an excellent example of *negative identification.*

Although the main theme traces the change in Harry's object of identification away from Falstaff and toward the king, secondary themes focus on the issue of identification in these two latter characters. The king, who had veered away from his true identity, comes back to it. Falstaff, on the other hand, is confused by Harry's abandonment of him and alternates between a failure to recognize Henry's new identity, refusing to believe it, and finally himself trying to identify with the new Henry, Prince of Wales.

The play opens with the king lamenting the failure of Harry to identify with him. Not long after this, young Harry lets us know that his life of carousing with thieves and ribalds is only temporary and that he will, before long, throw off his "negative identifications" and "be himself." Harry goes on to explain his strategy—that by providing a contrast between his old irresponsible behavior and his new unexpected reformation, he will be seen in an even better light than if he had always shown an exemplary character (Act I, Scene 2, lines 219–241). This revelation is immediately followed by a scene in which the king confesses that he himself has not been as strong as he might, but that he too intends to change (Act I, Scene 3, lines 5–9). There is a similarity, then, in the intentions of father and son. Unknown to each other, they both announce that they are about to change character, to become themselves.

The issue of identification continues in the next act. Harry, who is always referred to as "Hal" by Falstaff, requests that Falstaff play the role of his father, the king (Act II, Scene 4, lines 411–412). However, when Falstaff attempts to portray the king as subscribing to his own hedonistic values, Hal rejects this characterization of his father and berates Falstaff (Act II, Scene 4, line 77). Here begins the rejection of the identification with Falstaff. Hal himself then plays the role of the king, in which his identification with the king, although only in play-acting, is made clear, and his rejection of Falstaff's values is made overt.

The turning point of the drama occurs in Act III when the king rebukes the prince for his errant ways. Harry acknowledges that he has "wandered" and again suggests that he may change. The king continues, explaining how he attained his status—that he purposely kept himself out of public view so that, on the few occasions when he appeared, people would look in awe of him (Act III, Scene 2, lines 46–59).

The similarity between this passage, in which the King describes his strategy for attaining his position, and that noted earlier, in which Harry discloses his strategy for gaining the good opinion of men (Act I, Scene 2, lines 219–241) is striking. Like his father, Harry plans to enhance his image by use of a contrast effect. For the father, the contrast is between absence and presence; being rarely present, he is (hopefully) valued more. For Harry, the contrast is between irresponsibility and unexpectedly honorable behavior; his reformation will thus be all the more impressive. This similarity, not recognized by either father or son, is an excellent example of identification in which a strategy with which to approach life is shared unconsciously.

This, then, is the second time father and son have revealed unconsciously shared similar intentions, after their earlier separate announcements that they are about to change character (Act I, Scenes 2 and 3).

In the next scene Hal has a sharp change in attitude toward Falstaff, who is criticized, ridiculed, and cast off. Hal's announcement of his good relationship with his father (Act III, Scene 3, lines 203–204) comes as a surprise and marks the beginning of Hal's change in object of identification. This change in identification becomes clearest in Act V, where, for the first time, Harry refers to himself as "the Prince of Wales" (Scene 1, line 86).

This proclamation of royal identity is immediately echoed by his father, who also, for the first time, refers to Harry as the Prince of Wales (line 101), thereby securing the identification. In this same dialogue Harry offers to defend his father in battle, and he rejects his old friend and former object of identification, Falstaff.

The new identification is further highlighted in the next scene in which the king's adversary, the Earl of Worcester, also designates Harry as the Prince of Wales (Scene 2, line 46). This change, however, has not been recognized by Falstaff, as is made clear in Scene 3; three times, Falstaff continues to refer to the Prince as "Hal" (lines 45–55)—that is, in terms of his previous identity.

At the opening of Scene 4, the royal son again refers to himself as the Prince of Wales and then defends his father by fighting Lord Douglas. The prince is successful in chasing Douglas off, thereby reversing roles with his father and identifying with the king as protector. The king responds that the prince has restored himself to the king's good opinion, because he has shown that he respects his father's life. In this battle Harry twice more identifies himself as the Prince of Wales (lines 63 and 67).

Falstaff, however, still clings to the old relationship. He continues to refer to the prince as "Hal" (line 75) and then makes one last attempt to reestablish the bond of identification through a reversal in their roles. Although the prince has already killed his enemy, Hotspur, Falstaff appropriates the prince's action as his own, claiming that he, Falstaff, has killed Hotspur. The prince seems to recognize and accept this reversal of roles between the two of them, perhaps out of recognition of the reversal in his own relationship with his father (Act V, Scene 4, lines 161–162).

This maneuver is followed, however unconvincingly, with an attempt on Falstaff's part to identify with the new Harry, that is, with the noble prince. Falstaff proclaims that he will give up his gluttony and drinking and live as a nobleman should (Act V, Scene 5, line 68).

Thus, as the play unfolds, Harry's identification with his father strengthens, whereas his identification with Falstaff weakens. The latter, in a parallel refrain, repeats the course followed by the prince; Falstaff usurps the behavior of the identification figure (Harry) as his own and then declares that he will adopt his values and status as well. This mirroring or imitation of the prince by Falstaff, which borders on parody, serves to highlight the important change that has taken place in the prince.

With the establishment of the prince's positive identification with his father, Part 1 of the play ends. The king makes explicit his recognition of Harry as his son, and the two of them go off together to fight further battles in Wales.

The problems of identification are not over, however, as is revealed in *Henry IV, Part 2*. The play begins with the king repeatedly questioning the whereabouts of Harry. Thus we are informed that the identification with the king, brought about in Part 1, may not be secure. This tenuousness is made clear as the king laments that Harry has again fallen in with his carousing friends. It is left to the Earl of Warwick to explain to the king that his son needs to try out several different identifications before restoring his identification with the king (Act IV, Scene 4, lines 74–78).

The final scene of this act opens with the king lying in bed, dying. Harry arrives; thinking that his father has already died, he expresses his sorrow but also illustrates the defensive function of identification. By assuming his father's crown and its attendant strength, Harry's sorrow is requited (Act IV, Scene 5, lines 37–47).

The king, not yet dead, mistakenly interprets Harry's actions (i.e., his taking of the crown as his own) to be evidence of his son's greed and his wish for the king's death. But when Harry is found crying and in sorrow (Scene 5, line 84), it is clear to the audience that his grief over the loss of his father is genuine. When the king doubts this grief, Harry replies that his life has been guided by the strategy he proposed in Part 1: to make the world incredulous by his change in identification. The king is convinced. The prince then accepts and honors his father and what his father has "given" him—that is, he upholds that with which he has identified (Act IV, Scene 5, lines 221–223).

In the last act the prince, who has now become Henry V, speaks to his three mourning brothers and again explains how the defense works. Through the continuing identification of the prince with his father, Harry the old king lives on in Harry the new king; the lost father is restored and sorrow is changed into happiness (Act V, Scene 2, lines 59–61).

In the next scene Falstaff learns that Hal is now Henry V. He believes they still have a close bond, which he demonstrates in the manner in which he addresses the new king—as "King Hal" and "Royal Hal" (Act V, Scene 5, lines 45), not recognizing the inconsistency in identification of the two appellations. But Falstaff's attempts at connection are denounced by Henry V, who then turns on Falstaff with a viciousness that shows us how much energy is needed to sever the former identification and how what once was loved is now despised (Act V, Scene 5, lines 51–63).

To sum up: In the course of the two parts of the play, we see the struggle of the adolescent Harry, who has, as part of his development toward adulthood, rejected his paternal identification and looked outside the family for new objects of identification. After trying out these other patterns of life, he restores his identification with his father. This identification, however, is modified by other qualities lacking in his father, which Harry has acquired through his adolescent explorations. Finally, the defensive function of identification is demonstrated: Harry's sorrow over the loss of his father through death is abated through the possession of his father within himself.

As secondary themes, the king and Falstaff illustrate issues related to identification from the point of view of the object of identification. At the beginning of the play, the king has lost his position as the identified-with object and sees that some adjustment in his character is needed. At the end of the play, it is Falstaff who has lost out in this struggle: No longer an object of Harry's identification, Falstaff is befuddled. In contrast to the king, who became more himself when faced with the loss of Harry's identification, Falstaff attempts to reestablish the connection by trying to be more like the son. Thus we are shown the divergent reactions of parents when faced with the loss of the adolescent's identification.

Finally, in a general sense, the drama demonstrates how the development of identification is a long, often circuitous process that bounces forward and slides backward. It alerts us, as well, to the pain involved in the process for parent and child alike, and to the great psychic effort involved in severing old identifications. As is so often true, Shakespeare "knew it all."

Don Quijote

The tale of *Don Quijote* also centers on the theme of identification. However, the theme is presented as a farce, perhaps because the developmental issues involved are too close to the developmental level of the reader.[23]

The story begins with the description of a middle-aged gentleman named Quixada who has become obsessed with reading books about the knights of old.[24] This preoccupation has resulted in his abandoning other activities, including the care of his estate. In fact, he sold off sections of his land to buy ever more books about knights, reading and collecting all that could be found. He read night and day until his mind became so confused that he began to think of himself as a knight and to imitate the behavior of knights.

In *Don Quijote* we see the quintessential identification of a man with his poetic heroes, presented as an aberrant psychological process. The portrayal of the identification with a romantic knight is made comic through Quixada's actions: He adopts a suit of armor made partially from cardboard, mounts a bedraggled horse (whom he renames *Rozinante*, thereby marking the horse's change in identity), and assumes a new name for himself: Don Quijote de la Mancha.

Don Quijote then sets off to right the wrongs of the world. In this enterprise he is notoriously unsuccessful, creating more problems for those he would save. When the world cannot tolerate the antics of Quijote, which are guided by his identification, he is punished. To restore himself, he turns to passages in his knight books for comfort, thereby displaying the defensive function of his identification. For example, when he is discovered by a peasant lying on the ground, beaten and broken, the don's reaction to his misfortune is to speak to the peasant with verbatim speeches from the characters in his books. In this way his identification helps preserve his self-esteem.

The family believes they can cure Quixada by burning the books with which he identifies. Once they have destroyed all the knight books, they realize that the other volumes in his library might offer further possibilities for identification (such as shepherd or poet) and should also be eliminated. Thus the process of identification is continuously remarked upon and caricatured.

As the tale proceeds, it becomes evident that the burning of the books fails to undo the identification, for it has been internalized. Quijote's life as a knight continues; he acquires a squire, Sancho Panza, and the two of them set off to fight windmills.

CLINICAL EXAMPLE

Although we generally think of identification as involving the development of psychological characteristics, the defense is most easily seen when it occurs through physical manifestations. One dramatic example of this is the appearance of "stigmata" on the bodies of the religiously devout. Here the identification with Christ and his physical torment is so complete that the body of the worshipper changes to become the same as that of the figure of identification.

This type of identification, manifest in the sharing of a physical symptom, occurred in a middle-aged woman who consulted with me. The patient, successful in her profession and married with a family, had lost her mother during her early adolescence. After a long illness, her mother had died from cancer of the thyroid when the patient was 12½ years old. Although as a younger woman she had been aware of an underlying identification with her artistic mother as a motivating force for her interest in the arts and artists, and in her decision to move from her native Chicago to Washington, DC, where her mother had lived as a young woman, the power of this identification did not become apparent until later in her life. Having postponed childbearing while pursuing her career, her first child was not born until she was 35 years old—"coincidentally" the identical age of her own mother when my patient was born.

She had enjoyed good health throughout her life, although the death of her maternal aunt from cancer during her young-adult years contributed to my patient's lingering fear that she might, like her mother, develop cancer. Thus her anxiety about the possibility of a cancerous tumor was considerable when, at the age of 47, she became aware of a "lump" in her throat and experienced difficulty swallowing. Although external physical examinations by her physician and X-rays following a barium swallow revealed no pathology, the sensation of a growth in her throat remained over a period of 3 months. Because of her conviction/fear that there was some pathological growth around the area of her thyroid gland, she traveled to a large medical center to consult with a specialist in endoscopy, who would be able to look into her throat to determine definitively whether or not there was a tumor. The results of an examination by this physician, renowned in his field, would convince her.

His findings revealed no physical pathology. Instead, he offered a diagnosis of "globus," adding, presumably out of consideration for the feelings of the patient, that it was not necessarily "globus hystericus." My patient, being somewhat knowledgeable about matters psychological and having some familiarity with the concept of psychosomatic disorders, understood the meaning of the physician's remarks. Reassured that this was not cancer, the symptom remitted about 75% within the first week after her visit to the endoscopist and was 100% gone within 2 weeks. It was at that point that she realized that the symptom began on the exact day her daughter had pointed out that it was her "half-birthday"; on that day, her daughter had reached the age of 12½ years. According to this roundabout way of reckoning time, this meant that the daughter was the age of the patient at her mother's death, which made the patient the exact age of her own mother when she had died.

Here we see illustrated a double identification—the patient with her mother and with her daughter. The sensation of a lump in her throat was an obvious identification with the mother's cancerous tumor, whereas her identification with her teenage daughter provided the unconscious time clock for the emergence of the psychosomatic symptom.

THE USE OF IDENTIFICATION IN PROJECTIVE STORIES

Manifestations of identification in projective stories may occur at all ages but occur most frequently during adolescence and adulthood. In fact, it is not uncommon for the entire plot of an adolescent's story to revolve around issues of identity and identification. When identification occurs in the stories of young children, we sometimes see examples of the more primitive identification processes.

The following story was written by a 17-year-old 12th-grade girl in response to TAT Card 1. The picture on the card shows a young boy sitting at a table, on top of which rests a violin.

A little boy facing a violin. His parents have forced him to play the violin, when he'd rather be outside playing baseball. He is sitting looking at his violin and thinking. He is wondering why his parents are making him do something he doesn't want to do. He is frustrated because he is too young to be able to express his own view on things, but he isn't too young to think of them. Bigger people than he are always telling him to do things that don't make sense. Why do his parents want him to sit inside on a beautiful day and play a violin?— As he gets older he will either realize that his parents were trying to help him. He will see that what they were doing was for his own good. He will practice his violin diligently and become quite interested and good at it. Or, because his parents made him play the violin, he decides that he hates it, and shuts out any interest of the violin or music. It was his parents' interest, and not his to begin with, so he figures it's stupid.

This story nicely portrays a number of themes involving identification and, in a sense, illustrates the course of its development. Almost immediately, the storyteller goes to a central conflict between the child's wish for pleasure and the parents' imposition of rules and restrictions. It is, of course, in the mind of the storyteller that this conflict between unrestricted gratification and adult demands is taking place. As such, it indicates that the parents' mores have been internalized, and the internalization of adult demands is one aspect of identification. The way the demands are portrayed in the story indicate that they have not yet been fully integrated into the self ("He is wondering why his parents are making him do something he doesn't want to do"). Rather, they appear as an introjected other who is engaged in a struggle with the pleasure-seeking self. Despite the noticeable differentiation of self and other at this point, it soon becomes clear that the boy is not yet ready to separate from the other ("He is too young to be able to express his own view"); the focus stays on what the "bigger people" tell him to do. These controls that govern his behavior, however, continue to be experienced as alien to his own self (they "don't make sense"). Secondary identification, which involves a change in the ego whereby the values and sanctions of the identified-with figure becomes one's own, has not yet occurred in the young boy.

The story continues, raising the issue that, for secondary identification to occur, the boy must grow older. He then adopts the parents' point of view; he sees that "what they were doing was for his own good." His behavior now is governed by this identification; he gives up his pleasure-seeking orientation and acquires the capacity for work (he practices "diligently").

The storyteller then takes us one step further in the ongoing process. Not content to leave the boy in a state of secondary identification, she raises the issues of separation and individuation once more. Whereas when he was younger, the boy was only able to *think* about being different, now he is able to *act* on rejecting the parents' views. He "shuts out any interest of the violin" and works to differentiate himself from his parents by devaluing their interests ("he figures it's stupid"). Taken as a whole, the story can be understood as representing the stages of identification from introjection through adolescent individuation.

A rather different outcome occurs in a story written in response to the same TAT picture (Card 1) by a 17-year-old girl in the 11th grade.

> *This boy, John, is a very talented young musician. Constantly on the road, performing. He has played at such renowned places as Carnegie Hall and Denver Athenaeum. Even though he's only 4. John was practicing one day when he stopped, looked at his violin, and started to think. "Why do I practice 6 hours a day? I am always on the road and never get a chance to make friends my own age." He begins to wonder if he wants more from life than just music, music, music. John goes and starts to talk to his mother. They have a long talk. And when John leaves the room he feels as his mother does. Now John is concert master of the Vienna orchestra. . . .*

This story again focuses on several aspects of identification. It begins with a young boy who already shows evidence of having modified his own ego to include an orientation toward a profession ("musician"), the work ethic ("constantly on the road, performing"), and status as judged by adult standards ("Carnegie Hall and Denver Athenaeum"). There is no suggestion here that these activities are ego-alien, imposed by (introjected) adults. Rather, they seem to represent what the child feels himself to be. The first hint of possible tension comes when we learn that this working professional is but 4 years old. There is a sense of dissynchrony here; 4-year-olds are not expected to have yet identified so strongly with the adult world. We have, then, a case of precocious identification. As the story progresses, the boy begins to move into the next phase in the identification process—namely, to question the values acquired through secondary identification ("Why do I practice . . . ?"), and to begin the second individuation process. To do this, he expresses the need to turn to persons outside of his family ("a chance to make friends my own age"). As the disengagement from the earlier identification proceeds, he experiences the sense of insufficiency that accompanies the loosening of all ties; he "wonders if he wants more from life than just music."

It is at this point, however, that the forward progress in the course of identification comes to a halt, for the boy goes back to his mother rather than continuing to separate from her. That this regressive path might be followed has been foreshadowed by the earlier recognition that this boy's attainment of secondary identification was precocious; the ego structures needed to support further development may have been bypassed. Lacking the necessary inner strength for progression to the next phase of identification and the disengagement from the parents, the boy instead falls back to the earlier attachment to his mother. As they talk, the regression continues, until, when he leaves the room, "he feels as his mother does." Although he had been on the brink of the second individuation process of adolescence, he regresses back to the point of nondifferentiated merging with mother; their feelings are indistinguishable. The story's ending indicates that John remains fixated at this early level of primary identification throughout his life.

Yet another way in which issues involving identification may be expressed in projective stories occurs in the following example written by an adolescent boy. On first reading, the story may be understood as symbolic of a growing boy's concerns about his sexuality. In a broader sense the story reflects concerns about the process of identification, including the discovery of masculine sexual identity, as it is passed down from one generation to the next.

> At the age of 12 Ethan lives with his mother. His father died many years ago and all he has left of him is this violin. John sits and looks at it, puzzled by its strange shape. From time to time he plucks at its strings with his fingers. As time passes, he becomes fascinated with it. He soon discovers that it is not an ordinary violin. By picking it up and bracing it to his neck and just by resting the bow on its strings, his hand seems to move by itself and make beautiful sounds. He does not reveal his discovery to anyone. The more John played, the better things began to sound, until one day he picked up an ordinary violin and found that he could play it also. His mind and body had coordinated themselves after having played so much that they were now at home with any violin. So John found peace with his instrument and had a good life making and playing violins.

This story begins with a boy who is on the verge of puberty. He has been without a male identification figure for many years. However, his deceased father left him a (male) legacy. This is problematic for the boy, who, without a (male) model, is puzzled about how he is to use it. As the boy gets older, he increasingly focuses his interest on the enigmatic masculine object.

Then, as though his inheritance from his father guides him, he is able to use his hand to produce pleasure from this male legacy. Initially, this activity is carried on in secret. However, with time and more experience, the boy is able to reveal his masculinity in public. His masculine psychological identification is established and coordinated with his masculine physiology and drives. The development of this stable identification allows him to continue his life in a happy and productive manner.

Although identification is more likely to appear in the stories of older children, the following story, told by a 4-year-old boy in response to TAT Card 17BM (a man clinging to a rope), illustrates the use of incorporation, a primitive precursor of identification.

> *He's climbing on a rope. He's trying to get up onto a beanstalk. He saw a mean, big, old giant. The giant gets his muscles to make his bread. He said, Fe, fi, fo, fum, I smell the blood of the Englishman. I'll grind your muscles to make my bread. And he does. Then, he gets the giant's muscles, and now he's a giant.*

This story, which includes elements from a well-known childhood folktale, is constructed around the conflict between the young, growing boy and the big, powerful adult. The youth wants to succeed; he is trying to get ahead in life. But the old giant is mean and tries to destroy him by robbing him of his strength. It is in the storyteller's idea of how this conflict between young and old is resolved that we see the primitive use of incorporation. First, it appears that the giant will win by taking the boy's muscles, grinding them into bread, and then, presumably, eating the bread. Through oral incorporation, the giant will have destroyed the boy's strength and added to his own. This latter possibility—that through incorporation the individual acquires the characteristics belonging to the object incorporated—is made clearest in the turnabout that occurs at the end of the story: The boy gets the giant's muscles and thus becomes a giant. Although there is some confusion in this story about who is incorporating whom, the message is clear: Through eating the foe one acquires his strength.

CONCLUDING REMARKS

The length of this chapter indicates the greater complexity of identification, compared to denial and projection. It is a defense that has been defined in many ways, reflecting both its defensive and adaptive functions. Its development from the early components of incorporation, introjection, and imitation, through primary and secondary identifications, to the disruptions of old identifications during adolescence to form an individually chosen identity, is a process that occupies human life from birth to adulthood. The process is intimately connected with the development of the self, of self-esteem, and of the ego-ideal. It guarantees the continuity from one generation to the next; it is what parents and society "pass on" to their children.

In folktales, as in children's literature, identification is most likely to occur in one of its developmentally earlier forms, such as incorporation or imitation. These processes, we may speculate, are more recognizable, or familiar, to the intended audience and thus hold their attention. Likewise, in the projective stories that children themselves produce, it is the earlier components of identification that are likely to appear. Not until later adolescence are the characters of Prince Hal and Don Quijote likely to gain an interested audience—one that intuitively understands the developmental process being portrayed. Likewise, it is at this stage that the more mature components of identification begin to emerge in the adolescent's projective stories.

PART III

Defense Mechanisms in Action

*I*n this next section we see how defense mechanisms are continually in action, whether this involves dealing with stress or accommodating life changes over time. The first chapter discusses the use of defenses and children's pathology; the remaining four chapters present the extensive research that has been carried out in the past 15 years with normal, nonclinical groups of adults.

Chapter 6 presents empirical evidence supporting the theoretical premise that stress, trauma, and psychopathology increase the use of defenses by children. This evidence comes both from carefully controlled laboratory investigations and from studies based on "real-life" experience. Chapter 7 explores how stress also influences defense use in adulthood. Especially striking is the repeated finding that threats to the "self," or to personal identity, produce a decided increase in defense use. Also striking is the demonstrated relation between stress-induced autonomic nervous system reactivity and the use of defenses.

Chapter 8 turns to the question of the relation between defense use and other dimensions of personality, as well as the relation between defense use and IQ. In Chapter 9 the question of gender differences in defense use is considered, along with the related question of whether the use of the same defense might have different consequences for the two genders. Where gender-based differences are found, alternative explanations are considered.

Finally, Chapter 10 considers the long-term consequences of defense use. The chapter presents studies in which the same group of individuals has been followed over a period of years, thus allowing us to study defense and personality *change*. Considered here is how earlier defense use predicts personality and behavior in later years, and the related question of how early personality may contribute to later defense use.

CHAPTER 6

Defenses in Childhood
Stress and Psychopathology

One of the defining characteristics of a defense mechanism is that its use should increase in times of stress. In this way a child is protected from becoming too anxious, too upset—often about situations or circumstances over which he or she has no conscious control. At that moment, there is little a child can do about failing a school test or not being chosen for the baseball team. Disappointment, loss of self-esteem, and anxiety are expectable reactions, but the use of defense mechanisms can reduce the force of these feelings. For example, disappointment about not being chosen could be reduced through the mental maneuver reflected in denial ("I didn't really want to play) or projection ("They're afraid I'll show them up") or identification ("The cool people in my class don't get involved in baseball; soccer is the thing").

Again, this is what theory says: The use of defense mechanisms will increase when a person feels anxious or is threatened by loss of self-esteem. Anecdotal and clinical evidence of this phenomenon is plentiful. In this chapter I describe two experimental studies specifically designed to test the hypothesis that when children are stressed, they increase their use of defenses. Then we move from the laboratory to real life and consider children who are known to be experiencing psychological difficulties to see how these difficulties affect their use of defenses. Finally, we consider the question of whether the use of defense mechanisms does protect children from psychological upset.

STUDIES OF CHILDREN'S DEFENSES IN RESPONSE
TO EXPERIMENTALLY INDUCED STRESS

To test the hypothesis that stress increases defense use, my student and I studied the effects of success and failure on children's use of defenses in an experimental study (Cramer & Gaul, 1988). We created a situation in which the examiner had control over whether children would be successful or not in their performance of a simple task. This task, which was explained to the children as a test of their perceptual–motor ability, involved placing a marble on a rollway track and timing how long it took for the marble to reach the bottom of the track. Children were told to "try hard" to get the marble to roll fast, so that they could equal the time that "most kids" could make. In fact, there was no way a child could actually influence or control the marble's speed. The experimenter, using a conspicuous stopwatch, then timed the child's attempts. On a random basis, half of the children were told that they had beaten the standard time, and half were told they had not beaten the time. An assessment of their feeling state both prior to and after the experience of success or failure indicated that those who had "failed" were experiencing an increase in the negative emotions of sadness or anger. At the end of the study, the children in the failure condition were given an additional trial, in which they were "successful," so that all children left the study feeling satisfied.

Having determined that this procedure was successful in temporarily changing a child's emotional state, we proceeded to the main study. The question being investigated here was whether the experience of failure and the ensuing negative emotional state would influence the use of defenses.

The study included 64 children from second and sixth grades, who were brought into the laboratory one at a time. They began the study by telling stories in response to TAT pictures in the usual fashion. After coding these stories for defense use, two groups of children were created, matched for their preexperimental defense use. Two weeks later, the examiner returned and explained to each child that they were going to be tested on their perceptual–motor ability, using the rollway apparatus. As in the pilot study, the experimenter held a stopwatch to measure the time between the marble drop and its exit at the bottom of the rollway. All children were told that if they beat a specified time, they would win a big gold paper award, with their name on it, which they could place on an "honor board." Each child was given two tries to beat the standard time.

According to plan, the examiner told half of the children that they had been successful and half that they had *not* beat the time and therefore could not put their name on the honor board. Immediately after this, the children were asked to tell stories in response to a new set of pictures; these were subsequently coded for defenses. Next, every child in the failure condition was given another chance at the task; this time, every child was successful and was given the award for the honor board. In this way no child left the study feeling unhappy.

The hypothesis was that children in the failure condition would show greater defense use than those in the success condition. Remember that the two groups were equal in defense use prior to the experiment.

The effects of experiencing success and failure are presented in Figure 6.1. The children who experienced failure used more *denial* and more *projection* than did those experiencing success. In other words, they used the defenses that we expect children of that age range to use. *Identification*, a defense not yet fully developed in children of this age, was not increased. However, closer examination of the results showed that the use of identification was increased for children in the success group. Although not predicted, this finding suggests the possibility that success and self-esteem promote the use of a more mature defense, or, possibly, that the experience of failure interferes with the use of this more mature defense.

Further, looking more closely at the findings from this study, we noted that the experience of success or failure affected the two age groups in different ways. For the younger children, failure increased their use of the age-appropriate defenses of denial and projection. For the older children, the experience of success *decreased* their use of these lower-level defenses and tended to increase their use of the more mature defense of identification. Thus, depending on the child's age, it appears that negative life experiences

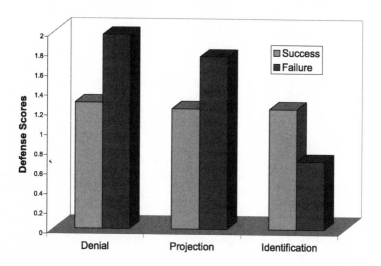

FIGURE 6.1. Children's study: Effects of success and failure. From Cramer and Gaul (1988); reprinted with permission from the *Journal of Personality*.

result in an increased use of lower-level defenses, and that favorable life experiences support the use of mature defenses.

The findings of a study by Smith and Rossman (1986) support this assertion. In an experimental investigation in which children experienced a stressful situation, 10-year-old boys, who ordinarily did not use the defense of denial as often as did the 6- and 8-year-old boys in the study, were found to increase their use of denial and become more similar to the younger boys as a result of the stress experience. Overall, the results of these studies support the hypothesis that stress increases the use of defenses in school-age children.

In another laboratory investigation the effect of peer rejection on defense use was studied (Sandstrom & Cramer, 2003a). Information about the popularity of fourth-grade girls was obtained from their classmates. In the sample selected for study, about half of the girls were of average or high popularity, whereas half were either rejected or disregarded (neglected) by their classmates. We hypothesized that girls who had a background of nonacceptance by peers would be especially sensitive to a further experience of rejection. In contrast, girls who were secure in their peer relationships were expected to be less distressed by a single occurrence of rejection. In turn, we expected the nonaccepted girls to react with greater use of defenses after being rejected, as compared to the secure girls.

Each child was brought into the laboratory. After responding to a few questions and telling several TAT stories, they were told that there was another girl in a room down the hall, and that later they would be able to play a game with her using "closed-circuit TV." The other child was actually a peer actor whose message had been prerecorded on videotape, but it was played for each girl as though it were a live transmission. When it was time to play the "game," each girl filled out a script to describe herself and then "transmitted" this message, via a video camera, to the peer. In response, the peer described herself, using a similar (prerecorded) format. Then the study participant asked the peer if she would like to play a game. The peer, via the prerecorded message, responded by rejecting the offer to play. After the child experienced the staged peer rejection, she told another set of stories to different TAT cards.

The stories that were told prior to, and subsequent to, rejection were then coded for the use of defenses; the coder had no knowledge of the girls' social status. As predicted, we found that the girls in the nonaccepted group used more defenses (denial and projection) after rejection than did the secure group, even though the two groups had not differed in defense use prior to rejection. The finding that children in the rejected and neglected categories do not differ significantly from popular children in DMM defense use, *in the absence of a rejection experience*, has also been reported by Rausch (1994).

A further analysis of the Sandstrom and Cramer (2003a) findings confirmed that the rejection experience affected the nonaccepted and peer secure girls differently, causing the former to increase their use of defenses. The nonaccepted girls reported experiencing increased stress after the rejection, and this increased stress was the mediating link between their social standing (the degree to which they were liked or disliked) and their use of defenses. The lower their standing, the greater the stress increased, and the greater the stress increased, the greater their postrejection use of defenses. In contrast, the peer secure girls were less stressed by the rejection experience, and this stress was unrelated to their subsequent use of defenses.

These findings suggest that children who have repeatedly experienced rejection and disregard from their peers have developed ways to protect themselves from the negative emotional consequences through the deployment of defenses. When yet another rejection occurs, their defense system is aroused, and those defenses that are available, depending on the child's age, will be activated. It also seems likely that a circular pattern becomes established in these children, such that their use of defenses interferes with their ability to engage in positive social interactions with their peers, which in turn further contributes to their social isolation.

CHILDREN'S DEFENSES IN RESPONSE TO "REAL-LIFE" STRESS

In addition to these laboratory studies showing that experimentally created stress increases defense use in children, it has also been possible to test this idea using stress from "real-life" situations. One of these studies involved the death of a child from a lightning strike. Another study investigated children growing up in HIV-positive families, where the threat and occurrence of death were constantly present. A further investigation focused on maltreated children. Finally, the effect of economic and family stress on defense use is considered.

The first study (Dollinger & Cramer, 1990) was based on a group of early adolescent boys who had been playing soccer when a severe thunderstorm came up; several bolts of lightning hit the playing field. One boy was killed and several others were knocked to the ground. Dr. Steven Dollinger, a child clinical psychologist from Southern Illinois University at Carbondale, was called on to evaluate the children affected by this tragedy. As part of the evaluation he had the boys tell TAT-like stories to two pictures depicting lightning. Subsequently, I evaluated these stories for the presence of the three defenses of denial, projection, and identification. Dr. Dollinger then related these defense scores to his previous assessment of psychological upset in the boys, based on clinical interviews.

The results indicated that boys who had higher total defense scores—especially higher scores for the age-appropriate defense of projection—manifested less upset than boys who had lower scores. In other words, the use of defenses, as assessed from TAT-like stories, was successful in protecting the boys from psychological upset—a finding that is again consistent with prediction from theory.[1]

Although the findings show that high defense use was associated with less overt upset, it is important to note that the defense assessment occurred a relatively short time after the disaster. During the period closely following a disaster, higher defense use may be a valuable initial reaction, allowing the individual more time to recover from confusion and to assimilate the trauma more gradually. This is especially true when the situation that caused the trauma cannot be controlled by the individual, as is the case with a lightning strike. However, the continued use of strong defenses may have subsequent negative effects, such as misinterpretation of reality, lack of self-understanding, and poor interpersonal relationships.

In fact, although these highly defended boys reported less psychological upset, there was evidence for such negative consequences of strong defense use. In a further study, the boys were asked to self-report on their fears about storms, death, and bodily perforation (fears more directly related to the lightning strike), as well as fears about sleep, embarrassment, and animals (Louisville Fear Survey; Miller, Barrett, Hempe, & Noble, 1972). At the same time, their parents provided information about sleep disturbances and somatic complaints. It might seem expectable that if a child had fears and was able to acknowledge them, then the child's report would correlate with the parents' report of problems. However, boys who were using more defenses would be likely to disavow fears, although their parents would report evidence of psychological disturbance. For this reason, the agreement between the child's self-reported fears and the parent ratings were expected to be greater for the boys who used fewer defenses.

To test this hypothesis, the boys' total defense scores were used to divide them into a high-defense group and a low-defense group (median split). Boys with high-defense scores reported somewhat fewer fears than did those with low-defense scores, consistent with the idea that the use of defenses protects the child from fears. Then, for each group separately, the boys' self-report scores for each of the fear categories were correlated with their parents' report of sleep disturbances and somatic complaints. High-defense boys' self-reports showed little agreement with their parents' ratings of disturbance. However, for the boys with low defense scores, those who reported having fears were rated by their parents as showing disturbance, whereas those who reported no fears were rated by their parents as not showing disturbance. An obvious interpretation of these results is that the high-defense boys misrepresented or denied their fears in their self-reports—that is, that the same defense that protected them from experiencing psychological upset about the lightning strike was also operating when they reported on a broader set of fears.

In the second study involving a tragic life event, 30 children who had younger siblings who were HIV-positive, and more than half of whom had lost one parent to the AIDS virus, were assessed for DMM defense use (Silverman, 1999). These children live under the constant daily stress of illness and the threat of death of their sibling. The participants, ages 9–18 years (mean = 15 years), came from a low-income background; 57% were African American, 37% Hispanic, and 6% Native American. In addition to the TAT stories, the examiner also administered the Youth Self-Report (YSR) version of the Child Behavior Checklist (Achenbach, 1991).

The DMM defense use of these children was found to be markedly different from that of the normative groups (Cramer, 1987; Porcerelli et al., 1998). These stressed children used denial twice as frequently as would be expected, and they used the more mature defense of identification less than half as often as would be expected. Although these results may reflect developmental delays, it is also likely that they result from a psychological regression due to the trauma experienced. Interestingly, the scores of this group on the self-report Achenbach scales did not differ from the data of the normative control group for this measure. In fact, males reported fewer somatic symptoms, and females reported fewer anxious/depressed symptoms than would be expected from normative data.[2]

The stress resulting from maltreatment in childhood has also been found to affect the use of defenses mechanisms (Finzi, Har-Even, & Weizman, 2003). Children ages 6–12 who were physically abused ($n = 41$) or neglected ($n = 38$) were compared with children who were not maltreated ($n = 35$). Participants' use of various defense mechanisms was assessed with the Ego Defense Scale (Pfeffer, 1986). The abused children used regression, denial, projection, repression, and introjection more frequently than the neglected group, who in turn used these immature defenses more often than the control group. In contrast, the control children were more likely to use the more mature defenses of sublimation, intellectualization, reaction formation, and undoing.

When their defense use was related to their self-reported scores on the Achenbach measure, the results for the defenses of denial and projection were similar to those found in the lightning strike study (Dollinger & Cramer, 1990). Those who had higher use of projection reported fewer externalizing symptoms; those who had higher use of denial reported fewer anxious/depressed symptoms and fewer attention problems. For these children, the use of projection and denial protected them from experiencing (or reporting) psychological upset. However, the use of identification was positively related to the externalizing symptom scale and to the presence of thought problems. Thus, in contrast to the reality-distorting defenses (projection, denial), this defense, which was used infrequently, did not protect the children from psychological upset.

Another kind of real-life stress occurs in connection with family strife and socioeconomic deprivation. Undesirable life events and increased psychological distress have been found to be associated with lower socioeconomic status in a number of population samples in the United States (McCleod & Kessler, 1990). Given this situation of increased stress as related to socioeconomic status, we might expect that adolescents from lower socioeconomic backgrounds would have greater need for the use of defenses, and that the experience of long-term stress would predispose them to rely on more immature defenses.

A study with nearly 1,500 Finnish adolescents, ages 14–20 years (mean age = 16.8 years) confirmed this expectation (Poikolainen, Kanerva, & Lonnqvist, 1995). These students were given the DSQ-72; their scores on the three factor scales were related to socioeconomic status, loss of father and/or mother through death or absence, grade point average, and gender. The results indicated a linear relation between the use of "neurotic" defenses and social class; the lower the economic level, the greater the use of neurotic defenses. In addition, loss of father was negatively related to the use of neurotic defenses. In contrast, the use of "mature" defenses was unrelated to stress factors. However, for boys in the sample, the use of "immature" defenses was related to the combination of both stress factors— low economic level and loss of father.

A further study of the relation between defense use and family environment, as assessed from a self-report true/false questionnaire (Thienemann, Shaw, & Steiner, 1998), was carried out with 106 female adolescent patients evaluated at a university teaching hospital (mean age = 15.9 years). Regression analyses indicated that scores for immature defenses were positively predicted by family conflict and achievement orientation and negatively predicted by independence. In contrast, scores for mature defenses were positively predicted by family "cohesion" and negatively predicted by "moral/religious emphasis." A further analysis indicated that scores on the Beck Depression Inventory positively predicted the use of immature defenses and negatively predicted mature defenses, and that the relation between the adolescent's level of depression and maturity of defense use was stronger than the relation with family environment. However, there was no significant relation between defense endorsement and diagnosis.

Related to the findings linking socioeconomic status stress with defense use, Vaillant and McCullough (1998) offered some evidence that the use of immature defenses by *adults* is not the result of growing up in a low socioeconomic status family. Rather, they argue that low socioeconomic status in *adulthood* is the result, not the cause, of using immature defenses.

This view, however, leaves open the question as to why some of the men continue to use lower-level defenses, whereas others do not. Vaillant and McCullough hint at genetic differences being the explanation.

Although Vaillant and McCullough found that adult defense immaturity was not related to childhood socioeconomic status, the studies of children reported above consistently demonstrate that stress, whether the result of laboratory interventions or real-life events, increases the use of defenses—especially lower-level defenses in younger or economically disadvantaged children. In turn, the use of these defenses then protects children from further psychological upset.

OBSERVATIONAL STUDIES OF THE RELATION BETWEEN CHILDREN'S DEFENSE USE AND PSYCHOLOGICAL PROBLEMS

Concurrent Studies: DMM

Several studies have demonstrated that normal, nonpatient children who are experiencing daily psychological stress will make greater use of defenses. This point was demonstrated in a study (Sandstrom & Cramer, 2003b) in which 95 children, ages 9–10 years, were evaluated by their parents on the Child Behavior Checklist (CBCL; Achenbach & Edelbrock, 1983), a well-standardized questionnaire that assesses the psychological adjustment of the child. From this information, each child's standing on scales assessing various psychological problems, such as anxiety, aggression, and withdrawal, was determined, as well as summary scores for internalizing and externalizing problems. In addition, each child provided self-report measures of depression and anxiety. The scores on these measures were then related to defense use, based on DMM coding of the children's TAT stories. The results of the study showed clearly that use of the immature defense of denial was greater among those children who were experiencing psychological difficulties. Parent-reported internalizing and externalizing problems and child-reported social anxiety and depression were all significantly correlated with the use of denial. Neither the age-appropriate defense of projection nor the defense of identification, which is not yet prominent in the defenses of children of this age, was related to measures of psychological problems. Interestingly, those children who had begun to use the more mature defense of identification gave evidence of higher self-esteem, as assessed by a measure of perceived self-competence (Harter, 1982). This defense was not related to indications of maladjustment, whereas denial was not related to perceived self-competence.

However, these findings suggest some specificity in the relation between maladjustment and defense use. For a group of fourth graders, the use of projection is normative; we expect children of this age to use this defense. What differentiates the problem-affected children is not the use of this age-normative defense but the use of a less mature defense—a defense that is normative for younger children. As is discussed in Chapter 10, psychological difficulties in early childhood are likely to result in the child's increased use of the defense that is available at that age—that is, denial. Subsequently, this defense may become ingrained in the child's personality and continue to be used long after the time it is usually relinquished. I am suggesting, then, that the relation between the psychological problems revealed on the CBCL and the use of denial by fourth graders was relatively longstanding, having begun at the time that denial was an age-appropriate defense.

In contrast, the use of identification, a defense typically associated with an older age, was found to occur in conjunction with perceived self-competence and self-esteem, but not with pathology. As in the experimental study of success and failure described above (Cramer & Gaul, 1988), this finding again suggests that self-esteem allows the child to relinquish less mature defenses and to advance on the pathway of defense mechanism development.

A further way of considering the relation between children's internalizing/externalizing problems and defense use is suggested by studies that relate such problems to the way in which aggression is externalized by boys and girls (Crick, 1997). Those who used gender non-normative forms of aggression had more psychological problems, which in turn we would expect to be related to greater defense use. This work is discussed further in Chapter 9.

Concurrent Studies: DSQ

Similar findings relating defense use and internalizing/externalizing problems have been reported in a study of adolescents (Evans & Seaman, 2000) ranging in age from 15 to 18 years of age. On the basis of their defense scores on the DSQ-78, the participants were divided into two groups: those who used immature defenses and those using mature defenses. Each group then self-reported on various psychological problems, yielding two overall measures of internalizing and externalizing symptoms (Youth Self-Report; Achenbach, 1991). They were also assessed for their self-reported competence and self-worth, using Harter's (1982) scale. The findings of this study demonstrated that those adolescents using immature defenses were characterized by a greater number of internalizing and externalizing symptoms, as compared to those who used mature defenses. At the same time, mature defense use was associated with higher perceived self-competence and higher global self-worth.

These results from a group of adolescents are quite consistent with those from the grade-school children and demonstrate, again, that immature defense use is associated with psychological problems, whereas mature defense use is associated with positive self-regard.

Further evidence for the relation between defense use and psychological adjustment in adolescents comes from two investigations of normal high school students. In the first investigation (Erickson, Feldman, & Steiner, 1997), students filled out the self-report DSQ-78 and were rated on the DSM-III-R Global Assessment of Functioning Scale (GAF) on the basis of psychiatric interviews covering school, work, play, family, and friends. GAF ratings were made on a continuum ranging from health to psychological illness. Subsequently, the 19 defenses assessed with the DSQ were correlated with GAF ratings. Four of the immature defenses (projection, regression, passive aggression, and splitting) were related to lower GAF scores, and two of the mature defenses (affiliation and sublimation) were related to higher GAF scores. When these six defenses were entered into a regression analysis to predict GAF, only regression, among the immature defenses, was significant for predicting poor GAF; both of the mature defenses were significant for predicting healthy GAF. These findings raise the question of whether the attempt to use 19 different defense rating scales, the majority of which consist of two or three items, is meaningful or useful.

This question was further investigated by Erikson et al. (1997). For a subsample (n = 81) of the adolescent group, their three defense factor scores (Immature, Mature, Prosocial), which were based on a factor analysis of the DSQ-78 using the extended adolescent sample, were used to determine the relation between GAF score and defense use, as this relation contrasted with the relation between GAF and two coping strategies.

As would be expected from the data of the larger study, two of the three defense factor scales were correlated with GAF. Mature defense scores were positively related and Immature defense scores were negatively related to GAF, as was Avoidance coping. Neither the Prosocial defense factor, nor the Approach coping factor was related to GAF. Further, these relations were significant only for females, for whom a regression analysis additionally indicated that only the Immature defense and Avoidance coping factors were uniquely significant predictors of GAF. The relative independence of these defense and coping factors for predicting GAF supports the theoretical position that the two types of adaptational processes are distinct, representing unconscious automatic mechanisms, on the one hand, and conscious, volitional strategies on the other (see Chapter 1 for a discussion of this issue).

In another investigation (Muris, Winands, & Horselenberg, 2003), more than 400 adolescents (range = 12–17 years) from the Netherlands completed the adolescent version of the DSQ-40 and the DSM-IV-

Psychopathology Questionnaire for Youths (PQY) syndrome scales (Hartman et al., 2001). The results indicated that scores on the Neurotic defense factor were related to symptoms of various anxiety disorders, including separation anxiety, obsessive–compulsive disorder (OCD), panic disorder, somatization, and depression. Self-reported use of defenses comprising the Immature factor were related to oppositional defiant disorder, conduct disorder, schizophrenia, and substance abuse. The report of Mature defense use was not related to pathological syndromes.

The relation between defense use and psychological problems was also demonstrated in a group of 7- to 10-year-olds. A modification of the DSQ-78 for use with children, the REM-Y (Yasnovsky et al., 2003), was completed by the children, and this self-report measure was related to a self-report measure of anxiety. The results showed that both the Immature and Mature defense factors were positively correlated with level of anxiety.

LONGITUDINAL STUDIES

I suggested above that psychological problems from preschool years would predict defense use at a later age. This prediction has been validated in three investigations. One of these (Cramer & Block, 1998) is described in Chapter 10. Briefly, this study found that psychological disturbance in 3-year-olds predicted use of the defense of denial (on the DMM) 20 years later. Marginally, this early disturbance was related to later use of projection. In contrast, there was a slight relation between early positive adjustment and later use of identification.

The second study followed the development of preschool Israeli children who had been exposed to missile attacks during the 1991 Gulf War (Wolmer, Laor, & Cicchetti, 2001). At the time of the attacks, parents had described their children (ages 3–5 years) using the CBCL (Achenbach & Edelbrock, 1983). Five years later the parents reported on the children's use of defenses, using the CADS (see pp. 334–335 for a description). As in the previous study, in which DMM defenses and CBCL were assessed concurrently, the Israeli study demonstrated that psychological disturbance during the earlier years subsequently predicted defense use in middle childhood. Similar to the previous findings, psychological disturbances—early internalizing and externalizing symptoms—were related to the later use of denial ("Self-oriented" defense factor). In this study early disturbance was also related to later projection ("Other-oriented" defense factor). In contrast, and again in agreement with the previous study, early psychological disturbance was not related to the later use of identification (Mature defense factor).

Yet another study demonstrating that earlier defense use can predict psychiatric status in subsequent years comes from an investigation of "at-risk" children (Shabad, Worland, Lander, & Deitrich, 1979). In this study children ages 7–18 years who were known to be at risk for future psychiatric problems, due to having a parent currently hospitalized for a psychotic illness, were administered a set of TAT cards that were subsequently scored for several characteristics, including the use of denial. Follow-up was conducted 10 years later and psychiatric status was determined. Those children who had evidenced greater use of denial in the earlier years were subsequently more likely to show major psychiatric problems requiring hospitalization or intensive outpatient therapy, as compared to the other at-risk children whose later development appeared normal.

PATIENT STUDIES

If defense use is greater in children experiencing psychological stress, then this pattern should be evident in children with known psychiatric problems. This hypothesis was investigated in a study that contrasted two groups of early adolescents who had psychiatric diagnoses of differing degrees of severity (Cramer & Kelly, 2004). One group consisted of 37 young adolescents who had been diagnosed as having a conduct disorder; the second group of 30 adolescents had been given the less serious diagnosis of adjustment reaction. Among the defining characteristics of conduct disorder are the findings that these adolescents often suffer from a developmental lag, showing evidence of immature functioning, failure to understand social situations, lack of empathy toward others, and "failing to see" the implications of their behavior. These characteristics suggest that conduct disorder would be associated with the defense of denial, which is immature for an adolescent and which contributes to the failure to understand the meaning of behavior. In addition, along with developmental lag, the characteristic lack of empathy of this group suggests that they may be deficient in the use of the defense of identification.

In contrast, adolescents with an adjustment reaction disorder would not be expected to demonstrate developmental lag. The psychological problems associated with the diagnosis of adjustment reaction are based on stressful current experience. Prior to this stressful time, the adolescents would be expected to have traversed the developmental pathway in an age-appropriate fashion and should be expected to be using the defense of identification, which is characteristic of this age.

A comparison of the two groups of adolescents confirmed these predictions. The youths with conduct disorder used more denial (DMM) than the adjustment reaction group, who used more identification (DMM) than the conduct-disordered group.

Similar findings were reported by Hernandez (1999). Comparing three groups of Hispanic and African American early-adolescent boys who had been diagnosed as conduct disordered (n = 19), depressed (n = 17), or normal (n = 18), he found that boys with conduct disorder used more denial (DMM) and less identification (DMM) than either of the other two groups. Yet another study, involving incarcerated female juvenile delinquents, found that their overall level of defense use, assessed by the California Psychological Inventory (CPI)-based Joffee and Naditch (1977) scales, was significantly higher than that of an adolescent control group of similar age and gender (Bartek, Krebs, & Taylor, 1993).

In an Israeli study (Laor et al., 2001) children ages 6–18 years, with various diagnoses that included separation anxiety, OCD, and depression, were assessed for defense use through their parents' report on the CADS.[3] These patients were compared with a group of normal children of similar ages on each of the three CADS defense factors and on each of the individual defense scales. The results from children and adolescents of this extended age-range sample demonstrated clearly that the psychiatric group made greater use of projection and other-oriented defenses, greater use of self-oriented defenses, and less use of identification and other mature defenses, as compared to the normal group.

A further study compared hospitalized and nonhospitalized child psychiatric patients (ages 6–12 years) with nonpatients of comparable ages (Pfeffer, Plutchik, & Mizruchi, 1986). The most frequent diagnoses for the inpatients were conduct disorder and borderline personality disorder (BPD); the most frequent diagnoses for the outpatients were adjustment reaction and specific developmental disorder. Defense use was determined from interviews with the child and parents, using the 3-point scales of the Ego Defense Scale to code 11 different defense mechanisms (Pfeffer, 1986). The results indicated that total defense use was significantly greater in the patient sample. In particular, projection, repression, intellectualization, displacement, and regression significantly differentiated the three patient and nonpatient groups, with the latter two defenses being the best predictors of need for psychiatric hospitalization.

Another study comparing hospitalized and healthy adolescents (average age = 16 years), using the Ego Defense Scale, determined defense use in three different diagnostic groups: schizophrenia, major depressive disorder (MDD), and OCD (Offer, Lavie, Gothelf, & Apter, 2000). The results showed that all three patient groups used regression, denial, projection, and repression more than the normal group; the patients also used sublimation less than the normal group. The only diagnosis to be differentiated from the others by use of defenses was the OCD group, who used reaction formation and undoing more than did the groups of patients with schizophrenia or MDD, consistent with the early formulation of Freud (1926). Interestingly, there were no gender differences in the use of defenses, nor did gender have any effect on the correlation between defenses and negative emotions. For both males and females, projection and regression correlated with anger, whereas displacement, reaction formation and undoing all correlated with state anxiety.[4]

In another report of this research (Gothelf et al., 1995), adolescent patients with anorexia were contrasted with the groups of patients with MDD, OCD, schizophrenia, and BPD, and with the group of normal adolescents. As in the previous study, all groups of patients, including those with anorexia, had higher defense scores on the Ego Defense Scales for regression, denial, projection, and repression. Notably, the patients with anorexia used more intellectualization than the adolescents in the normal group and more sublimation than the patients in the other groups. The authors note that this unusual combination of immature and mature defenses in patients with anorexia might help explain how patients with such severe pathology can manage to function successfully in school and other activities.

Studies of other psychological disorders in adolescence have also found evidence that psychopathology is associated with the use of immature defenses. A study from the Stanford University Eating Disorder Program found that adolescent girls who were depressed or who had eating disorders were more likely to use immature defenses (DSQ; Bond et al., 1983) and less likely to use mature defenses than control girls matched for age and socioeconomic status (Steiner, 1990). A 6-year follow-up of these young women with anorexia and a control group found that those who continued to have psychiatric problems used immature defenses more and mature defenses less than did the control women, both initially and at follow-up (Smith, Feldman, Nasserbakht, & Steiner, 1993). In contrast, the previous girls with anorexia who had no psychiatric disorder at follow-up (35% of the group) did not differ in defense use from the control group, either initially or at follow-up. Further, the use of more mature defenses at the time of the original diagnosis was a positive predictor for better outcome 6 years later. The latter finding is striking because none of the physical factors identified at the initial diagnosis, such as age of onset, duration of illness, height, or weight, were associated with outcome status (i.e., continuing disorder vs. no disorder). Another short-term (1-year) follow-up study of adolescent girls with anorexia (Sohlberg & Norring, 1989, as cited in Smith et al., 1993) also found that defense maturity was the best predictor of outcome status.

Subsequently, the Stanford patient group was expanded by adding adolescent girls with diagnoses of "psychosomatic disorder," including anorexia, bulimia, depression, and anxiety disorder, matched for ethnicity and socioeconomic status with a group of control participants (Steiner & Feldman, 1995).[5] In addition, incarcerated male adolescents with a diagnosis of delinquency were included along with control participants (whose socioeconomic status was higher). Using the DSQ to assess defenses, the results were consistent with the earlier study. Patients used more immature defenses and fewer mature defenses than did the normal controls. Specifically, girls with psychosomatic disorders were less likely to use mature defenses and more likely to use neurotic defenses (e.g., denial, projection) than were control girls. Delinquent boys also used fewer mature defenses than the controls; the two groups did not differ in their use of neurotic defenses, but the delinquent boys used more immature defenses than did the control boys.

Further discriminant analyses were undertaken to determine if defense use could correctly classify the adolescents into their known diagnostic groups (pathology vs. control). Using this approach, the DSQ defense scores correctly classified 61% of the girls, slightly better than chance; the scores on mature defense were most successful in accomplishing this classification. For boys, the defense scores successfully predicted actual diagnostic group at a slightly better rate (65%), with the greatest success being the prediction of normalcy (80%), as compared to delinquency (50%). Success in distinguishing between the two groups was primarily due to scores on the immature and mature defenses.

A revision of the DSQ for adolescents was created by Feldman, Araujo, and Steiner (1996) to assess the use of 17 defenses classified as *immature* (denial, projection, regression, somatization, repression, and others), *prosocial* (altruism, reaction formation), and *mature* (suppression, humor, affiliation, sublimation, anticipation). This version of the DSQ was used to study 107 female adolescents who were psychiatric inpatients with various diagnoses, the most frequent being eating disorders (56%) and major depression (32%) (Shaw et al., 1996). These patients also completed a self-report measure assessing four dimensions of temperament, conceptually derived from the work of Thomas and Chess (1980) in the New York Longitudinal Study. The defense styles endorsed by these hospitalized adolescents were then related to the four dimensions of temperament. Regression analyses indicated that the use of immature defenses was positively predicted by activity level and negatively predicted by adaptability. Prosocial defenses were positively predicted by the temperament dimension of attentional focus. Mature defenses were positively predicted by the temperament dimension of adaptability.

A further study of hospitalized adolescents demonstrated the relation between defense use and the externalizing/internalizing symptom scales of the YSR (Noam & Recklitis, 1990). Nearly 200 adolescents with various nonpsychotic diagnoses (e.g., conduct disorder, anxiety disorder) were studied for the relation between defense scores on the DMI and the internalizing/externalizing scales of the YSR. Interestingly, in this patient sample boys and girls did not differ for scores on any of the five DMI defense scales, as contrasted with earlier DMI adolescent findings (Cramer, 1979; Levit, 1991). However, girls reported (on the YSR) having more symptoms, suggesting the possibility that the girls were less defensive than the boys in acknowledging psychological disturbance—an idea that is supported by the findings of a study by Dollinger and Cramer (1990; discussed later). Alternatively, the girls may have actually been experiencing greater pathology. At any rate, when the girls' defense use was correlated with the YSR scales, TAO and projection were positively related to externalizing symptoms, whereas TAS was positively related to internalizing symptoms. In contrast, both PRN and REV were negatively related to both externalizing and internalizing scores, indicating that girls who self-report using these defenses also self-report fewer psychological problems. For boys, TAO was positively related to externalizing, and TAS was positively related to internalizing. The only other significant relation was the negative relation between REV and externalizing symptoms. In general, these results are consistent with the idea that those who use defenses that place problems outside of the self, such as projection and TAO, will manifest more externalized, aggressive behaviors. In contrast, those who place problems within the self through the use of defenses such as TAS and REV will display more internalized, depressive, or self-destructive symptoms.

Both theory and prior research have suggested that defenses involving turning aggression toward the self are related to depression and suicidal behavior (cf. Cramer, 1991a). To test this hypothesis using the adolescent version of the DMI, defense use in hospitalized adolescent girls who had attempted suicide (n = 52) was compared to use in nonsuicidal hospitalized girls (n = 87) (Borst & Noam, 1993). The suicidal girls were significantly higher on the TAS scale and on the internalizing symptom scale from the YSR (Achenbach & Edelbrock, 1983), as predicted.

In another report from this research group (Recklitis, Noam, & Borst, 1992), inpatient adolescent boys and girls (mean age = 14 years) with a diagnosis of conduct disorder, affective disorder, or mixed (both conduct and affective disorders) were divided into three groups: those who had attempted suicide within the past 6 months (attemptors: n = 68), those who had thought of, but not attempted, suicide (ideators: n = 27), and those who had neither attempted nor thought of suicide (n = 105). Defense use was assessed with the DMI. The results indicated that TAS was more frequent in the attemptors and ideators, whereas REV was more frequent in the nonsuicidal group. It also turned out that attemptors were more prevalent in the mixed diagnostic group. When this fact was accounted for, only TAS differentiated the attemptors from the nonsuicidal group.

The relation between defenses and suicidal behavior was also investigated in a follow-up study in which preadolescent patients (mean age = 10 years; range 4–17 years) who had been hospitalized for attempting suicide (n = 25) were contrasted with patients who did (n = 28) or did not (n = 16) report suicidal ideation as well as with a nonpatient control group (n = 64) (Pfeffer, Hart, Peskin, & Siefker, 1995). All participants (73% male) were assessed for defense use at the time of initial hospitalization and again 6–8 years later, using the Ego Defense Scale (Pfeffer, 1986). Defense scores were then related to suicide status.

Unfortunately, the interrater reliability for the 11 defense scales was very low in this study, ranging from .15 to .46; only repression reached an acceptable level (kappa = .82).[6] Perhaps related to this issue of scale reliability, only the repression scale was successful in predicting subsequent suicide attempts. For patients who had previously attempted suicide, during the follow-up period there was an inverse relation between initial repression scores and time until a new suicide attempt occurred. This same pattern of a negative relation between initial repression and subsequent time to suicide attempt was found for the other patient groups and for the nonpatient group.

The four subject groups were also compared for total defense use (number of different defenses rated). At the initial assessment all three patient groups had higher scores than the control group but did not differ from each other. At the follow-up assessment 7 years later, those who had not attempted suicide during the follow-up period had lower total defense scores (used fewer defenses) than those who had attempted suicide either before or during the follow-up period.

CONCLUDING REMARKS

Taken as a group, these studies show that children who are under stress or experiencing psychological problems increase their use of defenses. Whereas temporary stress increases the use of age-appropriate defenses, long-term stress is related to greater use of immature defenses and less use of mature defenses. Regardless of the defense measure used, adolescent psychiatric patients are found to use more immature and fewer mature defenses than nonpatients.

Theory explains this increase as an attempt, on the part of the psyche, to protect the child from further anxiety and psychological upset. In some cases this increased defense use, if continued for an extended period of time, may create further psychological difficulties by distorting the child's perception of reality or interfering with the development of satisfactory relationships with others. However, in the short term, the use of defenses should provide some positive benefit to the stressed child (e.g., Dollinger & Cramer, 1990; Silverman, 1999).

How are defenses, stress, and psychopathology interrelated? Defenses may be thought of as a link between the developing ego and the potential for psychopathology. When age-appropriate defense development is delayed or inhibited, it is more difficult for the child or adolescent to deal with the life tasks being experienced in that period of development. In this case there is an "age–stage dysynchrony" (Noam, Recklitis, & Paget, 1991). The use of age-inappropriate—that is, developmentally immature—defenses then interferes with the child's ability to integrate cognitive, emotional, and behavioral processes. In turn, this decreased integration contributes to maladaptive behavior.

A significant question here is whether undue stress results in delayed ego development, including the failure of more mature defenses to develop, or whether ego (and defense) immaturity results in an increased experience of stress. Put another way, does adequate ego development support the development of more mature defenses, or does the development of more mature defenses facilitate ego development, such that fewer stressful situations are encountered? It seems likely that both processes occur—that is, ego development supports the development of mature defenses and the presence of mature defenses decreases the deleterious effects of stress on ego development.

Support for the idea that healthy ego development facilitates the development of more mature defenses comes from two studies with grade-school children. In the first, an experimental intervention of success increased the children's use of the mature defense of identification, as compared to children in the failure condition. Additionally, the results of an observational study (Sandstrom & Cramer, 2003b) supported this idea: Children with higher self-competence were more likely to use the defense of identification. Although these findings are suggestive, more work on this issue is needed. As pointed out by Noam et al. (1991), the investigation of ego development, defenses, and symptomatology "should produce important insights for developmental psychopathology" (p. 326).

A related question is whether the use of defenses is associated with greater or lesser psychological disturbance. That is, does the use of defenses serve a protective function, reducing the likelihood of psychological disturbance, or does defense use promote further psychological difficulties?

Research findings suggest that the answer to this question depends on two factors. First, whether or not defenses are helpful or hindering depends on the time frame being considered. When defenses occur as a reaction to a currently stressful situation, their use protects the child from experiencing psychological upset. In contrast, the use of defenses—especially immature defenses—as an ongoing, continuing process, although presumably serving a protective function of one sort, is likely to result in other psychological difficulties. When this situation continues over a longer period of time, we find a positive association between defense use and psychological problems.

The second factor relates to the assessment methods used. Using self-report measures to assess either defense use or indications of psychological disturbance may yield different results from studies in which these ratings are made by an independent observer. This difference was demonstrated in the lightning strike study (Dollinger & Cramer, 1990), in which the self-report of psychological fears and anxieties by children who had high defense levels did not agree with their parents' report. A similar discrepancy between child and parent report for defense use was found by Yasnovsky et al. (2003). Using the REM-Y to assess defenses, the researchers reported that the agreement between parent and child for immature defenses was modest ($r = .36$), and there was virtually no relation between self-report scores of mature defenses and parent report for the same defenses ($r = .03$).

Apart from these measurement issues, I am suggesting that the relation between defense use and pathology may vary over time. The only way to test this hypothesis is to conduct longitudinal studies that examine both the course of defense development and its relation to psychological functioning over a period of years. This type of research is difficult to carry out, but it would yield answers to questions as yet unanswered.

CHAPTER 7

Stress and Defense Use in Adulthood

Thus far we have focused primarily on children's use of defenses—how they develop, how they relate to psychological disturbance, and how they help the child adapt to unfortunate experiences. We turn now to the question of how stress influences the use of defenses in adulthood.

As with children, theory says that the use of defense mechanisms should increase when the adult is under stress. From the theory of defense mechanism development, we should expect that the defenses that increase will be those appropriate to the age of the individual. If we are studying late adolescents or young adults, these will be the defenses of projection and identification.

To study the relation between stress and defense use in a controlled research setting, it is necessary to expose the participants to experimentally created stress. In all of the studies in which stress is purposely created, each participant is carefully debriefed at the end of the session. The purpose of the study is explained, as is the reason for the stress intervention. It is also explained that stressful information provided as part of the experiment was, in fact, bogus. Any questions or concerns of the participant are carefully addressed.

STRESS AND DMM DEFENSE ASSESSMENT

In keeping with the assumption that a threat to self-esteem will increase the use of defenses, three experiments were conducted using different types of self-esteem threat. The first challenged students' creativity; the second challenged their intellectual curiosity; the third challenged their sex-role orientation. Two further studies investigated the effect of a threat to sexual identity on the use of defenses. Each of these studies found that a threat to self-esteem or a challenge to sexual identity increased the use of defense mechanisms.

An initial investigation of the relation between stress and defense use in adulthood employed an experimental paradigm in which the self-esteem of college students was temporarily challenged (Cramer, 1991b). The participants in this study—late adolescent students who had been accepted into a selective, small liberal arts college—generally prided themselves on their intelligence and creativity. One would expect, then, that if this important part of their self-image were challenged, they would increase their use of defenses—especially those defenses that are age appropriate.

The study was carried out with 80 college students. Each student was brought into the lab by an attractive, slightly older female experimenter. The student was requested to lie down on a small bed; at the foot of the bed was a large TV camera, focused directly at the student. The experimenter turned on the camera, then sat in a chair behind the head of the bed, where she could see the student but the student could not see her. She explained that this was a study of creative imagination, that the student would be asked to create stories in response to a series of pictures, and that the stories would be evaluated for evidence of imagination.

Each student was then presented with four pictures, one at a time. The stories were tape-recorded. After each story, the experimenter made some neutral comment such as "Okay" or "All right." This procedure was continued for eight stories for half of the students; however, for the other half of students, the experimenter became very critical after the fourth story. For example, after the fourth story, she said, "These stories are really terrible. They are some of the worst that I have ever heard. Please try a little harder." After the fifth story, she said, "This is still pretty bad. See if you can't do better." This type of criticism continued after the sixth and seventh stories.

After the eighth story, as a check to determine if the students were actually being affected by the experimental manipulation, two kinds of information were gathered. First, students were asked at the end of the study to indicate how they had felt on arriving and how they now felt, at the end. These data showed that at the beginning of the study the emotional state of the to-be-criticized group did not differ from the control group, but by the end the criticized students reported feeling angry and/or anxious. Second, we looked for indications of angry, aggressive feelings in the stories the students had told. Whereas the criticized and control groups did not differ prior to criticism, the criticized students evidenced significantly more aggression in their stories after being criticized. As part of the debriefing, students were then given an explanation about why the experimenter had been so critical, and they were assured that their stories were, in fact, just fine.

After the stories were transcribed, the four stories that were given prior to criticism were coded for defense use, and the two groups of students—those who later would be angered by criticism and those who were not criticized—were compared. As Figure 7.1 illustrates, the two groups did not differ in defense use prior to criticism. However, after the criticism intervention, the groups were markedly different. Students who were stressed in this way increased their use of *projection* and *identification*, as compared to the nonstressed students, as may be seen in Figure 7.2. As with the stressed children, it is the age-appropriate defenses that are increased.

Another experimental study created stress by challenging college students' intellectual capacity. The DMM approach was used to assess the effect of this stress on defense use (Tuller, 2002). Participants were randomly assigned to an experimental group and a control group and told stories in response to three TAT cards (1, 8BM, and 3BM). In this baseline measure the two groups did not differ in their use of denial, projection, or identification. After the third story had been told, participants in the experimental group were presented with a series of six mathematical problems to be solved mentally, under conditions of time pressure. Following this stress experience, both groups told stories in response to three more TAT cards

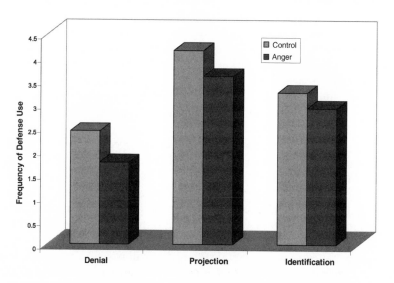

FIGURE 7.1. College students prior to intervention: Anger and control groups.

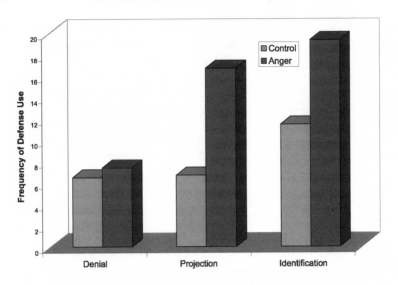

FIGURE 7.2. College students: Effects of anger on defense use.

(17BM, 13MF, and 6BM). A comparison of the experimental and control groups indicated that DMM defense use was greater in the stressed group for denial ($p < .04$), projection ($p < .009$), and identification ($p < .03$). The results also showed that defense use increased from prestress to poststress in the experimental group but decreased in the control group.

The studies discussed in the preceding material created stress and a threat to self-esteem by challenging the students' sense of their own creativity and intellectual ability. A third investigation was devised in such a way that students' sex-role orientation would be challenged (Cramer, 1998a). In discussing the process of identity formation, Erik Erikson wrote: "Identity formation, finally, begins where the usefulness of identification ends" (1968, p. 159). The implication here is that if identity is challenged, the adolescent will revert to the use of the defense of identification, which should thus increase. Thus, for theoretical reasons, we expected that a direct challenge to gender identity would be especially likely to increase the use of the defense of identification.

During this study, male and female college students were told either that they had a strong masculine sex-role identity or a strong feminine sex-role identity, creating four experimental groups. Initially, as each student entered the laboratory, he or she was told: "This is a study of imagination. You will be asked to write several stories that will be evaluated for their evidence of imagination." The student then wrote stories in response to three pictures. At this point the student was given the Bem Sex Role Inventory

(BSRI), a paper-and-pencil questionnaire that has been well standardized and used in many studies of sex-role identity. After completing the inventory, the examiner explained that it measured sex-role identity and that she would score it and tell the student his or her score. The examiner then left the room, presumably to do the scoring, and returned with a computer printout with the student's presumed score and a detailed, but confusing, table of statistics. The student, whether male or female, was told that on this "highly reliable and widely used test," he or she had received either a very high masculine score or a very high feminine score. At that point the student was invited to discuss the findings with the examiner. After some discussion, the student was again asked to create three more stories in response to three different pictures. At the end, for a manipulation check, all students were asked how they had felt when they arrived and how they felt during and after the study. In debriefing, the purpose of the feedback was explained, and the fact that their scores had been made up and were not real was emphasized.

The stories were coded for defense use. Although prior to the sex-role feedback, the four groups did not differ, after the feedback, the two groups that had been given cross-sex feedback—males told they were feminine and females told they were masculine—showed significantly higher identification scores than those shown by the sex-consistent groups. Also, to a lesser extent, the cross-sex males used more projection than the sex-consistent males; the same increase in projection was seen for the cross-sex females. But it is primarily the defense of identification that was affected by a threat to identity—as would be predicted from theory (see Figure 7.3).

Further examination of the findings was equally informative. Because the participants had completed the BSRI, a measure of their actual sex-role identity was available. Some students were found to be highly sex-stereotyped as masculine or feminine, whereas others were minimally stereotyped. Using this information, it was possible to divide the male students into a high-masculine sex-typed group and a low-masculine sex-typed group. We hypothesized that the high-masculine sex-typed group would be more upset by being told they had a female orientation than would the low sex-typed group. In turn, this increased upset should result in the high-masculine sex-typed group making more use of the defense of identification than would the low-masculine sex-typed group.

When the two male groups (high- and low-masculine sex-typed) were compared for defense use prior to the experimental feedback regarding sex-role orientation, they did not differ. However, after feedback suggesting a feminine orientation, the men who were highly sex-typed made the greatest use of identification.

In a similar way, the female students were divided into two groups on the basis of their masculine sex-typed scores. Although they did not differ

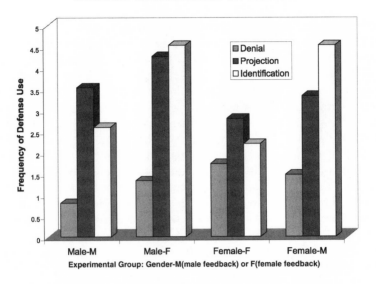

FIGURE 7.3. College students: Threat to gender identity.

in their use of identification prior to the feedback, those women who were low on masculine sex-typing but were given masculine feedback used more identification than those given feminine feedback. Thus, overall, the increased use of identification was primarily due to those students for whom the contrived gender feedback was in conflict with their personal sex-role identity.

The idea that a threat to sexual identity would increase defense use was studied in a different way in the doctoral research of Jason Luciano (1997, 1999). He reasoned that some of the TAT pictures—those that portrayed heterosexual couples in close or intimate interaction—would be likely to arouse anxiety in gay men because the intimate relationships portrayed in these pictures are in conflict with their sexual orientation. Thus these TAT pictures should be expected to elicit greater use of defenses than would neutral pictures, and should elicit greater use of defenses for gay men than for heterosexual men.

Luciano (1997) confirmed these expectations in an initial study: Gay men and heterosexual men told stories in response to three TAT cards known to elicit themes of heterosexual sex and romance, and in response to two control cards that did not display a heterosexual relationship. The results indicated that whereas gay and heterosexual men did not differ in their use of defenses in response to the control TAT cards, they did differ on the heterosexual cards. In particular, the gay men used significantly more identification on all three cards, as compared to the heterosexual men.

They also used more denial and projection on one of the heterosexual cards (Card 10), which depicts a particularly close physical relationship between a man and a woman.

These findings are consistent with the assumption that a picture that conflicts with one's sense of self will arouse anxiety when one is requested to tell a story about that picture, and, in turn, the use of defense mechanisms will increase. Again, the increase in the defense of identification is most striking.

The second study by Luciano (1999) confirmed and extended these findings by investigating the effect of a challenge to the identity of deaf men as well as to gay men. For the deaf to communicate with others in sign language, it is necessary that they be able to establish eye contact with the other person and have free use of their hands. Being asked to tell a story in response to a picture that violates these requirements (e.g., the characters do not have eye contact and do not have free use of their hands) would challenge the identity of a deaf person as one who is able to communicate with others.

This second study thus included both gay and heterosexual men; half of each group was deaf, the other half had normal hearing. All participants told stories in response to TAT cards portraying heterosexual relationships, to TAT cards violating the communication requirements of deaf people, plus two neutral cards. Each deaf participant told his stories to the examiner using sign language; these signing sessions were videotaped and subsequently given to a qualified sign-language interpreter who voice-interpreted each story into a recorder; each story was then transcribed. The hearing men also told their stories to the examiner, and these were subsequently transcribed. An initial test showed that the defense coders were unable to identify group membership (heterosexual/homosexual; deaf/hearing) from the narratives provided, assuring that the defense ratings would not be influenced by such knowledge.

The results of this study are striking in demonstrating the specificity of the defense mechanism effect. An initial comparison showed that gay men did not differ from heterosexual men in overall level of defense use—that is, when defense scores were summed across all nine stories. Likewise, deaf men did not differ from hearing men when this comparison of total defense use was made. Rather, as before, the gay men had higher defense scores for all the TAT cards depicting heterosexual romantic situations, but they did not differ from the heterosexual men for stories told in response to the TAT cards depicting violation of deaf communication or the neutral cards. Similarly, the deaf men had higher defense scores for the communication violation cards than did the hearing men, but they did not differ on the other cards. Strikingly, for the one TAT card that challenged both sexual orientation and hearing status (Card 4 depicts a man and woman in physically close relation, with the man's face turned away), the greatest use of defense mechanisms was found in the group of men who were both gay and deaf, whereas the least use of defenses for this card occurred with the heterosexual hearing group. This finding demonstrates that a dual challenge to personal identity results in even greater use of defense mechanisms.

Once again, a challenge (or challenges) to the person's identity increased his use of defenses, and, as before, it was especially the defense of identification that increased.

OTHER STUDIES OF STRESS AND DEFENSE USE

A different experimental approach to demonstrate that defense use increases when personal identity is challenged was used in a study by Schimel, Greenberg, and Martens (2003). This study showed that the use of a defense not only increases when self-esteem is threatened, but also that the defense mechanism *protects* self-esteem by removing disturbing thoughts from conscious awareness. In this study students' self-esteem was challenged by giving them contrived feedback that psychological testing had shown them to have a high level of repressed hostility or a high tendency toward dishonesty. Then, using a cleverly designed task, the students were given the opportunity to project (attribute) this undesirable trait to another person. Those who had been given high anger or dishonesty feedback showed higher levels of projection of this trait onto a contrived, ambiguous target person than did those who had been given low anger or dishonesty feedback. An indirect assessment of students' anger, or a measure of their acknowledged dishonesty, indicated that those who had been given the opportunity to project the trait were less likely to express the trait now, as compared to those who had not had the opportunity to use projection. In other words, the undesirable trait had become less accessible—that is, less likely to be acknowledged as part of the self. In this sense the defense of projection was successful in that it functioned to maintain the students' self-esteem. Interestingly, projection of the specific trait of anger or dishonesty did not affect the attribution of other negative traits to the target. That is, the arousal of concern about the specific traits did not lead to an overall negativity about the target person but was highly specific to the manipulated undesirable trait of anger or dishonesty.

An earlier study by Newman, Duff, and Baumeister (1997) also found that individuals who were generally more defensive were more likely to project (attribute) traits to others that they found to be personally unacceptable. That is, by using projection they defended their self-concept, or self-esteem, by perceiving in others the traits they wished to deny in themselves. Importantly, this study also demonstrated that awareness of the use of projection undermined its effectiveness, in agreement with the results of the Cramer and Brilliant (2001) study discussed in Chapter 2.

Yet another experiment by Maner et al. (2005) used film clips to arouse either the emotion of fear (need for self-protection) or sexual interest. Then white college students were shown portraits of 16 black and white males and females, some of whom were more attractive than others. The students were told that the people in the pictures were trying to conceal their emotional state and that the students' task was to decide what emotion was being covered up. For each portrait, students rated the degree to which the target was sexually aroused, angry, frightened, or happy.

Students' reactions showed that when fear had been aroused, they were more likely to perceive anger in the faces of the black males but not in the other target faces. Also male students who had been sexually aroused were more likely to perceive sexual arousal in the faces of the attractive white females. In both cases the perception of the other three emotions was unaffected by the arousal condition, similar to the findings of Schimel et al. (2003).

An additional and important finding of this study was that even when no arousal condition was used, students with a preexisting concern about self-protection were more likely to perceive anger in the black male portraits, and students with a preexisting attitude of engaging in unrestricted sex were more likely to perceive sexual arousal in the attractive white female pictures. In this latter case, the experimental arousal served to enhance an already existing phenomenon: that is, the underlying motives or attitudes of individuals will influence their perception of selected targets when there is some "fit" between the perceived emotion and the target.

It should be noted that the experimentally aroused sexual motive was directly projected onto the target, who was seen as sexually aroused. However, the experimentally aroused fear resulted in the perception of a different emotion—anger—in the target. This latter result does not illustrate projection in the strict sense of that defense, but it is clearly a related phenomenon. The authors refer to this attribution of emotions that are different from but still related to one's own emotions and expectations as "functional projection."

Finally, using bogus personality test feedback, it has been demonstrated that such a threat to self-esteem increases the use of defense mechanisms (Grzegolowska-Klarkowska & Zolnierczyk, 1988, 1990). In addition, when the personality traits that were erroneously reported were more central to the individuals' representation of themselves, there was a greater increase in the use of defense mechanisms, as compared to a threat to traits that were more peripheral.

All of the studies discussed above demonstrate how external stress, whether in the form of criticism, intellectual challenge, feedback that conflicts with biological gender, sexual orientation, or threats to self-concept, result in an increased use of defenses. It is assumed that such stress increases anxiety, and that anxiety prompts the use of defenses. We do have the participants' self-reports in some of the studies that the stress experience increased their negative affect. It would be nice, of course, to have some independent assessment that would demonstrate that an increase in internal anxiety actually occurred, following the stress experience, and that it was linked to the increased use of defenses. In fact, such a mediating link was demonstrated earlier in the study of children who differed in social status (Sandstrom & Cramer, 2003a; see Chapter 3). For the nonaccepted children, self-reported stress was the mediating link between the experience of rejection and the use of defenses.

PHYSIOLOGICAL CONCOMITANTS OF DEFENSE USE

A more forceful demonstration that defense use is linked to change in internal states that was brought on by external stress comes from a study of young adults (Cramer, 2003a). In this study the participants were exposed to a series of stressful mental challenges; then they told stories in response to six TAT pictures. During both procedures, their blood pressure and skin conductance were monitored. Subsequently, the stories were coded for defense use and the resulting scores were related to the two autonomic nervous system measures, both of which are known to be related to stress and anxiety.[1]

The use of autonomic nervous system measures to assess stress has the advantage of measuring a response system that is not normally under the conscious control of the individual, and so may be free of possible self-report biases. This feature suggests that autonomic reactions might be related to another type of stress response that is out of the conscious control of the individual: the defense mechanism. According to theory, psychological stress will activate the use of defense mechanisms; the greater the stress, the greater the need for defense. Because stress also activates the autonomic nervous system, an increased use of defenses should be related to heightened physiological arousal. The use of defenses then protects the individual from the conscious experience of anxiety, although arousal on the physiological level continues. Indeed, in an early paper Alexander (1939) used this formulation to explain certain psychosomatic illnesses—namely, that defenses against the expression of negative emotions could be a cause of physical illness. More recently, work by Pennebaker, Barger, and Tiebout (1989) has supported a similar thesis. Thus demonstrating a clear relation between stress-induced autonomic reactivity and the use of defenses would provide further support for the theoretical assumption that increased stress results in an increase in the use of defenses.

In this study (Cramer, 2003a),[2] after each participant was attached to psychophysiological recording equipment, he or she spent 10 minutes relaxing and then a baseline measure of diastolic blood pressure (DBP) and skin conductance level (SCL) were taken. Next the participant was given three stressful tasks. The first required him or her to count backwards by 13s from 609 for a 1-minute period, with pressure for speed and accuracy. The second task required the participant to rapidly complete sentence stems with emotionally evocative themes of sexuality, aggression, or dependency (Shedler, Karliner, & Katz, 2003). The third task required the participant to devise stories in response to TAT pictures. Performance of these three tasks was accompanied by increased autonomic nervous system reactivity, as compared to the resting baseline, indicating that the tasks were indeed stressful.

The fact that participants were being assessed for defense use from their TAT stories at the same time that they were being stressed made it possible to relate the magnitude of the autonomic nervous system stress response to the level of defense use. In general, it was expected that greater physiological arousal would be related to more defense use. Further, two specific predictions were made based on previous research showing that DBP increases when cognitive work is required, whereas SCL increases when emotional inhibition is required (e.g., Assor, Aronoff, & Messe, 1986; Dozier & Kobak, 1992; Gray, 1975; Lacey, 1967; Obrist, 1981; Pennebaker & Chew, 1985). On this basis, an increase in DBP was predicted to be related to greater use of the defense of identification, which is cognitively the most complex and thus requires the most cognitive work of the three defenses studied. Second, an increase in SCL was predicted to be related to an increase in the use of denial, which functions to inhibit the recognition of troublesome thoughts or emotions. No specific predictions regarding the use of projection were formulated.

The results generally confirmed the predictions. Not only were defense mechanisms related to autonomic reactivity, but different defenses were found to be associated with different patterns of autonomic response. A strong increase in DBP was associated with a greater use of identification. In contrast, high use of projection was associated with a lower DBP level, suggesting that the externalization of thought and emotion reduces the internal cognitive workload. The relation between SCL and defense use was more complex. Although increased SCL was positively related to high use of denial, it was also related to low use of identification. Of the two defenses, low identification was the more powerful predictor of SCL. Overall, however, this study clearly demonstrated that the use of defense mechanisms was significantly related to internal physiological changes that come about when a person is stressed.

Notably, this study also demonstrated that *pre*stress DBP and SCL were not related to subsequent defense use. A similar result was found by

Blaess (1998); prestress DMM defenses were not related to stress-induced SCL. The joint results indicate that the relation between DMM defense use and SCL occurs only during the time that individuals are experiencing stress. Because both defense and SCL are aroused in response to stress, it makes sense that it is under stress conditions that a relation between the two reactions is found.

A different experimental intervention was used by Tang (2002) to investigate the relations among emotional arousal, defense use, and SCL. In this study the arousal method involved presenting explicitly sexual images to the women participants and did not require any work or activity on their part. Rather, they sat quietly and viewed the images. The study also included a control group who were presented with neutral images. All participants told TAT stories both prior to, and after, viewing the images; these stories were coded for defense use with the DMM.

The results showed that watching the sexual images was emotionally arousing, as seen both in the women's self-report and in an increased SCL. Prior to viewing the images, the sexual image group had lower total defense scores, as compared to the control group; after viewing the sexual images, they increased their use of defenses and had higher defense scores than the control group. This change (interaction) was statistically significant. An interesting concomitant of this result was that for women in the sexual image group, the greater their use of defenses after viewing the images, the *less* the self-report of anxiety. As in the lightning strike study (Dollinger & Cramer, 1990) and the anger/dishonesty projection study (Schimel et al., 2003), this finding indicates that defense use does decrease the subjective experience of psychological upset. Also the results again demonstrated a correlation between autonomic reactivity and the use of defenses. For women in the sexual image group, there was a correlation between the use of (DMM) projection and SCL. Taken together, these findings suggest that anxiety increases autonomic nervous system reactivity, which in turn prompts the use of a defense, which is then followed by a reduction in experienced anxiety.

The connection between projection and SCL was not found in the Cramer (2003a) study. This difference may reflect the fact that only females participated in the sexual image study. Additionally, it may be a function of the different tasks involved in the two studies. In the stress task study, participants were required to actively produce solutions to challenging tasks, and defenses were assessed concurrently. In the image study, participants passively viewed the images, and defense reaction was assessed after the viewing was completed.

A further study of young-adult participants (Shedler et al., 2003) focused on the relation between coronary reactivity and defensiveness, as assessed from responses to sentence stems. Here it was found that persons with higher coronary reactivity were characterized by "illusory mental health"—that is, they self-reported that they had no psychological difficulties, whereas other test results indicated that there were problems. Further, those with illusory mental health were more defensive on the sentence stems, thus demonstrating again the connection between stress, increased autonomic nervous system reactivity, and defense use.

The studies reported above focused on demonstrating that when stress increases autonomic nervous system reactivity, there is an increase in the use of defense mechanisms. They did not, however, demonstrate a relationship between defense use and level of autonomic nervous functioning under everyday, nonstress conditions. Such a relation might be expected, based on the belief that psychophysiological symptoms are associated with emotional maladjustment (e.g., Alexander, 1939).

A large-scale population study of 667 participants from the Nova Scotia Health Survey investigated the relation between resting blood pressure (DBP and systolic blood pressure; SBP) and defenses, based on the Q-sort profile of the Adaptive Defense Profile (ADP) (see Chapter 16) (MacGregor, Davidson, Barksdale, Black, & MacLean, 2003). Blood pressure was assessed twice during a home visit and twice during a clinical visit. In each case the reading was taken after a 10-minute rest period and prior to any interview procedure, so that BP would not be affected by current stress. When this nonstress BP was related to nonstress maturity of defense use, the results indicated that more mature defense use was associated with lower SBP for all age and sex groups. However, DBP was related to defense use only among older women (mean age = 68 years); for this group mature defense use was related to lower DBP. Younger women and men of all ages did not show a relation between defense use and resting DBP. These findings are consistent with those of the Cramer (2003a) study, in which resting DBP was not related to defense use; all of the participants in that study, males and females, were young adults, age 23.

Another investigation studied the relation between defense use assessed between ages 20 and 47 and hypertension (SBP, DBP) at age 70 in a group of men who had been followed since graduation from Harvard College (Vaillant & Gerber, 1996). Consistent with other findings, there was no relation between this earlier defense use, assessed under nonstress conditions, and subsequent nonstress hypertension level.

"REAL-LIFE" STRESS AND DEFENSE USE

The studies described above used experimental paradigms that were explicitly designed to increase stress. The role of defenses in "real-life" stress has also been investigated (Ungerer, Waters, Barnett, & Dolby, 1997). On the assumption that the arrival of a new baby will place considerable stress on a husband–wife relationship, the marital satisfaction of couples was assessed before and after the birth of a baby. The participants in this study were selected on the basis of their defense use prior to the baby's birth, such that they represented the lower, middle, and upper third of DSQ-36 mature and immature defense scores. The findings indicated clear relations between defense use and subsequent ability to navigate the transition to parenthood. For fathers, those who relied on immature defenses reported more marital dissatisfaction at 4 weeks and 12 months after the baby was born. For mothers, the same relationship was found, but only at 12 months, suggesting that mothers' marital satisfaction shortly after birth was based on factors other than their defense mechanisms, but that these became increasingly important as the time from birth lengthened.

There were some gender differences in the *specific* defenses that predicted poorer marital adjustments. For men, who are often characterized as less emotionally expressive and more likely to downplay emotions than women, the defenses of denial and rationalization predicted negative change when comparing pre- and postbaby satisfaction. For women, defenses involving passivity, isolation, and negative self-evaluation were the significant predictors of marital dissatisfaction.

Interestingly, in contrast to the role of other personality variables, including trait anxiety and locus of control, hierarchical regression analyses indicated that the defense measures were the only variables to significantly predict *change* in marital satisfaction. Generally, the earlier assessment of immature defenses predicted negative change—that is, poorer marital adjustment—after the baby was born. Moreover, in contrast to some other studies, the individual measures of defenses, such as projection, passive–aggression, denial, and acting out, were better predictors of level of adjustment than were the summary scales (e.g., Immature).

Another study relating real-life stress to defense use was carried out with women who had been sexually abused as children (Romans et al., 1999). In this study women (mean age = 46 years) from the community who reported having been sexually abused as a child ($n = 171$) were contrasted with those reporting no sexual abuse ($n = 179$). A comparison of these two groups indicated that the abuse group had higher scores on projection, displacement, passive–aggression, and autistic fantasy defenses; they also scored higher on the DSQ Immature defense scale. Those women who had experienced chronic abuse (abuse occurring more than 10 times) also scored lower on the DSQ Maturity scale, as compared to the no-abuse women. The abuse group was then subdivided into three groups on the basis of increasing severity of sexual abuse: (1) nongenital (touching breasts/buttocks), (2) genital touching without penetration, and (3) intercourse. Although the three DSQ factor scales (Immature, Neurotic, and Mature) were not related to severity of abuse (or to nonsexual physical abuse in childhood), there was a linear relation between severity and the use of four *individual* defenses: displacement, passive–aggression, somatization, and projection. The strongest link was found between severity of abuse and projection.

One other study related defense use, as assessed by the DSQ, to everyday life stress, based on the self-report of Daily Hassles (Kanner, Coyne, & Schafer, 1981; cited in Flannery & Perry, 1990). Using two different versions of the DSQ (DSQ-67 and DSQ-88), the reported life stress of adult college students (mean age = 31 years) was found to be positively correlated with the use of immature defenses.

CONCLUDING REMARKS

In this chapter we have seen further evidence supporting the second theoretical premise of defense mechanism theory: that the use of defenses will increase under conditions of stress. The introduction of a stressful intervention was shown to increase the use of defenses in 10 different experimental studies. As we saw with children in Chapter 6, it was age-appropriate defenses that increased in these studies with college students. Furthermore, challenge to these late adolescents' identity was especially associated with an increased use of the defense of identification. Also, as with children, it was demonstrated with college students that having awareness of the use of a defense rendered it ineffective.

We have also seen that stress-activated functioning of the autonomic nervous system is accompanied by an increase in defense use. These relations are complex and may be summarized as follows: Prestress physiological reactivity (diastolic blood pressure; skin conductance level) is unrelated to defense use during stress, and prestress defense use is unrelated to physiological reactivity during stress. However, physiological reactivity during stress is clearly related to defense use during stress, and there is some evidence that this defense use is associated with a decrease in self-reported anxiety. Under stress conditions, as well, different physiological measures of autonomic nervous system reactivity appear to relate to different defense mechanisms. Further, under nonstress conditions, one measure of cardiac reactivity (systolic blood pressure) was found to be related to immaturity of defense use. The interesting question that remains is whether, when stress occurs, the activation of defenses precedes, or is subsequent to, physiological reactivity. That is, does defense arousal prompt a physiological reaction, or does physiological arousal prompt the activation of a defense mechanism?

In real-life stressful situations the use of immature defenses is related to encountering more stressful situations. Again, the sequence of events is difficult to determine: Does the use of immature defenses increase the likelihood of encountering such situations, or does facing a greater number of stressful situations result in the use of immature defenses? The prospective study of marital reaction to the birth of a baby makes it clear that couples who used immature defenses prior to the birth were more likely to experience marital dissatisfaction 1 year later—that is, the use of immature defenses predicted subsequent maladjustment. In later chapters (10 and 13) I present further evidence that level of defense use predicts subsequent psychological functioning as long as 25 years later.

CHAPTER 8

Defenses and Personality

If asked to define personality, psychologists will respond in different ways. However, whether we conceive of personality in terms of traits, such as extraversion, openness, or agreeableness, or in terms of mechanisms of ego functioning, such as resiliency, control, or self-monitoring, or whether we think in terms of developmental maturity, such as levels of ego organization, stages of identity development, or stages of moral development—there are theoretical reasons to expect that defense mechanisms will influence, and be influenced by, these personality characteristics.

What kinds of connections might we expect to find between defense use and other aspects of personality? Consider first the defense of denial, an immature defense in the sense that it is cognitively simple and is characteristic of young children. When adults rely on denial, we might expect to find other indications of personality immaturity as well as signs of benign misperception or misinterpretation of life experiences. In contrast, reliance on projection might be expected to contribute to a worldview that is uneasy, with a focus on self-protection. Because projection is a defense especially predominant in adolescence, we might expect that an adult who relies on projection may be still involved in some of the issues that are characteristic of adolescents, such as concern about how one is perceived, hypersensitivity, and avoidance of those who are "different" (i.e., not in one's own clique); projection might also be expected to be related to strivings to separate from parents as part of adolescent identity development. Identification, the most mature of the three defenses, would be expected to be associated with other aspects of personality that demonstrate maturity and a well-functioning personality. Also, in that identification contributes to identity

161

development (Erikson, 1968), a meaningful relation between the two processes might be expected.

DEFENSES AND NARROW-BAND
PERSONALITY VARIABLES

I begin by describing the relation between defense use and a number of different personality characteristics in a sample of 90 young adults (age 23) who had been part of a longitudinal study beginning at age 3. I refer to this as the young-adult sample (Block & Block, 1980).[1] At age 23 the DMM was used to asses their use of defenses. In addition, experienced personality and clinical psychologists rated their personality and cognitive and emotional functioning using the 100-item California Adult Q-sort (CAQ; Block, 1971). Let us consider first what was found for the young adults in this age range who relied on the defense of denial (DMM).[2] The young men and women who relied on denial were found to be behaviorally unstable, unpredictable, unconventional, and rebellious. Further, their behavior was characterized as self-centered and narcissistic, and their thinking lacked clarity. Denial was also found to be positively associated with anxiety in both men and women.

This relation between denial and immature functioning has also been found in a sample of college students (Hibbard & Porcerelli, 1998). In this group use of the Pollyannish components of denial (DMM) were related to difficulties in interaction with others. This relationship of denial to interpersonal difficulties and to a dismissing attitude toward personal relationships was also found in a study of women by Hibbard et al. (2000). These findings are all consistent with the expectation that the use of denial by young adults occurs in conjunction with a personality that is characterized by immaturity.

Turning now to the relation between the use of projection and concomitant associations in personality, we again consider the findings from the young adults (Block & Block, 1980). In this group the defense of projection was the predominant defense style at age 23 and was related to a number of behavioral and personality characteristics. As is discussed in Chapter 9, there were marked differences between young men and women in the relation between projection and personality. These findings are briefly summarized in the following paragraphs.

Extensive use of projection by men was related to an interpersonal wariness, hypersensitivity, and mistrust. Additionally, measures of both anxiety and depression were correlated with men's use of projection, although regression analyses indicated that their use of projection was primarily associated with anxiety rather than with depression. In contrast, the use of projection by the young women in this sample was indicative of quite a different picture. Perhaps the most striking finding here was that, for these women, the use of projection tended to be related to adaptive behaviors. These women were described as cheerful, expressive, and socially skilled. Further, the use of projection by women was negatively related to depression. In a different sample of men and women college students, the use of projection was found to be a predictor of narcissism (Hibbard & Porcerelli, 1998), a finding also reported in a study of Asian women (Hibbard et al., 2000).

Finally, we consider the relation between the use of identification and personality in the young-adult sample. The first striking finding was that, for males, the use of identification was unrelated to CAQ personality descriptors and to ratings of anxiety and depression. However, men who used identification were found to be lacking in self-esteem and to have low ego control. For the women in the sample, there were significant relations between use of identification and personality. As is discussed in Chapter 9, women who used identification were described as socially competent and less depressed than those who use little identification.

These findings were repeated in a separate study (Hibbard et al., 2000). Women who used more identification had positive relationships with others, a secure attachment style, and reported more positive affect. Thus women who rely on the more mature defense of identification—that is, women who have moved along the developmental continuum of defense use—tend to show other indications of maturity and adjustment. In a further study of first-year college students, identification on the DMM was positively related to narcissism (Narcissism Personality Inventory [NPI]; Cramer, 1995), a result also found with Asian women (as measured by the O'Brien Multiphasic Narcissism Inventory [OMNI]; Hibbard et al., 2000).

The assumption that the use of immature defenses would be accompanied by other indications of personality immaturity, whereas mature defenses would be found in connection with indications of healthy adjustment, is also supported by studies using alternate methods of defense assessment. For example, the relation between defense use and narrowband personality variables has also been studied using the Mature and Immature scales of the DSQ-36 (Whitty, 2003). In a sample of individuals ranging in age from 17 to 70 years ($n = 120$), the Mature defense scale correlated positively with self-reported internal locus of control and higher self-esteem, whereas the Immature scale correlated with self-reported external locus of control and lower self-esteem. Self-esteem was also found to be positively related to the DSQ-40 Mature defense scale and negatively related to the Neurotic and Immature scales in a group of women ($n = 354$, mean age = 46 years), half of whom had been sexually abused as children (Romans et al., 1999).

A further study with the DSQ-40 (n = 128) related defense use to several other self-report personality dimensions (Mulder, Joyce, Sellman, Sullivan, & Cloninger, 1996). The Immature defense scale was associated with low scores on the personality dimensions of self-directedness and cooperativeness. The Neurotic defense scale was associated with low scores on self-directedness and novelty seeking. The Mature defense scale was associated with the ability to accept uncertainty and global identification.

Mature defense use assessed by the Adaptive Defense Profile (ADP) has also been found to be related to positive personality characteristics (Davidson, MacGregor, Johnson, Woody, & Chaplin, 2004). College students (n = 133) with higher scores on the ADP (more mature defenses) received higher observer ratings for empathy and competence and lower scores for self-rated hostility. In a second, large population sample (n = 667), higher ADP scores again were related to higher observer-rated competence and to lower scores on the hostility scale. Higher ADP scores in this sample were also found to be positively related to self-reported optimism (MacGregor, Davidson, Rowan, Barksdale, & MacLean, 2003).

DEFENSES AND THE BIG FIVE PERSONALITY FACTORS

Thus far we have been considering the relations between defense use and a variety of "narrow-band" personality characteristics. Extensive research has shown that many personality variables may be subsumed within five broad factors (John & Srivastava, 1999; McCrae & Costa, 1999): Neuroticism, Extraversion, Agreeableness, Openness, and Conscientiousness. These factors can be assessed in several ways, including ratings by others and self-report. To the extent that the five factors represent important and stable aspects of personality, we might expect to find a relation with the use of defenses.

Two studies have investigated the relations between the Big Five factors of personality and the use of defense mechanisms. One of these (Cramer, 2003b) studied 155 men and women from the San Francisco Bay Area. This group of adults had participated in a longitudinal study begun in 1928–1932 at the Institute of Human Development, University of California, Berkeley.[3] I refer to this as the early-adult sample. The defenses of early-adult participants were assessed when they were approximately 30 years old. Adult Q-sort-based scales were used to measure the five personality factors; defenses were assessed using the DMM. The first finding with this adult group is noteworthy because it contradicts the assumption and the findings that the use of denial will be associated with indications of personality immaturity. Although this group did use the defense of denial, and at a level comparable to late-adolescent or young-adult groups, their use of denial at age 30 was not related to any of the of the Big Five traits of Neuroticism, Extraversion, Openness, Agreeableness, and Conscientiousness. One possible interpretation of this finding—that denial is unrelated to personality traits in early adulthood—is that the defense has become unimportant for adult personality functioning. This possibility seems unlikely, however, given that, as is discussed in Chapter 10, at the subsequent ages of 45 and 60 years,[4] both very high and very low use of denial at early adulthood by these same individuals was significantly related to four of the Big Five traits. Apparently, personality functioning is increasingly influenced by denial as adults grow older.

In contrast to denial, both projection and identification were related to Big Five personality traits in the 30-year-old group. Projection predicted low Agreeableness (men) and low Conscientiousness (women). Projection was also curvilinearly related to Extraversion; both very high and very low use of projection predicted high Extraversion. Also, for higher IQ males (mean = 135), the use of projection predicted higher Neuroticism.

The relation of identification to Big Five traits was entirely determined by IQ level. For individuals with lower IQs (male mean = 113; female mean = 109), the use of identification predicted higher Extraversion. Similarly, identification in concert with lower IQ predicted greater Agreeableness (women) and greater Conscientiousness (men). In general, then, the importance of identification for predicting adult personality is moderated by IQ level. Identification appears to play a compensatory role in individuals with lower IQs, fostering more positive personality outcomes. This issue of the relation between defense use and IQ is discussed further in a later section of this chapter and again in Chapter 10. The issue of gender as a moderator of the relation between defenses and personality variables is discussed in Chapter 9.

Another study of defense and Big Five traits was based on outpatients who were participating in group therapy (Soldz, Budman, Demby, & Merry, 1995). The Big Five factors were assessed by using scales based on the patients' self-ratings of 50 bipolar adjective scales. Using the DSQ-88, three factor scores (Immature, Mature, and Withdrawal[5]) from this group of participants were used to assess defense use. The results showed that Immature defense scale scores predicted low Agreeableness, low Conscientiousness, and high Neuroticism, whereas Mature defense scale scores predicted Extraversion, Openness, and low Neuroticism.[6] The Withdrawal scale scores predicted low Extraversion and low Openness.

The findings of these two studies showing the relation between defense use and Big Five personality factors are not difficult to understand. Immature defenses, including projection, are associated with disagreeableness: A person who expects others to act hostilely or to harbor various negative characteristics is likely to behave in an unpleasant way toward people in general (low Agreeableness). Similarly, a person who attributes responsibility to others (i.e., externalizes blame) is likely to exhibit less responsibility for his own actions (low Conscientiousness). Finally, a person who projects hostility and responsibility is likely to show evidence of psychological maladjustment (high Neuroticism).

An alternative to the Big Five set of personality variables was developed by researchers at the Institute of Human Development, University of California, Berkeley (Haan et al., 1986). Based on factor analyses of the Q-sort items across multiple age groups, six higher-order factors were identified that characterized personality dimensions. At age 30, these six dimensions were found to be correlated with DMM defenses. Those who relied on projection were assessed as being both Outgoing and Undependable; those who relied on identification were seen to be Self-Confident, Cognitively Committed, and Outgoing (Cramer & Tracy, 2005).

DEFENSES (DMM) AND IDENTITY DEVELOPMENT

We turn now to a consideration of the relation between defense use and another aspect of personality: the process of identity development. The interest in identity and its development in adolescence was fostered by Erik Erikson's (1968) seminal writings that described how an adolescent moves from a state of uncertainty and confusion about personal identity that includes values, goals, sexuality, and future career (termed *diffusion*), through a period of searching and trying out alternatives (termed *moratorium*), to finally reaching an *achieved* identity based on previous exploration of options and eventual commitment to a personally chosen way of life. In some cases an alternative route to commitment may be followed, in which the adolescent moves from diffusion directly to commitment, without spending time or effort to explore available alternatives. Such a foreclosed identity is constructed by adopting the values, interests, and goals of someone else—generally a parent or other authoritative figure or, occasionally, some charismatic leader or cult group. These four identity states were differentiated by Marcia (1966) in terms of their standing on two dimensions: exploration (sometimes referred to as "crisis") and commitment. The diffused identity is characterized by little or no involvement in exploration, although some attempts may be made sporadically, and by low or absent commitment. The moratorium identity is in the midst of exploration but has not made a commitment. The foreclosed identity has made a commitment but has not engaged in exploration. Only the achieved identity has both engaged in exploration in the past, and made a commitment, based on that exploration.

The relation between identity status and defense use was studied in the group of young adults from the San Francisco Bay Area (Cramer, 1997a). Their standing on the four identity statuses was determined from observers' Q-sort ratings.[7] These four identity scores were then related to DMM defense scores.

Previous research studies have shown that a number of distinctive personality characteristics are associated with each identity status. One consistent personality finding for the different identity statuses is based on the relation between crisis and anxiety. Persons in the identity status experiencing the most crisis (moratorium) are found to be the most anxious, whereas those who have never experienced crisis (foreclosed) are reported to be the least anxious. One way in which anxiety may be controlled is through the use of defense mechanisms (A. Freud, 1936). Identification, a defense mechanism especially characteristic of late adolescence, also contributes to the development of identity. As quoted earlier, Erikson wrote, "Identity formation, finally, begins where the usefulness of identification ends" (1968, p. 159). Projection is also typically used by adolescents, and denial has been found to show a small increase in use during late adolescence (see Figures 2.1 and 2.2, p. 27). Because it has been shown experimentally that the use of age-related defenses increases when self-esteem decreases (Cramer, 1991b, 1998a; Cramer & Gaul, 1988), we might expect both the diffused and moratorium identity to be associated with increased defense use. From this viewpoint, adolescents who are experiencing the crisis associated with the process of identity development (moratorium and diffused) will have greater need for the use of defense mechanisms in order to control the anxiety and low self-esteem associated with that crisis. On the other hand, persons in the identity statuses for whom self-esteem is high and anxiety is low (achieved and foreclosed) will have little need for the use of defenses.

To test the hypothesis that defense mechanisms will be used more by individuals at the moratorium and diffusion levels of identity development, DMM defense scores were correlated with scores representing the four identity statuses. As predicted, there was a significant positive relation for moratorium with the use of both denial and projection and for diffusion with the use of denial. The picture was rather different for the two identity statuses without crisis present. The achieved identity status was unrelated to the use of defenses, whereas the foreclosed status showed a significant *negative* correlation with the use of denial and projection (see Figure 8.1).

Further study of the relation between identity status and defense mechanisms in the group of young adults suggested the existence of a transitional condition between moratorium and achieved identity. The use of identification was most evident in those individuals who were moving from moratorium to achieved identity—a finding that is consistent with Erikson's statement that the process of achieving identity is significantly contributed to by the defense of identification. In contrast, maintaining the moratorium

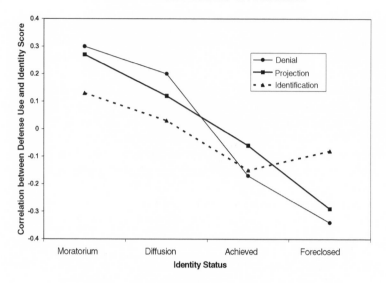

FIGURE 8.1. Identity status and defense mechanisms.

identity (and a transitional diffusion–moratorium identity) in young adulthood was associated with the less mature defenses of denial and projection but not with identification.

The present findings also go beyond demonstrating an overall relationship between identity status and defenses to provide information about the personality characteristics that define the identity statuses, as these relate to defense use. Two personality characteristics are associated with defense use in all four identity personalities. The first of these—having a clear, consistent personality—is a defining characteristic of the achieved and foreclosed identities; the absence of this characteristic defines the moratorium and diffused identities. Significantly, the presence of this characteristic is associated with low use of defenses. The second characteristic—being unpredictable and changeable—is a defining characteristic of the moratorium and diffused identities; presence of this characteristic is associated with high use of defenses.

These findings are also relevant for the issue of the relation between personality immaturity and defense use. The finding that the immature defense of denial was associated with diffusion in these young adults suggested that individuals who remain in the earliest state of identity development in young adulthood are developmentally less mature in other areas of personality as well. For the diffused status, the use of denial and projection was related to the presence of personality features associated with immaturity and instability, and to the absence of personality features associated with psychological maturity. For example, defense use in this group was associated with uncontrolled, lax behavior and the *absence* of incisiveness, dependability, predictability, self-enhancement, productivity, as well as the *absence* of interpersonal generosity, availability and warmth.

On the other hand, in the moratorium identity, defense use was associated more with rebelliousness than with immaturity. Thus personality characteristics such as noncompliance, deviousness, and fluctuating moods were related to defense use, as was the absence of conservativism, conformity, conventionality, overcontrol, moralism, and self-satisfaction. Overall, the most striking finding and best summary of the relationship between identity status and the use of defense mechanisms is to note that the use of defenses is a linear function of the degree of crisis associated with an identity status[8] (see Figure 8.1).

The study just discussed was based on a group of 23-year-olds for whom the achieved identity status was most characteristic. A further study of the role of defense mechanisms in identity development in a younger group produced highly similar results and provided the opportunity to discover how identity development and *change* were related to defense use (Cramer, 1995, 1998b). A large group of students were enlisted into a study of identity just as they entered college. In many ways this age group is ideal for studying the relation between developing identity and the use of defense mechanisms. Late adolescence, and especially entry into college, is a period of life in which the adolescent is separating from parents, old friends, and others who have provided psychological support for many years and been a source of self-esteem. The need to separate from early relationships is increased as part of healthy development, but this need also creates a situation in which the adolescent loses these sources of self-esteem. The loss of parent-based support is then replaced by forming new attachments to people who will provide similar support as well as by a self-generated narcissism in which the adolescent turns the admiration and idealization once focused on the parents back onto the self (Blos, 1962). Nevertheless, the process of separating from parents and moving toward a separate identity is difficult. Questions of "Who am I?" and "Who will I become?" remain unanswered for some time and may contribute to anxious uncertainty during this period of searching for an identity. When self-directed narcissism fails to quell anxiety, the use of defense mechanisms may increase.

To study the interrelations among identity status, narcissism, and defense use at the moment that adolescents were first entering college, students were recruited to participate in an assessment of their identity status during their "freshman days"; they also completed an assessment of their use of defense mechanisms (DMM) and of narcissism (NPI). As a first step, the current identity status of each student was determined. Most students were at the moratorium stage of identity development, with a sizeable group also in the diffusion stage. A smaller number was characterized as having a foreclosed or achieved identity.

When identity status was related to defense use, the findings were consistent with the young-adult study. For students in the moratorium and diffusion groups, the anxiety associated with these statuses resulted in stronger use of all three defenses: denial, projection, and identification. At the same time, narcissism in these students was quite low.

For those adolescents whose identity status indicated a commitment to goals and values—that is, those in the foreclosed and achieved identities—there was a strong reliance on narcissism to protect self-esteem. Importantly for the foreclosed identity, this narcissism was defensive in nature and included feelings of entitlement and exploitativeness. Anxiety was generally low in this group, resulting in low use of defenses. In contrast, the students with achieved identity were characterized by adaptive narcissism based on realistic pride and self-confidence. This latter group had less reason to feel anxious and made little use of defenses.

Overall, this study demonstrated that late adolescents, who are in the process of identity development, rely on two different psychological processes to maintain self-esteem during these stressful years. For those in the earlier, anxiety-filled statuses of diffusion and moratorium, defense mechanisms are brought into play to protect the self. For those who have made a commitment and are no longer anxious, positive self-regard is supported through narcissism—defensive narcissism in the case of the foreclosed identity, adaptive narcissism for the achieved identity. In other words, there is a reciprocal relationship between the use of ego defenses for maintaining self-esteem, on the one hand, and the presence of narcissism on the other.

However, in studies based on developmental hypotheses, it is difficult to make conclusive judgments about developmental processes from a single assessment of functioning. In the case of identity studies, we assume that adolescents in the achieved status have moved further along the developmental pathway of identity development than those in the moratorium status. Based on the study just described, we further assume that this movement is associated with a shift in the defense mechanism/narcissism balance. However, a much more convincing demonstration of this developmental process would be to follow the same individuals over a period of time and show that actual persons change in the way hypothesized on the basis of the single-occasion assessment. These thoughts suggested that a follow-up study would be informative. I predicted that if the use of defenses by moratorium and diffused students occurs in response to the heightened anxiety of these statuses, then for those students who subsequently advance to the achieved status where anxiety is low, there should be a decrease in defense use because anxiety associated with identity uncertainty should have decreased. At the same time, I hypothesized that those students who moved from noncommitted to the achieved identity status would show an increase in adaptive narcissism but not in defensive narcissism. These predictions were tested 3 years later when these students became members of the senior class (Cramer, 1998b).

Although a quarter of the original sample of students was unavailable for follow-up, 75% did participate in the second study. An initial check indicated that there were no differences in personality variables between the participants who continued in the study from freshman to senior year and those who did not continue.

Each senior class student completed the same set of personality assessment measures that they had completed on entry to college. A comparison of their scores over the 3-year period indicated that a significant number had moved from the moratorium to the achieved status. As before, the use of defenses was greater for those in the diffused and moratorium statuses, but the difference with the committed statuses was significant only for projection. Regarding the main hypotheses, the results showed that, indeed, students who had moved from moratorium to achieved status now had lower DMM defense scores than students who remained in the moratorium status.[9] Further, an increase in scores for achieved identity was related to an increase in narcissism, especially in adaptive narcissism. These findings are striking: I was able to successfully predict the relations among changes in identity, defense use, and narcissism over a 3-year period. In turn, the study points to the importance of defense mechanisms for understanding identity development. Further evidence of the role of defense mechanisms for identity change in adulthood is discussed in Chapter 10 (see pp. 216–217) (Cramer, 2004).

Thus far we have considered the role of defense mechanisms in identity development. Clearly, there are other important factors that contribute to this development. One of these is the parent–adolescent relationship. As described by Erikson (1968), the development of identity is influenced in important ways by identifications with significant others. This point suggests that identification contributes to identity in two ways. One way is the developmental process of identification that begins early in life, when the child begins to imitate parents' gestures and speech. This process continues as the child mimics the adults' activities through fantasy play and the adolescent adopts certain parental interests and values. This developmental process of identification, of which the adolescent may be aware, differs from the second way the defense of identification contributes to identity development. In contrast to the developmental process of identification, the defense of identification involves a process that occurs outside of awareness and functions to reduce anxiety and protect self-esteem.

It is thus of interest to consider the degree to which each of these types of identification contribute to identity development. In the work described so far, we have considered identification only as a defense. In a subsequent study, we also considered the contribution of developmental identification and the possibility that the interaction of the two types of identification might contribute to identity development. The clearest description of the findings is to note that both the DMM defense of identification and identification with parents, as well as their interaction, differentially predicted the four identity statuses. However, the nature of these relationships differed for males and females. The specific findings, as determined by gender, are discussed in Chapter 9.

Although the issue of identity is generally considered to be important for the late-adolescent period, identity and defense use have also been studied during adulthood (Cramer, 2004), where we find that the relation between identity status and defense use is different, and is moderated by IQ to a significant degree. In an investigation based on the early adults of the Berkeley longitudinal study, DMM defense use at age 30 was correlated with identity status at that time. The results indicted that none of the three defenses, individually, was significantly related to identity status. However, the interaction between the defense of identification and IQ was a significant predictor of identity status. At lower levels of IQ, identification was positively related to both the achieved and the foreclosed identity status. At higher levels of IQ, identification was a negative predictor of both identity statuses. Thus the defense of identification appears to play a compensatory role for individuals with lower IQs, fostering their development of a committed identity.

OTHER APPROACHES TO THE INVESTIGATION OF IDENTITY AND DEFENSES

A different way of looking at identity is to consider the role that an individual plays within her nuclear family. The children's Role Inventory (Potter & Williams, 1991) has been used to assess four different family roles: *hero* (appeasing and helping other family members); *mascot* (expression of repressed emotions of others in the family; may include being the family clown); *lost child* (avoidance of interaction with family members); and *scapegoat* (opposition to family norms and parental expectations). Although all of these roles are considered to be dysfunctional, interfering with the development of individual identity, only the hero role ($n = 179$) was found to be significantly related to defense use. Based on the four-factor version of the DSQ-88, the "adaptive" level defense scale was positively correlated with the hero role ($r = .28$) (Randolph, Anderson, Smith, & Shipley-Clark, 2003). The mascot role was also correlated with the adaptive defense level ($r = .22$), but a smaller number of individuals in this category ($n = 41$) prevented statistical significance. The lost child role was related to both the maladaptive action level ($r = .35$) and image-distorting level ($r = .20$) of defense, but again the small number of college students falling into this category ($n = 9$) prevented these correlations from being statistically significant. Overall, the results are consistent with the point of view that a more adaptive identity—in this case, the hero role—is associated with more mature defense use, whereas a less adaptive identity—in this case, the lost child role—is associated with immature defenses.

Two studies have investigated the relation between defense mechanisms and racial identity (Nghe & Mahalik, 2001). African American college students ($n = 30$) were assessed for their developmental level of racial identity, using the Black Racial Identity Attitudes Scale (Helms, 1984). This Likert-scale questionnaire provides a score on five black racial identities considered to represent increasingly mature statuses. The "preencounter" status, associated with devaluing black people and culture and seeing whites as superior, is considered relatively immature. The "encounter" status is characterized by confusion and anger in response to strong negative experiences with white people or positive experiences with African Americans. The "immersion" status involves a rejection of earlier identity statuses, immersion in African American culture, rejection of white people and institutions, with anger at both whites and preencounter blacks. Two more sophisticated identity statuses may follow. The "emersion" status involves moving to a more positive, internalized worldview that includes exploration of African culture and self and a positive sense of unity with other African Americans. The final status, "internalization," is characterized by a rejection of racism, an ability to establish relationships with white associates when this is merited, and an ability to consider white culture for both its strengths and weaknesses (Helms, 1990).

Scores on these racial identity statuses were related to defense scores on the DSQ-40 and on the DMI. Canonical correlation analyses indicated that preencounter and encounter identities were positively associated with the Neurotic DSQ scale, the DMI-PRN and REV, and negatively associated with DMI-projection and TAO. A second canonical root showed that the immersion status was associated with the DSQ Immature defense scale, whereas the emersion status was positively associated with the DSQ Mature scale. Overall, the findings suggest that a more mature racial identity status is associated with the use of more mature defenses.

In the second study the use of DMM defense mechanisms was studied in Asian ($n = 69$) and white ($n = 83$) women (Hibbard et al., 2000). Defense use was related to a measure of acculturation (the Asian Self-Identity Acculturation Scale: Suinn, Acuna, & Khoo, 1992) and to several criterion measures expected to be related to defenses on theoretical or empirical grounds. The results demonstrated an interesting relation for the Asian women between acculturation to American society and the DMM defense of identification. The greater the acculturation (i.e., loss of Asian identity), the lower the identification score. In addition, acculturation was positively correlated with projection (DMM) for Asian women. Importantly, although white women scored higher on denial (DMM), the DMM was found to be equally valid for the two ethnic groups. In fact, the predicted correlations between DMM defense scores and the criterion variables, including attachment style, narcissism, positive affect and interpersonal behavior, were actually stronger for the Asian women.

DEFENSES AND EGO DEVELOPMENT

In keeping with our expectation that the use of immature defenses will be related to other indications of personality immaturity, we turn now to a study in which defense use was related to level of ego development. As described by Loevinger (1976), an important function of the ego is to control impulse expression; the manner in which this is accomplished is a feature that defines the level of ego development. Given that one of the functions of defense mechanisms is to modulate impulse expression, we would expect to find a relation between ego level and defense use.[10]

To describe the nature of the relation between ego development and impulse control and the relevance of this relation for the use of defense mechanisms, Loevinger's stages of ego development may be divided into three groups based on the dimension of impulse control. The first group includes the impulsive and self-protective stages[11]; here there is minimal conscious control of impulses; anxiety around the expression of these impulses takes the form of feared consequences ("objective anxiety," A. Freud, 1936). Thinking is simplistic and organized around dichotomies: good/bad, yes/no. For adults who remain at these early stages, troubles are located outside of the self and blame is externalized (Cohn, 1991; Loevinger, 1976). The simplistic thought processes involved suggest that low-level defense mechanisms would predominate. Denial, a defense that is based on dichotomous thinking in which a negative marker (*no, not*) is attached to an anxiety-arousing perception[12] in order to turn it into something less threatening, should be typical. In the self-protective stage, in which negative affect is externalized onto others, followed by mistrust of others (Loevinger, 1976), projection also should be characteristic.

The second group includes the conformist and self-aware levels. The conformist stage of ego development signals a major change in the control of impulses. In this stage there is a conscious recognition of the need to control impulses, although the source of this control is seen as external to the self: Social norms control behavior. The advent of this conscious control, based on external sanctions, replaces the need for unconscious mechanisms of control—that is, for defense mechanisms. The self-aware level is a transition period. Conscious control of impulses based on external rules continues, replacing the need for defense mechanism use. From the perspective of impulse control, the transition involved here is from conscious control based on external rules to conscious control based on internal dictates. Rules are internalized but not yet fully integrated into the ego.

The third group includes the conscientious, individualistic, and autonomous stages. With the beginning of the conscientious stage, the conscious control of impulses is based on internalized standards of conduct. Impulse control is maintained through conscience, but conscience is still closely tied to external sanctions and moral realism. This stage is followed by the individualistic level; internal control of impulses continues, but the moralism of the preceding stage is replaced with a conscious awareness of inner conflict. To the extent that this conflict can be tolerated, there is little need for defense use; to the extent that awareness of conflict creates anxiety, defenses may be called into play. Finally, at the autonomous stage, there is a capacity to acknowledge and consciously cope with conflict, "rather than ignoring it or projecting it onto the environment" (Loevinger, 1976, p. 23). At this stage, the role of lower-level defense mechanisms, such as denial and projection, should be minimal.

This analysis suggests that the relationship between defenses and ego level may be curvilinear, an idea supported by evidence that the relation between impulse control and ego level is curvilinear, not linear (e.g., Starrett, 1983; Lorr & Manning, 1978). When impulse control is weakest and impulsivity greatest, as at the lowest impulsive and self-protective ego levels, then the need for defense mechanisms use will be greatest. However, when the ability for conscious control and delay of impulse expression is greatest, as at the conformist and self-aware levels, then the need for defense mechanisms is least. At the highest ego levels, when impulse control has become less rigid, the need for defenses may increase somewhat. In other words, the relation between defense mechanisms and ego level should be the inverse of that between impulse control and ego level—that is, U-shaped.

At this point becomes necessary to consider a further ego function that may be important for understanding how defenses function in adulthood to influence personality. It may be that some personality characteristics are influenced by an interaction between defenses and IQ. For example, we have considered evidence that the defense of denial is related to immaturity in an adult; one reason a person may be immature is that he has limited intellectual resources—that is, a lower IQ. In this case the defense of denial may be a developmental match for the IQ level and may facilitate adaptation appropriate to this person's level of functioning. Put another way, if the IQ is insufficient to promote successful adaptation, defenses may play a needed compensatory role.

This possibility was investigated by considering both defense mechanisms and IQ as possible predictors of ego level. In the sample of young adults (age 23) from the Bay Area (Block & Block, 1980), ego level was assessed using the Sentence Completion Test (SCT; Loevinger & Hy, 1970), a frequently used, reliable measure of Loevinger's concept of ego level. Both the Wechsler Adult Intelligence Scale—Revised (WAIS-R) IQ and DMM defense mechanism use were related to ego levels. In this sample, IQ and defense mechanisms were not correlated.

The results indicated that the lowest levels of ego development (preconformist), in which impulse control is lacking, were related to use of the lower level defenses of denial and projection and to lower levels of IQ. These findings are consistent with Loevinger's description of these ego levels as characterized by simplistic, dichotomous thinking and the externalization of blame. Because previous research has shown that impulse control and the ability to delay gratification are weak at these levels (Westenberg & Block, 1993), whereas impulsivity is high (Roznafsky, 1981; Starrett, 1983), I interpret the present findings to indicate that, at the preconformist levels of ego development, the lower-level defense mechanisms function to protect the individual from experiencing the affect, or anxiety, associated with the presence of uncontrolled impulses.

In contrast, beginning with the conformist level of ego development, the use of denial and projection were negatively related to ego level, and IQ was unrelated. Again, the findings are consistent with Loevinger's description of the conformist and self-aware levels, in which impulses are controlled through conscious adherence to external rules and social norms; the findings are also consistent with previous research that reported a decrease in impulsivity at these stages (Roznafsky, 1981; Westenberg & Block, 1993). If impulses are successfully controlled from without, there is no need for defenses. Behavior that is based on the adherence to rules rather than rational evaluation is reflected in the absence of a relation between ego level and IQ. Overall, it appears that the importance of external control at these levels supersedes the role of internal ego functions of defense and intelligence in managing impulse expression.

However, beginning at the conscientious level, external sources of impulse control are internalized to form an inner conscience, reducing the importance of external controls. The findings show that at this ego level, the function of intelligence becomes more important and the role of defenses less important. Again, these findings fit with theory. At the conscientious level and higher, cognitive functioning becomes increasingly complex: The ability to deal with uncertainties increases and the capacity for self-evaluation develops. The appearance of such higher forms of thinking would be expected to be related to level of intelligence. At the same time, the progressive freeing of impulses from the rigid controls of conscience is accompanied by some increase in defense use.

The curvilinear relation between defense use and ego level described above can be seen in Table 8.1. Each of the three defenses demonstrates increased use at both the lower and higher levels of ego development, with less use in the middle levels (conformist, self-aware, conscientious). A test of this curvilinear relation (quadratic trend) was significant for denial and projection and borderline significant for identification. In contrast, the relation between ego level and IQ is linear.

The relation between defenses and ego level is made more complex when we consider the interaction of intelligence with defenses. Using multiple regression analyses, *high* levels of ego development were associated either with high intelligence and low use of denial, or, alternatively, with low intelligence and high use of denial. In contrast, *low* levels of ego development were associated with high intelligence and high use of denial or

TABLE 8.1. Means (and Standard Deviations) of Defense and IQ Scores by Ego Level

	Defense[a]			
Ego level	Denial	Projection	Identification	WAIS-R[b]
Impulsive + self-protective (n = 7)	7.43 (5.44)	14.71 (5.99)	5.43 (2.99)	110.57 (18.81)
Conformist (n = 8)	3.50 (2.20)	7.00 (3.82)	5.38 (2.77)	103.88 (12.81)
Self-awareness (n = 33)	5.52 (5.11)	8.45 (4.11)	4.70 (3.00)	114.81 (14.31)
Conscientious (n = 32)	4.62 (3.25)	11.25 (8.84)	3.97 (2.36)	118.81 (10.89)
Individualistic + autonomous (n = 9)	8.44 (4.64)	12.77 (8.08)	6.44 (3.00)	114.78 (9.54)
Trend analysis				
Linear	.46	.01	.10	4.57*
Quadratic	6.62**	6.27**	2.97†	.36

Note. From Cramer (1999c); reprinted with permission from the *Journal of Personality.*
[a] df = 1 and 84; [b] df = 1 and 82.
†$p < .10$; *$p < .05$; **$p < .01$.

with low intelligence and low use of denial. At average levels of IQ, denial was unrelated to ego development.

The interaction of intelligence and projection in relation to ego level produced a somewhat different picture. Here ego level was predicted primarily by IQ. However, within the low IQ range, strong use of projection was associated with higher ego levels. In contrast, at high IQ levels, both low and high use of projection was associated with lower ego levels,[13] whereas moderate use of projection was associated with higher ego levels.

These interesting interactions between defense and IQ in predicting ego level may be understood by considering the "fit" between defense and intellectual level. The results of the study show that denial, a low-level defense, is related to higher ego development at low levels of IQ but not at mid and high levels of IQ. Developmentally, this pattern makes sense. Denial is a defense that "fits" with lower levels of intellectual development. Owing to their lesser cognitive capacities, young children do not "see through" the defense of denial (see Chapter 2). Lesser cognitive capacities allow this defense to function effectively and to protect children from excessive negative affect. The continued use of an age-inappropriate defense such as denial at higher mental ages, however, is unlikely to be successful and would be expected to interfere with ego development, as found in this study. At lower mental ages, however, the continued use of denial is developmentally more appropriate and contributes to ego development. In a similar way, low IQ may be compensated by the use of the more mature defense of projection, which then supports ego development.[14]

In sum, this study demonstrated that IQ and defenses were related to level of ego development. Whereas intelligence was related to ego development in a linear manner, the relation between ego level and defense was found to be curvilinear. This curvilinear relation was consistent with the theoretical description of the locus of impulse control that characterizes each ego level: Ego stages characterized by low internal impulse control showed stronger defense use; ego stages characterized by external control of impulses showed the least use of defenses; and ego stages characterized by internal control showed a moderate use of defenses. The explanation for this last, seemingly inconsistent, result is found in the interactive effects of defense and IQ in predicting ego level; defenses are used at high ego levels in relation to low IQ.

The relation between defense use (DMM) and ego level has also been demonstrated for children. In a study of grade schoolers (grades 4–6; $n = 94$), those who were using the more mature defense of identification were at a higher level of Loevinger's ego development ($p < .01$) (Avery, 1985). Although not statistically significant, those who relied on denial were found to be at a lower level of ego development.

The relation between ego level and defense use has also been demonstrated using the DSQ-88 to assess defenses (Bond, 1992). The defense scores of a group of 200 patients and nonpatients were related to their ego development scores on Loevinger's (1976) Sentence Completion Test. Consistent with the DMM study just reported, use of "immature" defenses ("maladaptive action" defenses) was found to be associated with low levels of ego development, as were "image-distorting" and "self-sacrificing" defenses. However, the "Adaptive" defense scale was positively related to ego level. This finding differed from the DMM results in which there was no clear-cut relation between identification and ego level. Likely, this disparity reflects the difference in defenses that constitute the DSQ Adaptive scale (Suppression, Sublimation, and Humor). Also important, this study did not take IQ into account when assessing the relation between defense use and ego level.

DEFENSES AND IQ

In three studies reported above, we have seen that IQ is a moderator of the predictive power of defense mechanisms. These findings raise the larger question of the relation between IQ and defense mechanisms. Information on this question may be gleaned from several studies in which both variables were assessed.

Overall, the findings indicate that IQ and defense use are unrelated in children and adolescents. In a study that assessed the use of denial and projection (DMM) by 122 grade-school children (ages 6–11), there was virtually no relation with IQ ($rs = -.03$ and .01) (Cramer & Brilliant, 2001). A study of early adolescents (ages 13–14) found that defense maturity, based on Haan's Q-sort defense measure (Haan, 1977), did not correlate with IQ; for late adolescents (ages 16–18), the relation was marginal ($p < .08$) (Hart & Chmiel, 1992). Also, as described previously, there was no relation between IQ and DMM defense use in the sample of 23-year-old young adults (Cramer, 1999c). However, IQ was a significant moderating variable in the relation between defense and ego level.

Among older adults there is some evidence that IQ and defense use are related. For the 155 adults from the Institute of Human Development intergenerational study, defense use in early adulthood (ages 30 and 37) was significantly related to IQ in middle adulthood (ages 40 and 47) (Cramer, 2003b, 2004). Specifically, all three of the DMM defenses (denial, projection, and identification) were significantly correlated with WAIS IQ (Wechsler, 1955). More important, in this sample, IQ was found to be a significant moderator of the predictive relations between defenses and identity status (Cramer, 2004) and between defense use and Big Five personality factors (Cramer, 2003b), as discussed previously. Similarly, in a sample of hospitalized adults, IQ was found to moderate the relation between DMM defense use and symptom change following treatment (Cramer, 2005; see Chapter 13).

An additional study of community participants (n = 99; mean age = 34 years) who were recruited from ads placed in local media also demonstrated some relation between DMM defense use and IQ, as estimated from the Vocabulary subtest of the WAIS-R (Blaess, 1998). In this study Vocabulary IQ was significantly related to the use of identification (p < .01), but there was no relation with denial, and the correlation with projection, although positive, was not significant. However, in Vaillant's (1993) studies, there was no significant relation between IQ and his composite measure of defense maturity in samples of adult men and women.[15]

CONCLUDING REMARKS

The assumption that the use of immature defense mechanisms is related to other indications of personality immaturity is well supported by the research literature. Whether we look at narrow-band personality characteristics such as narcissism, optimism, or empathy, or more broad-band dispositions such as the Big Five factors, the evidence is consistent in showing that the use of immature defenses is related to less favorable personality characteristics. In contrast, the use of mature defenses is found to be related to the presence of favorable aspects of personality. These findings are consistent across different measures of personality and different methods of assessing defense use.

The relation between level of ego development and defense use is especially interesting given that defenses, in theory, are an ego function. My research shows that just as impulse control is related to ego level in a curvilinear fashion, so is defense use. At immature ego levels, defense use is strong; at higher ego levels, where external control predominates, defense use is low (i.e., not needed to control impulse expression). At the most mature levels of ego development there is some increase in defense use, but, significantly, the degree depends on IQ level. For individuals with lower IQs, strong defense use appears to support their attainment of higher ego levels, whereas the reverse is true for individuals with higher IQs. More specifically, for individuals with low IQs, the use of either a mental-age-appropriate defense (denial) or a chronologically characteristic defense (projection) is positively related to level of ego development. However, for individuals with higher IQs, the use of a developmentally inappropriate defense (denial) is related to low levels of ego development, and deviation from the group norm in magnitude of projection, in either direction, is associated with lower levels of ego development.

Defense use has also been found to be related to identity. In general, more mature levels of identity, whether psychosocial, racial, or familial, are related to the use of more mature defenses. The most immature identity statuses—diffusion and moratorium—are associated with strong defense use, presumably related to the high level of anxiety and low self-esteem that characterize these identity statuses. In contrast, individuals in the foreclosed and achieved statuses, who are not anxious and have high self-esteem and thus have less need for defenses, show less defense use. This shift in defense use as a function of identity development was demonstrated by following a sizeable group of students from the beginning to the end of the undergraduate college years.

The relation of defense use to identity development in somewhat older individuals is found to depend on IQ. For early adults (age 30), reaching the more mature, committed identity statuses (achieved, foreclosed) was predicted by the interaction between the defense of identification and IQ. The combination of lower IQ and strong use of the defense of identification supported an achieved or foreclosed identity, whereas the reverse was true for individuals with higher IQs. As with ego development, identity development in individuals with lower IQs is enhanced by the use of defenses.

Curiously, most current studies of personality overlook IQ as an important variable to be included in the investigation. If IQ is included, it is used to match groups, thus controlling for, or eliminating, possible effects related to IQ. Yet the assessment of intelligence and the development of the IQ measure represent the earliest success by psychologists to measure complex psychological functioning, and the IQ measure continues to be the best standardized procedure among our battery of assessment procedures. Moreover, an assessment of IQ as part of the diagnostic battery is considered important by clinicians of varying theoretical positions, and the concept of IQ is more familiar to the general public than are many of our other clinical constructs.

The studies that have included IQ bring to the fore two important issues for understanding defense mechanisms. First is the finding that IQ is unrelated to defense use earlier in life (childhood, adolescent, and to some extent, in young adults) but may be related for older adults. Although this finding may indicate that intelligence and defenses develop on two separate, unrelated tracks during childhood, it may also be due to the adjustment of IQ measures for chronological age. That is, it might be that measures of mental age during childhood, rather than IQ, would show a relation with defense use, in the manner that would be expected from a developmental point of view: namely, that lower mental age would be associated with the use of immature defenses such as denial, and higher mental age with mature defenses such as identification. However, when children with the same mental age but different chronological ages are collapsed into one group, their IQs will differ. A given mental age for an 8-year-old will yield a different IQ than the same mental age for a 10-year-old, and thus a possible relation between intelligence and defense use will be obscured.

The second point is that, when assessing the relation between defense use and personality in adults, it is important to determine whether IQ moderates the effect of defense. Failure to account for possible differences in defense effect at different levels of IQ may lead to a false conclusion that defense is unrelated to personality factors. The role of IQ as a moderator in the relation between defense mechanisms and personality change is discussed further in Chapter 10.

CHAPTER 9

Gender Differences and Defenses[1]

Up to this point, we have considered defenses and personality without much regard for gender. However, an obvious question is whether males and females use the same or different defenses. In my previous book (Cramer, 1991a), I reviewed clear evidence that defense use differs by biological sex. However, more recent investigations are not always so clear on this question. Reasons for this disparity might include the use of different defense measures, social change, or the role of previously unconsidered moderating factors.

In addition to the possibility that males and females might differ in the particular defenses that they employ, it is also possible that using the *same* defense may have different gender implications. Certainly this is true for other aspects of personality. A man who is assertive, forthright, and demanding may be seen as a strong leader, whereas women who demonstrate the same characteristics may be characterized as "bitchy" (Fiske & Stevens (1993).

Curiously, the theoretical literature on defense mechanisms has ignored, by and large, the idea that gender differences in personality might result in gender differences in defense use. Defense mechanism theory has also failed to consider the possibility that the employment of defenses may have different consequences for the two genders. These omissions are true both for classical psychoanalytic theory (e.g., A. Freud, 1936; Fenichel, 1945) as well as for contemporary treatises (e.g., Cooper, 1998; Cramer, 1991a; Vaillant, 1976, 1993).

In this chapter, I consider three questions:

1. Do males and females (children and adults) differ in their use of defense mechanisms?
2. Does the relation of specific defenses to other personality variables differ for males and females?
3. If defense use is found to differ for males and females, is this difference a function of biological sex, or is there some other explanation?

To examine these three questions, I draw on studies in which defense use is assessed from the DMM, the DSQ, the DMRS, and, where especially relevant, from the DMI.

Among the psychoanalytic theories that investigate the general question of gender differences and personality, there are aspects that are relevant to the issue of gender and defense. For example, both Freud (1932) and Deutsch (1944) theorized that female sexual identity included a component of turning aggression inward, from which we might predict that females would be likely to use defenses such as turning against the self (TAS). Also, both Deutsch (1944) and Erikson (1964) emphasized that women's sexual identity is based on a proclivity to focus attention toward their internal world, whereas men's sexual identity involves an outward orientation. Extrapolating from these theoretical positions would suggest that females rely more on defenses that modify inner thoughts and feelings (such as denial, reversal, or reaction formation), even if this usage results in falsifying external perception, and on defenses that direct aggression inward (such as TAS). In contrast, males would depend more on defenses that locate conflict in the external world (such as projection or turning against the object [TAO]), even if this usage means falsely attributing inner motivations to that external world. In this chapter I examine empirical research relevant to these theoretical positions.

THE "MASCULINE" DEFENSES

The results from a large number of studies show that, when defense use is assessed by semistructured projective techniques (e.g., the DMI), adult men consistently use projection and TAO more frequently than adult women (Cramer, 1991a).

When defense is assessed from TAT narratives (DMM), some findings support the predictions. In two studies of upper-level college students, projection was more frequent in males than females (Cramer, 1991b, 1998b). However, a longitudinal study of college students is informative. Although the males and females did not differ at freshman year in their use of projection (DMM; Cramer, 1995), continuing study of these same college students indicated that by the time they became seniors, they showed the typical pattern: Males scored higher on projection (DMM) than females (Cramer, 1998b). The gender difference was also found in the Berkeley community study of early adults[2] (age 30 years), in which men scored significantly higher on projection (DMM) than women. A similar result has been found with children and adolescents and is discussed later.

However, not all research using the DMM approach to assessing defenses has found gender differences in the use of projection. Among the young adults (age 23 years) of the Block and Block (1980) longitudinal study,[3] males and females did not differ significantly in their use of projection (Cramer & Block, 1998). Similarly, a study of college students (mean age = 20 years, range = 18–50 years) found no significant difference between males and females for the use of projection (DMM; Hibbard & Porcerelli, 1998).

THE "FEMININE" DEFENSES

From theory, we expect that inwardly directed defenses, such as TAS, or defenses that function by changing inner affect or perception, such as denial, will characterize females more than males. As with masculine defenses, the research results largely support these predictions.

Research with the DMI (or similar assessment methods) consistently demonstrates that females use more TAS, are more likely to employ reaction formation, and, in some studies, are more likely to use reversal (REV; which includes both reaction formation and denial). (See Cramer, 1991a, for a review of these studies.)

Defenses as assessed from TAT narratives (DMM) also follow the pattern suggested by gender-based predictions. Among upper-level college students, females typically use denial more than males (Cramer, 1991b, 1998b); as in the case of projection, this difference between males and females was not statistically significant during the first year in college. Among older individuals (young adults and early adults), the use of the immature defense of denial is infrequent for either gender. Where there is a gender difference, it is in the predicted direction.

The third DMM defense, identification, is not easily characterized as either masculine or feminine; thus we might not expect to find gender differences in the use of this defense. The research findings regarding gender differences in the frequency of use of identification are mostly consistent. In various samples of college students, both upper and lower levels, and in samples of adults from the general population, men and women have not shown any difference in the employment of identification (DMM). However, a sample of college students studied by Hibbard and Porcerelli (1998) did find females to have higher identification (DMM) scores.

Interestingly, the majority of studies using the DSQ with adults do not consider gender differences, perhaps because large-scale studies such as the one conducted by Andrews et al. (1993), using both the DSQ-40 and DSQ-72 in a normal, nonpatient sample, failed to find gender differences for defense factor scales or for individual defenses.[4] This sample included 388 individuals ages 12–75 years, approximately two-thirds of whom were female. In another large-scale study with the DSQ-40, gender differences in Canadian college students were found for only three defenses; men scored higher on suppression and isolation, whereas women had higher scores on pseudoaltruism (Watson & Sinha, 1998). Males also scored higher on both the Immature and the Mature factor scales. In a further study that included both psychiatric outpatients and controls, men were found to have higher scores on both the Immature and Mature factor scales of the DSQ-36 (Spinhoven & Kooiman, 1997).

GENDER DIFFERENCES IN CHILD AND ADOLESCENT DEFENSE USE

Although adult gender differences in defense use may be explained by socialization processes that vary for males and females, gender differences are also found for children and adolescents. Significantly, these dissimilarities in defense use are greater for *young* children than for older children, whereas we would expect to find the opposite result if continuing social pressures were entirely responsible for gender divergences.

DMM

Employing the narrative DMM approach, the use of projection is higher among boys than girls. The difference is statistically significant only among the youngest children (mean age = 5 years, 8 months), but boys consistently use projection more than girls across childhood and adolescence. In contrast, girls employ denial more than boys. This difference is statistically significant only at the youngest age, but girls continue to use more denial than boys throughout childhood and adolescence (Cramer, 1987; Cramer & Gaul, 1988). In two samples of elementary schoolchildren, girls were found to use more identification than boys (Cramer & Brilliant, 2001; Cramer & Gaul, 1988). A similar trend was found in a third study comparing adolescent females and males (Cramer, 1987).

DSQ

In contrast to studies of adults, adolescents show gender differences in their DSQ defense scores. A study of 187 high school students (average age 16 years) indicated that females reported greater use of regression, reaction formation, somatization, and altruism, whereas males reported greater use of suppression and repression (Feldman et al., 1996). The authors interpret these gender differences as related to existing sex-role stereotypes. For the girls, negative emotions are turned into positive reactions (reaction formation), and stress is dealt with by helping others (altruism) and by converting it into physical symptoms (somatization). For the boys, dealing with conflict through suppression and repression is seen as fitting with the male stereotype of being unemotional.

A large-scale study of approximately 1,500 Finnish adolescents, using the DSQ-72, also found gender differences in defense use (Poikolainen et al., 1995; Tuulio-Henriksson et al., 1997). Females were found to score higher on the Neurotic factor scale at both ages 16 and 21 years. There were no gender differences found for the Immature scale at either age. In the initial publication of this study (Poikolainen et al., 1995), 16-year-old males were reported to score higher on the Mature scale; in the subsequent report (Tuulio-Henriksson et al., 1997), no gender differences in Mature scale scores were reported for either age 16 or age 21 years.

In another large-scale ($n > 400$) study, this time of Dutch adolescents using the DSQ-40, females also reported greater use of the defenses comprising the Neurotic factor, whereas males reported greater use of those on the Mature factor (Muris, Winands & Horselenberg, 2003).

DMI

Using the DMI (or similar assessment procedures), both early and late adolescents (grades 9–10 and 11–12) show the typical gender-related pattern. Boys use TAO and projection more than girls, whereas girls rely on TAS more than boys (Cramer, 1979; Levit, 1991, 1993). In addition, Levit found that adolescent girls (ages 14–19 years) scored higher on principalization (includes intellectualization, rationalization, and isolation) than did boys. Gender differences may also vary within the age range of childhood and adolescence. For example, older adolescent girls employed REV more than the boys of that age (Cramer, 1979). Likewise, in first- and second-grades, girls used REV more often than boys; the same pattern was found in fourth and fifth graders, but was no longer significant (analysis of results reported in Cramer, 1983). Also among younger children, first- and second-grade boys used TAO significantly more often than girls; the same pattern was found in the fourth- and fifth-grades, but was no longer significant.

THE IMPLICATIONS OF DEFENSE USE: GENDER-BASED DIFFERENCES

Differences in the frequency of defense use by males and females have been demonstrated. At the same time, both genders use a variety of defenses, albeit to a greater or lesser degree. In this connection, we may ask whether the use of the same defense by males and females has the same implication for their psychosocial functioning. For example, if projection is typically associated with males, whereas denial is typically associated with females, what are the consequences for males who rely on denial or for females who rely on projection?

In this section of the chapter we consider gender-based differences in the relation between defense use and personality functioning, examining this relation first for denial, then for projection, and finally for identification, as assessed by the DMM. We investigate this question in two different age groups: college students from a variety of different locations, and the young-adult group of 23-year-olds from the San Francisco Bay Area. Gender-based differences in the relation between defenses and the personality traits for older individuals are discussed in Chapter 10.

Denial

Among college students, are there different implications for males and females who use denial? Under nonstress conditions, denial is used infrequently by college students. Thus, in several studies, it is not surprising that the use of the defense of denial (DMM) did not show gender differences in relation to other personality variables. Neither for male or female students were personality variables such as narcissism, ego control, ego resiliency, depression, and anxiety associated with denial (Cramer, 1995, 2002a).

However, the use of denial did have different gender implications in the experimental study in which students' self-esteem was threatened by critical remarks made by the experimenter (Cramer, 1991b; see Chapter 7). When they were queried after the experiment, the students who had been criticized reported that they had become angered by the experimenter's remarks. This increased anger was also seen in the content of their TAT stories. This content consisted of anger directed outward for some students; for others, the content indicated anger directed inward. This direction of anger expression was then related to the use of defenses. Significantly, gender differences were found in the relation of anger expression to denial. Males who used the feminine defense of denial were less likely to direct aggression outward, a relation not found for the females. Rather, after criticism, females who used denial were more likely to direct aggression inward. In these college students the use of denial was thus related to a more feminine mode of anger expression for females and a less masculine mode for males.

For this age group we also asked whether DMM defense scores were related to the students' stage of identity development, as provided from an independent measure (Mallory, 1989) created to assess Erikson's (1968) four stages of identity: diffusion, foreclosure, moratorium, and achieved. In addition, we determined whether their use of defenses was related to their identification with their parents. In both cases, the possibility that gender functioned as a moderating factor was tested (Cramer, 2001). To assess the degree of identification with either the same-sex parent or the opposite-sex parent, each of the 172 male and female students was first asked to describe his or her ideal self using a set of 70 adjectives pertaining to personality, values, morals, attitudes, and intellectual functioning. Subsequently, each student used the same 70 adjectives to describe his or her same-sex or opposite-sex parent. The degree of similarity in the rating of each adjective for ideal self and for parent was used as a measure of parent identification: The more similar the ideal self to the parent—that is, the more the student ideally wished to be like the parent—the stronger the identification with the parent. This measure of parent identification was then related to the students' use of defense mechanisms. The results indicated that the use of denial was not correlated with identity status, nor with identification with parents, for either males or females (Cramer, 2001). However, as discussed below, both projection and identification were related to these variables.

The DMM was also used to assess defense functioning in the slightly older, more diverse sample of young-adult males and females from the Block and Block (1980) study. In contrast to the college students, the use of denial by these young adults was related to a large number of narrow-band personality characteristics (Cramer, 2002a). As discussed in Chapter 8, men and women who relied on the immature defense of denial showed a high degree of similarity in the way in which they were described. They appeared to be inconsistent and unpredictable, with an unstable personality. They were also characterized as showing a weakness in cognitive functioning, engaging in what might be termed "fuzzy thinking," and being unable to "see to the heart" of important problems. These men and women also had a strong egotistical quality; they were self-centered, self-indulgent, and self-dramatizing. The women, however, were rated as having some positive features that were not characteristic of the men, including being interesting, expressive, and initiating humor. For both men and women denial was associated with anxiety.

These results are also relevant to an issue raised earlier: that is, whether the use of an age-inappropriate defense such as denial would be associated with other indications of psychological difficulties. The findings indicate that this is, indeed, the case: Males and females who relied upon denial were characterized by ego instability, inability to delay gratification, and self-centeredness. Although these heavy denial users had shown gender differences in behavior at age 3 (see Chapters 1 and 10), by age 23 they were described in remarkably similar terms. The main difference at age 23 appeared to be that this combination of behavioral characteristics was more favorably perceived when it occurred in women than when it occurred in men, suggesting the possibility that aspects of this behavioral style fit more readily with a female gender stereotype.

Projection

In contrast to the findings with denial, there were clear gender differences in the way that projection relates to personality variables. Projection tended to be positively connected with depression in the college men but not found in the women. Instead, in the freshmen women projection was related to the positive, adaptive aspects of narcissism, including authority, superiority, and self-sufficiency (Cramer, 1995). This positive connection between projection and adaptive narcissism continued into the senior year of college (Cramer, 1998b). Consistent with this result was the finding that, for females, the use of projection was negatively associated with a measure of ego overcontrol, indicating that the women who used projection were not overly rigid or "uptight" in their psychological functioning.

Differences in the implications of the use of projection were also found in the experimental study (described earlier) in which students were purposely angered (Cramer, 1991b). Prior to criticism, the use of projection by both males and females was positively correlated with the outward expression of anger. In addition, projection was positively related to anger directed inward for females only. However, after criticism, this pattern changed. Now, there was a tendency for projection to be correlated with aggression directed inward for males, whereas for females, projection was correlated only with aggression directed outward.

Gender differences in the implications of the use of projection were also found in another study of 100 college students (Hibbard & Porcerelli, 1998). For the 49 women of the study, projection (DMM) was positively related to the Anger scales of the Symptom Checklist–90—Revised (SCL-90-R; Derogatis, 1989). This relation was not found for the 52 men in the sample; for the men the use of projection was related to a measure of pathological narcissism (O'Brien Multiphasic Narcissism Inventory [OMNI]; O'Brien, 1988); this relation was not found for the women.

In the study of defense use and parent identification, there was an interesting tendency for projection to be positively associated with females' identification with their mothers but negatively associated with males' identification with their fathers (Cramer, 2001). However, for both genders, projection has been found to be positively related to the moratorium status and negatively related to the foreclosed status (Cramer, 1995, 2001).

Striking personality differences were associated with the use of projection by men and women in the study of young adults. Men who relied on projection were described by expert observers as having a wary, paranoid style of behavior, being distrustful of others, transferring blame to others, evaluating the motives of others, and tending to be guileful, manipulative, and hostile toward others (Cramer, 2002a). This behavioral description of the males shares many features with the clinical description of the paranoid personality disorder (American Psychiatric Association, 1994). Thus men who show some of the behavioral characteristics associated with a paranoid personality are those who also make use of the defense of projection—the defense that characterizes this diagnosis (Freud, 1911; Vaillant, 1994). They also appeared both anxious and depressed. Also, similar to the college students, men who used projection tended toward a pathologically narcissistic personality.

In contrast, the young-adult women who relied on projection were described quite differently (Cramer, 2002a). Perhaps the most striking finding here is that, for these women, projection was related to healthy adjustment and adaptive behaviors. The women were seen as lively, positive, and extraverted, and were rated as *not* showing the interpersonal wariness and mistrust shown by the men. They did not transfer blame to others and did not see themselves as victims of others. In contrast to the men, the use of projection by women was unrelated to anxiety. Further, women who used projection were less likely to be depressed.

Table 9.1 shows these striking gender differences in the relation between the use of projection and personality characteristics. The first column lists the characteristics that are positively associated with the use of projection, first for men, then for women. Then the characteristics that are negatively associated with projection for men and for women are listed. In each case the correlation for the other gender is given in the third column. The striking differences in the implication of the use of projection for men and women are easily seen.

Further analysis of the defense indicated that, for women, the adaptive behaviors related to projection were due one facet of the DMM projection measure—namely, the externalization of anger and other negative emotions, consistent with the findings from the anger-inducing experiment (Cramer, 1991b). In contrast, for the men it was the DMM facets of suspicion and distorted thinking that were responsible for the relation between projection and behavior, consistent with the observation from the young-adult study (Cramer, 2002a).

Another investigation using the DMM to study college students again

TABLE 9.1. CAQ Correlates of Projection for Men and Women

CAQ item

Positive correlates for men	Men	Women
Tries to stretch limits	.47***	.06
Is unpredictable in behavior, attitudes	.44**	.01
Unable to delay gratification	.43**	.08
Evaluates motivations of others	.38**	−.11
Basically distrustful of people	.33*	−.25
Tends to be rebellious, nonconforming	.33*	.12
Is subtly negativistic	.31*	−.26

Positive correlates for women	Women	Men
Is facially, gesturally expressive	.37**	−.12
Initiates humor	.37**	.04
Is a talkative individual	.32*	.12
Concerned with philosophical problems	.31*	−.05
Has a rapid personal tempo	.30*	−.02
Skilled in social techniques, play, humor	.28*	.04

Negative correlates for men	Men	Women
Sympathetic, considerate	−.55****	−.28*
Dependable, responsible	−.51***	−.03
Behaves in ethically consistent manner	−.45**	.01
Has a readiness to feel guilty	−.34*	−.08
Overcontrols needs, impulses	−.33*	−.07
Liked and accepted by people	−.30*	.18
Has giving way with others	−.29*	−.07
Favors conservative values	−.29*	−.10
Submissive; accepts domination	−.29*	−.05
Arouses nurturant feelings in others	−.29*	.07
Judges self and others in conventional terms	−.29*	−.07

Negative correlates for women	Women	Men
Is sensitive to criticism	−.38**	.21
Creates/exploits dependency in people	−.33*	−.17
Extrapunitive; transfers blame	−.33*	.28
Vulnerable to threat	−.31*	.09
Feels cheated, victimized by life	−.29*	.18

Note. Male n = 45; female n = 46. From Cramer (2002a); reprinted with permission from the *Journal of Personality*.
*p < .05; **p < .01; ***p < .001; ****p < .0001.

found a striking difference between males and females for the implications of using projection (DMM; Pickens, 2002). In general, there were positive relations between the Minnesota Multiphasic Personality Inventory–2 (MMPI-2) defensiveness scales and DMM Projection for the males but negative relations for the females. For example, males showed a positive relation between Projection and the MMPI-2 Malingering scale, whereas for females, Projection and the Malingering scale scores were negatively related. The implications of this gender difference in the use of projection is examined later.

Identification

Identification is a frequently used defense by college students, especially as they are entering college, and there are gender differences in the implications of their using this defense. From the anger-induction study I found that under neutral, noncriticized conditions, females who used identification were more likely to direct aggression inward, whereas males who used identification were more likely to direct aggression outward (Cramer, 1991b), consistent with the normative description of feminine and masculine identity.

The use of identification was positively correlated with scores on the Narcissism Personality Inventory (NPI; Raskin & Terry, 1988) for freshmen females (Cramer, 1995). This relation was partly due to high scores on the Authority and Superiority subscales, which are generally considered to be positive, adaptive aspects of narcissism. However, the use of identification by these females was also associated with the Exploitative and Exhibitionistic subscales—narcissistic features seen as defensive and maladaptive. These relations were not found for males, and they were no longer in evidence for the females when they were restudied during their senior year of college (Cramer, 1998b). At that point males evidenced a negative association between identification and narcissism scores that was largely due to those aspects of narcissism that involve domination or control of others (Cramer, 1998b). For college men identification also tended to be positively connected to ego resiliency and negatively connected to alienation—associations not found for the females (data from Cramer, 2001).

In the study of the defense of identification, parent identification, and identity (Cramer, 2001), the defense of identification predicted the closeness of the male students' identification with their fathers. Also, the defense of identification by itself was the strongest predictor of the achieved identity status for college men. However, for college women the defense of identification was unrelated to identification with either father or mother. Rather, there was a reciprocal relation between the defense of identification and father identification in predicting an achieved identity, and between the defense of identification and mother identification in predicting foreclosed identity. Either strong defense identification or strong parent identification, but not both, predicted the identity status. Further, same-sex parent identification in both males and females moderated the effect of the defense of identification in predicting diffusion. For both genders, the combination of low identification as a defense with a weak same-sex parent identification predicted high diffusion, whereas low identification as a defense with strong same-sex parent identification predicted low diffusion.

It is noteworthy that moratorium was not predicted by the defense of identification, parent identification, or the interaction between these two variables for either males or females. This failure of moratorium to show reliable relations with other personality variables has been found previously (Cramer, 2001) and most likely reflects the inconsistency and changeability of personality associated with this status.

Identification as a defense also had different implications for men and women in the young-adult group (Cramer, 2002a). Women who relied on identification were described quite positively and appeared to be socially competent. They communicated well, were sought out for their ideas, and were at ease with themselves and others. In addition, they were less likely to be depressed than women who used little identification. Overall, they appeared mature and well adjusted. In contrast, there were few clear personality correlates of identification for the men in this sample. However, different from the women, those men who did rely on identification were characterized as lacking self-esteem and having low ego control. This lack of relationship between identification and personality in the males was not due to a difference in the incidence of identification in the men and women, although both groups used this defense less often than is typically found in samples of college students. However, the result is consistent with previous studies that have found that other defenses involving internalization—an aspect of identification—are more important in the functioning of women than men (Cramer & Carter, 1978; Frank, McLaughlin, & Crusco, 1984).

SYNTHESIS

Gender Differences in Defense Use and the Implications of Defense Use

Ample evidence demonstrates gender differences in defense use that generally conform to predictions made on the basis of psychodynamic theory, with males using externalizing and females using internalizing defenses. Comparable results are found using three distinctive paradigms to assess defense use. The diversity of these three methods lends assurance that the results are not method specific. Because the differences between boys and girls are stronger in younger than in older children, socialization does not appear to provide an adequate explanation for gender differences in defense use.

Not only are there gender differences in the use of different defenses; the implications of using the same defense differs by gender. In this section, I attempt to synthesize these reported findings based on two different participant groups: the young adults from the general population of the San Francisco Bay Area, and the students from a small New England college.

The findings for denial as a defense may be summarized by three general points:

1. College students (both males or females) do not use denial often, and it generally is not associated with their personality characteristics.
2. Both young-adult men and women from the general population who rely on denial have immature, egotistical, and unstable personalities, although the women who employ denial are perceived more favorably than the men.
3. In the case of handling anger, the use of denial by college men and women has different implications: Men who employ the feminine defense of denial do not show the typical male pattern of directing anger outward, whereas women who use the feminine defense of denial do show the feminine pattern of directing anger inward in response to criticism.

There are striking gender differences in the implications of using the defense of projection. The use of projection by men is associated with depression and anxiety. These men tend to be distrustful, blaming of others, hostile, manipulative, and pathologically narcissistic. On the other hand, as seen in the late adolescents and continuing into young adulthood, females who use projection are characterized by healthy narcissism, lively sociability, and positive adjustment. Furthermore, females who employ projection are positively identified with their same-sex parent, whereas males who rely on projection are negatively identified with their same-sex parent. Notably, when males who rely on projection are criticized, they direct anger inward; this tendency likely explains the positive association for males between projection and depression in both the college and the young-adult groups. These relations are not found for females. When criticized, females who rely on projection direct their anger outward, and they are not depressed.

The use of identification also appears to have different implications for the way males and females perceive themselves, and for the way they are perceived by others. Late-adolescent females who rely on identification are also narcissistic, showing both the adaptive and defensive types of narcissism. This connection, however, no longer holds as these young women mature to their last year in college. By young adulthood, women who use identification are seen as socially competent, mature, and well adjusted. The picture is rather different for males. Among late-adolescent males, identification is positively related to ego resiliency and negatively related to alienation. As they mature, those males who use identification are low in narcissism, especially the type involving domination and control of others. As young adults they also lack ego control. In a society in which male domination is rewarded, it is likely these associations contribute to the finding that young adult men who rely on identification are also lacking in self-esteem. Finally, for both genders the defense of identification is differentially related to individuals' sex-typed handling of anger: Males who use identification direct anger outward, but females who use identification direct anger inward. Identification is related to reaching an achieved identity for both genders, as suggested by Erikson (1968). However, this process occurs somewhat differently for males and females. For males there is a direct positive relation between the defense of identification and achieved identity; there is also a direct relation between the defense of identification and identification with father. For females, however, the defense of identification is related to achieved identity *only if* the woman's identification with her father is weak; otherwise, the defense of identification is not related to her identification with either parent.

Does Biological Sex or Sex-Role Orientation Determine Defense Use?

Having demonstrated all these gender differences in defense use and shown how gender moderates the relation of the defenses to other personality characteristics, I turn now to a complicating factor for understanding these differences. In an early study of defense mechanisms (Cramer & Carter, 1978), we discovered that defense use was determined more by sex-role orientation than by biological gender. Evidence for the importance of sex-role orientation could also be found in other early studies. For example, both males *and* females who were independently determined to have a masculine orientation made strong use of the masculine defense of TAO. Likewise, the feminine defenses of TAS and REV were found to occur most frequently among persons with a feminine sexual orientation, whether they were biologically male or female (Cramer & Carter, 1978; Evans, 1982; Frank et al., 1984; Gleser & Ihilevich, 1969; Lobel & Winch, 1986). Again, it appears that sexual orientation, rather than biological gender, was the important factor in determining these gender differences. However, the masculine defense of projection was found to be associated with a masculine orientation in males but not in females. Here a masculine orientation in consort with biological gender, rather than sexual orientation alone, was the critical factor for the increased use of projection (see Cramer, 1991a, for a review of these studies).

More recent work has continued to show that sexual orientation, or issues associated with gender identity, are significant determinants of defense use. Using different defense measures, different research paradigms, and different subject groups, there has been a series of findings that is consistent with this assumption.

For example, in a study of adolescents ages 14–19 (Levit, 1991), biological gender initially was shown to predict defense use on the DMI. As in other studies, boys used projection (PRO) and TAO more than girls, and girls used TAS and principalization (PRN) more than boys. Further study, however, indicated that the masculinity and femininity scores of these students, determined from the Bem Sex Role Inventory (BSRI; Bem, 1974), were a stronger predictor of defense use *in every case* than was biological sex. Thus having a masculine orientation, regardless of biological sex, was a positive predictor of the use of projection and TAO and a negative predictor of TAS. In contrast, having a feminine orientation, regardless of biological sex, was a positive predictor of PRN and REV and a negative predictor of projection and TAO. The finding for REV was especially interesting; by itself, biological gender did not predict the use of this defense.

One of the findings from this study initially seemed to contradict the gender-orientation hypothesis: Although girls scored higher on TAS, the Femininity scale score did not predict TAS. A further analysis of the Femininity scale suggested that it could be divided into two subscales: Passive-Dependent and Communal. A subsequent analysis, including both males and females, indicated that whereas the Communal subscale did not relate to TAS, the Passive-Dependent subscale was positively related—that is, this aspect of feminine sexual orientation was found to predict defense use. Overall, then, as was found for adults, adolescent sex-role orientation moderated the relationship between biological sex and defense use.

Further study of the relation between defenses and sex-role orientation suggests that the conflict about gender role is responsible for increased defense use (Mahalik, Cournoyer, de Franc, Cherry, & Napolitano, 1998). Men are highly socialized to eschew behaviors such as emotional expressiveness and same-sex affection, which are stereotypically considered to be feminine and if manifest by men may be a source of shame and guilt. Consequently, men are seen to develop a rigid masculine gender role that revolves around demonstrating success, power, and competitiveness. However, it is assumed that maintaining this gender role creates conflict in which emotions and affection that naturally occur must be blocked or concealed, much in the same way that defense mechanisms block or conceal other unacceptable feelings or wishes. In particular, to the extent that this gender role conflict reflects a lack of psychological development—that is, an unthinking, unconsidered acceptance of social stereotypes without further exploration and evaluation—it would be expected to be related to defense immaturity.

This expectation was confirmed in a study of college students and of men from the community (mean age = 26 years). Here a measure of gender role conflict was found to be related to defense use, as assessed by both the DSQ and DMI (Mahalik et al., 1998). Strong conflict was positively related to the use of DSQ immature defenses (including projection), and to a lesser extent, DSQ neurotic defenses. On the DMI, gender role conflict was related to projection and TAO. These findings are consistent with the assumption that men who have a strong need to maintain a stereotyped gender role are especially likely to use the defense of projection to avoid experiencing internal conflict regarding this role. The findings are also consistent with those of the study discussed in Chapter 7, in which the men who were most highly sex-stereotyped used more defenses when told that they had a feminine orientation, as compared to low-stereotyped men who were given the same information. In other words, the most defensive men were those for whom the contrived experimental feedback was in conflict with their sex-role identity.

An interesting parallel to the findings that cross-gender sex-role orientation is related to defense use comes from studies of aggressive elementary schoolchildren. Although children who engage in either overt aggression or relational aggression are likely to exhibit hostile attribution biases—that is, project hostility onto others—those children who show cross-gender forms of aggression (relational aggression for boys, overt aggression for girls) are found to have significantly higher levels of psychological maladjustment than is found in children who engage in gender-normative forms of aggression. That is, it is the presence of cross-gendered behavior (aggression) that is related to maladjustment.

Equally striking, it is the gendered form of aggression rather than gender *per se* that is related to type of maladjustment. Those children who engage in overt aggression, whether male or female, exhibit externalizing psychological problems; those who engage in relational aggression exhibit both externalizing and internalizing problems (Crick, 1997). Because other research (reported in Chapter 6) has found that DMM and DSQ defense use is greater among children with internalizing and externalizing problems, it seems probable that children who engage in cross-gender forms of aggression would manifest greater use of defenses.

A theoretical expansion on the idea that sex-role conflict is related to defense use has been proposed by Brody, Mudderrisoglu, and Nakash-Eisikovits (2002). Beginning with the assumption that there is a relation between the use of a particular defense and the type of emotion being experienced, Brody et al. hypothesized that the nature of this relation will differ for men and women, since the socially acceptable expression of emotions differs for the two genders. For example, the expression of externalizing emotions such as anger or aggression is acceptable for men but not for women. In contrast, internalizing emotions, indicating vulnerability, are acceptable for women but not men. Although the relations among DSQ defenses, externalizing and internalizing emotions, and gender in a study of 118 college students were not exactly as hypothesized and depended, to some extent, on whether the emotions were appropriate or inappropriate,[5] there were clear gender differences (Brody et al., 2002). The use of immature defenses by women was related only to the experience of inappropriate *externalizing* emotions (e.g., contempt, disgust). However, men who reported using immature defenses were more likely to experience inappropriate *internalizing* emotions (e.g., guilt, shame) as well as externalizing emotions. Again, the findings are consistent with the hypothesis that it is sex-role *conflict*—here evidenced by the occurrence of cross-gender-type emotions—that is related to defense use.

In answer, then, to the third question raised at the beginning of this chapter, the research findings suggest that it is not gender *per se*, but rather gender orientation, that is the critical factor in determining defense use.

In thinking about these differences, it is also interesting to contrast the description of the women who use the masculine defense of projection with that of women who use the more typically feminine defense of TAS (e.g., Cramer & Carter, 1978, 1991a; Gleser & Ihilevich, 1969; Massong, Dickson, Ritzler, & Layne, 1982).[6] TAS is associated with self-blame, low self-esteem, maladjustment, symptom distress, and suicide attempts for both men and women (e.g., Frank et al., 1984; Ihilevich & Gleser, 1986; Scholz, 1973; Vaillant, 1983). As discussed earlier, TAS is also positively associated with a feminine sex-role orientation, especially with passive–dependence (Cramer & Carter, 1978; Evans, 1982; Frank et al., 1984; Gleser & Ihilevich, 1969; Levit, 1991; Lobel & Winch, 1986). However, projection is negatively associated with a feminine orientation (Levit, 1991).

As these studies indicate, females who direct negative affect inward are more prone to psychological difficulties, especially depression. Using a defense that directs negative affect inwardly is also associated with feminine sex-role adoption. Thus there is a stereotyped sex-role configuration consisting of TAS, femininity, and depression. This configuration may garner a degree of social approval in women, for the "feminine" defense of TAS is *positively* correlated with social desirability in *women*; however, it is *negatively* correlated for *men* (Evans, 1979; Richert & Ketterling, 1978; Wilson, 1982).

These research-based findings also suggest a corollary: Women who fail to direct negative affect *outward* are more subject to depression than women who do direct negative affect outward. Support for this corollary is seen in the results reported: Minimal use by women of the externally oriented defense of projection was associated with depression, sensitivity to criticism, vulnerability to threat, dependence, feeling victimized, and a tendency to withdraw when faced with difficulties. In contrast is the configuration in which projection—that is, the externalization of negative emotions—is used by females. This usage occurs in conjunction with lively sociability, communality, humor, and poise, and with the absence of vulnerability, passivity, and depressive symptoms. Thus women who use projection are less likely to experience psychological difficulties; they may also be perceived as less feminine.

The implications of these findings are relevant for considering gender differences in psychopathology. Lewis (1985) has discussed the question of why depression is more often found in women, whereas paranoia is more often found in men. She argued that because women are more concerned about maintaining interpersonal relationships, they are more likely to inhibit the overt expression of aggression. Nevertheless, aggressive feelings are likely to arise in the normal course of events; at that point cultural disapproval of the outward expression of aggression by females increases the sense of shame and self-blame—emotions to which women are hypothesized to be more prone, given their greater sensitivity to the opinions of others. Thus women who conform to this at least partly socially based stereotype will be at greater risk for becoming depressed. If this analysis is accurate, it implies that women who are able to maintain sociability without undue inhibition of aggression and without excessive concern for the approval of others will be less prone to depression. In the young-adult sample, these are the women who use projection.

For men, on the other hand, competitiveness and independence are emphasized over cooperation, and there is less social condemnation for aggressive acts. Men are also encouraged to be emotionally detached, objective, and impersonal. Further, they are expected to dominate, which increases the likelihood of aggressive behavior. Lewis hypothesizes that this combination of factors increases their level of chronic, unresolved guilt, and "the way is thus paved for the development of paranoia (1985, p. 150).

In my research (Cramer, 2002a) with a relatively small sample, I noted that men who used projection were described as antisocial and lacking in attachment to others, focused on satisfying individual desires and expressing hostility both directly and through self-serving indirect maneuvers. Such behavior may set the stage for guilt and for possible retaliation from others, which in turn would create anxiety and, in the extreme, paranoia (Lewis, 1985). Such antisocial behavior also would likely cut the man off from attachment to others, which in turn might contribute to depression.

Thus the characteristics hypothesized by Lewis to contribute to the association between maleness and paranoia are consistent with the results for men who rely on projection, the defense associated with paranoia. These findings expand on Lewis's (1985) explanation for the gender differences in paranoia and depression by adding an additional gender-related hypothesis: that the defense of projection may contribute to the presence of paranoia in males but to the absence of depression in females.

CONCLUDING REMARKS

At the beginning of this chapter, I raised three questions that we are now able to answer. Males and females, both children and adults, do differ in their use of defenses. Further, the use of the same defense has different implications and relates to different personality variables for men and women. These differences, as they pertain to the defenses of denial, projection, and identification, have been described in some detail.

The third question—how to explain gender differences in defense use—led to a consideration of the importance of sexual orientation, as compared to biological sex. There is evidence from several different research studies that gender identity, and especially *conflict* around gender identity, is a more significant determinant of defense use than is biological sex. Sociocultural expectations are seen as important explanatory factors for these gender-related differences.

CHAPTER 10

Studying Defenses over Time: Longitudinal Studies[1]

As discussed in Chapter 2, a few studies have compared groups of individuals who differ in age for their use of defenses. The difficulty for the interpretation of such cross-sectional studies is that there are often significant cohort differences that may impact defense use. For example, Vaillant has found that individuals with high IQs live longer (Vaillant & Vaillant, 1990), meaning that differences in defense use in old age are confounded with differences in IQ.

To make a meaningful assessment of how defenses *change* with age, or to reliably determine how defenses and behavior influence each other over the course of development, it is necessary to follow the same group of individuals over an extended period of time. Then there are several ways in which we may examine the longitudinal course of defense mechanisms. First, because we conceptualize defenses as developing during the earlier part of life, we might follow the same group of children, adolescents, or adults over time, looking for changes in the defenses that they use. Alternatively, because defenses are understood to emerge in the context of the child's ongoing life experiences, and because these experiences may influence defense use at that time, we might study how childhood personality and experience influence later defense use. For example, a child who has experienced unusual stress during the period of development at which denial is the normative defense will be likely to make strong use of that defense, which may then continue as an ingrained part of the personality into adulthood. As a third strategy, we could study how previously established defenses are related to the presence of subsequent personality traits. Or, as a fourth strategy, we might ask whether previous defense use predicts subsequent personality change. In this chapter I examine each of these four approaches to studying defenses over time.

CHANGE IN DEFENSE USE OVER TIME

In taking a developmental perspective toward understanding defense mechanisms, we would expect to find changes in defense use as the young child grows older. Although this idea is consistent with cross-sectional findings from children ranging in age from 5 years to late adolescence, in order to clearly demonstrate defense change we would need longitudinal studies of the same children over time.

As reported in Chapter 2, such a longitudinal study was carried out with children between the ages of 6 years, 6 months and 9 years, 5 months (Cramer, 1997b). As predicted, the assessment of DMM defenses showed that the children significantly decreased their use of denial between ages 6 years, 6 months and 7 years, 3 months, and significantly increased their use of projection between ages 8 years, 0 months and 8 years, 8 months.

A second longitudinal study with the DMM followed late-adolescent students from the time they entered college until their senior year (Cramer, 1998b). There was evidence of consistency in defense use across this time period (for denial, $r = .33$, $p < .01$; projection, $r = .43$, $p < .001$; identification, $r = .26$, $p < .01$). However, there was also evidence for a significant decrease in the level of identification by the last year of college ($p < .06$), suggesting that this defense becomes less salient as the individual moves beyond the developmental period in which the issues of identity and identity confusion are paramount (Erikson, 1968). Other evidence supporting this view is presented in Chapter 2.

Defense change in late adolescence has also been assessed using the DSQ (Tuulio-Henriksson et al., 1997). In this study 516 Finnish high school students completed the DSQ-72 [2] in late adolescence (mean age = 17 years, range = 15–19 years) and again 5 years later (mean age = 22 years). The results indicated that scores on both the Immature and Neurotic defense scales decreased with age, but there was no significant difference in scores on the Mature scale.

One other study followed men from college age (in 1940) to adulthood, focusing on change in defense use over this period of time (Vaillant, 1976). Selecting 50 men from the Harvard College sample, Vaillant rated defense use based on his clinical interviews with the men at three points in time: prior to age 20 years, during the period between 20 and 35 years, and after age 35 years. The period between late adolescence and adulthood showed a decrease in the immature defenses of hypochondriasis, acting out, TAS, denial in fantasy, and reaction formation, whereas the mature defenses of altruism, sublimation, suppression, and anticipation increased with age. Somewhat surprisingly, dissociation (neurotic denial) continued to occur frequently in adulthood. It is possible that this finding is related to the great stress that had been faced by these men in connection with three major wars that occurred after their graduation from college. Other studies have shown that denial is commonly used by otherwise stable individuals when faced with extreme stress that is outside their own control (e.g., Hackett & Cassem, 1974).

PREDICTING OVER TIME FROM CHILDHOOD PERSONALITY TO LATER DEFENSE USE

If we hold the view that there is some continuity in the development of personality from early childhood to later adult functioning, it would then follow that early manifestations of personality disturbance may be expected to influence the later use of defense mechanisms. The basic idea here is that a child who is experiencing stress or psychological upset will make strong use of the defense mechanisms that are available at that particular age. Then, if these defenses are overly utilized, they may become an integral part of the child's personality, continuing in prominence beyond the time that they are usually relinquished. In a general sense, then, we might expect that early experience will affect later personality development and defense use. To investigate this question requires the study of longitudinal data.

The good fortune to access such data came to me through my association with Professor Jack Block of the University of California, Berkeley. As part of a longitudinal study carried out with San Francisco Bay Area children, ages 3 to 23 years (Block & Block, 1980), it was possible to relate the personality functioning of these children at age 3 with their defense use at age 23 (Cramer & Block, 1998). For the early age groups, the researchers asked the children's nursery school teachers to rate their personality, emotional, and cognitive characteristics, using the 100 items of the California Child Q-sort (CCQ)and other measures. At age 23, these now young adults told TAT stories that were audiotaped, transcribed, and then coded for the use of DMM defenses. From the theoretical expectations discussed above, it was hypothesized that the use of the immature defense of denial at age 23 would be predicted by evidence of personality disturbance and psychological upset at age 3. That is, it is assumed that preschoolers who were psychologically upset would react by using, and overusing, the age-available defense of denial. In turn, this defense might become a continuing part of their personality, retaining prominence beyond that period for which it was developmentally appropriate.

To test this hypothesis, the age 3 ratings on 100 CCQ items were related to age 23 defense scores, separately for males and females. In addition, a measure of "psychological upset" at age 3 was also related to age 23 defenses. The results indicated that, for males, 27 of the early childhood items significantly predicted the use of denial (DMM) at age 23, a finding far exceeding chance. As shown in Table 10.1, these items indicated that males who were relying on denial at age 23 years had been rated at preschool as (1) expressing feelings of low self-worth, (2) being emotionally labile and inappropriate, (3) lacking intellectual competence, (4) showing poor impulse control, (5) lacking prosocial skills, and (6) having poor interpersonal relationships. Also, they had been rated at preschool age as lacking in ego resiliency and appearing depressed. An overall measure of psychological upset at age 3 years also was a positive predictor of men's use of denial at age 23, whereas a measure of "no upset" was a negative predictor.

The findings were rather different for the females in the study. Although those who were still relying on denial at age 23 also showed signs of psychological difficulties at age 3, the nature of these problems differed from those of the males (see Table 10.2). As 3-year-olds, these young girls tended to withdraw from others, to avoid social interaction, to be involved in fantasy, and to rely on nonverbal communication—a somewhat schizoid picture.

Overall, the findings are consistent with the hypothesis that a preschool child who is experiencing multiple psychological difficulties would have extensive need to use the defense mechanism available at that age—

TABLE 10.1. Age 3 CCQ-Item Correlates with the Use of Denial at Age 23: Males

Positive correlates	Negative correlates
• Appears to feel unworthy	• Is competent, skillful
• Cries easily	• Is planful, thinks ahead
• Is unable to delay gratification	• Is attentive and able to concentrate
• Is inappropriate in emotive behavior	• Uses and responds to reason
• Overreacts to major frustration	• Is verbally fluent
• Is emotionally labile	• Shows concern for moral issues
• Tends to go to pieces under stress	• Can be trusted, is dependable
• Is easily victimized by other children	• Has high performance standards for self
• Tends to be sulky or whiny	• Is helpful and cooperative
• Is afraid of being deprived	• Develops true and close relationships
• Displays immature behavior under stress	• Tends to give, lend, share
• Has a readiness to feel guilty	• Is reflective
• Attempts to transfer blame to others	• Is considerate of other children
• Has bodily symptoms from stress	

TABLE 10.2. Age 3 CCQ-Item Correlates with the Use of Denial at Age 23: Females

Positive correlates	Negative correlates
• Withdraws under stress	• Is helpful and cooperative
• Has an active fantasy life	• Is eager to please
• Keeps thoughts, feelings to self	
• Is immobilized under stress	
• Shows specific mannerisms	
• Likes to be by herself	
• Prefers nonverbal communication	
• Has transient relationships with others	
• Daydreams	
• Tends to brood or worry	

the defense of denial—in order to protect the self. As that mechanism becomes ingrained in the personality, it continues as a significant defense even into young adulthood.

It was not expected that psychological characteristics at age 3 years would predict later use of projection or identification, because these defenses would not have been predominant at that early age. Consistent with this expectation, the number of correlations between preschool Q-items and the later use of projection and identification did not exceed that expected by chance. Nevertheless, there are some interesting differences between the few preschool characteristics that were related to later use of projection and those related to the later use of identification. Men who relied on projection at age 23 were earlier rated as having low self-worth, lacking competence, and having an external orientation. Women who relied on projection at age 23 were earlier rated as having low self-worth, being emotionally labile, and showing a tendency to somatize.

In contrast, the precursors for later use of identification portrayed positive characteristics rather than the negative personality characteristics associated with denial and projection. For the boys these precursors included both verbal and emotional expressiveness, self-assertiveness, and engagement of adults' interest in them. For the girls, these included self-assertiveness, self-motivation, comfort with self, and engagement of adults' interest in them. Although these connections are interesting, it should be underscored that relatively few personality characteristics at age 3 years predicted the use of projection and identification in young adulthood.

A second study that related preschool children's personality variables with later defense use was carried out by Wolmer et al. (2001). Israeli children who had been exposed to Scud missile attacks during the Gulf War were assessed by parent report at ages 3–5 years, using both the Achenbach CBCL (Achenbach & Edelbrock, 1983) to determine the presence of internalizing and externalizing symptoms and the Childhood Personality Scales (Cohen, Dibble, & Grawe, 1977) to measure five personality factors. Approximately 5 years later, the defense use of these children was assessed using the Comprehensive Assessment of Defense Style (CADS), a 50-item observer report questionnaire that evaluates 25 defenses and three defense styles, designated as Self-Oriented (including Denial), Other-Oriented (including projection), and Mature (including identification). These three factors were validated against the three scales of the DMM and were found to correlate with DMM scores in ways expected: Other-Oriented was positively related to DMM projection; Mature was positively related to DMM identification and negatively related to DMM denial.

The CADS factor scales were then related to the earlier measures of personality and symptoms. The resulting correlations demonstrated that preschoolers who had been characterized by poor capacity for attention, inability to modulate behavior, and low sociability at ages 3–5 years had higher scores on both Self-Oriented and Other-Oriented defenses at ages 8–10 years. Also, the presence of both internalizing and externalizing CBCL symptoms at ages 3–5 years predicted both types of defense use 5 years later. In addition, earlier apathy was found to predict later Self-Oriented defense use, whereas lack of verbal expressiveness was found to predict later Other-Oriented defenses. As in the Cramer and Block (1998) study, preschool personality did not predict the Mature defense scale.

These findings are consistent with the expectation that children who evidence psychological difficulties at ages 3–5 years continue to use immature defenses such as denial beyond the period at which they are age appropriate, as in the Cramer and Block (1998) study. In addition, although it was not reported in the Wolmer et al. (2001) study, it is likely that these distressed children continued to have psychological problems at ages 8–10 years, in which case the age normative defense for this period—projection—would be expected to be used in connection with these continuing psychological difficulties, as found.

A third study also investigated the relation between childhood personality and later defense use; in addition, this study examined the pathway from early personality to defense use to later personality and psychological adjustment at age 30 years (Cramer & Tracy, 2005). In this investigation 62 children who were studied intensively at ages 5–7 years, as part of the Berkeley Guidance Study at the Institute of Human Development, University of California, were followed over the next 25 years; at age 30 years, another intensive study of their personality was conducted. At this time they also told TAT stories, providing an opportunity to assess defense mechanism use (DMM) at age 30.

Based on a factor analysis of Q-sort responses at each age of assessment, six personality factors were identified that could describe personality both at early childhood (ages 5–7 years) and at early adulthood (age 30 years) (Haan et al., 1986). In the subsequent longitudinal study, the first question investigated was whether early childhood personality would predict later defense use; the second question was whether this defense use would predict early-adult personality and adjustment.

The findings relevant to the first question showed that three of the personality variables assessed at ages 5–7 predicted defense use 25 years later. Children who were characterized as "hostile" and "assertive" were more likely to rely on DMM Denial in early adulthood. Children who were characterized as "victimized" and "hostile" in early childhood were prone to rely on DMM Projection as early adults. Strikingly, then, childhood personality predicted the use of denial and projection 25 years later.

This finding is consistent with previous research showing that personality disturbance in very early childhood predicted adult use of denial, a defense that is age appropriate in very early childhood. However, in that study (Cramer & Block, 1998) very early childhood disturbance did not significantly predict adult use of projection or identification; these defenses would not have been developed at that early age. In the present study with somewhat older children (ages 5–7 years), for whom both denial and projection are likely to be active, we suggest that personality disturbances in these children—namely, feeling victimized and displaying hostility and assertiveness—resulted in the entrenchment of the defenses that are appropriate to that age period (denial and projection) as an enduring part of the personality.[3]

PREDICTING OVER TIME FROM DEFENSE USE TO LATER PERSONALITY/BEHAVIOR

An alternative perspective considers whether earlier defense use influences later personality or behavior.

Adolescent Studies

The relation between adolescent defense use and subsequent psychological disturbance was demonstrated with 516 Finnish adolescents (Tuulio-Henriksson et al., 1997). At ages 15–19 (mean age = 17 years) the students completed the DSQ-72. Five years later they again took the DSQ-72 as well as the General Health Questionnaire (Goldberg, 1972), a measure of psychiatric disturbance. Comparing their defense scores with subsequent psychiatric disturbance indicated that the use of immature defenses at the earlier age and an increase in Immature defense scores over the 5-year period were significantly related to psychiatric disturbance at the later date. For females, but not males, earlier scores on the Mature defense scale were associated with subsequently lower scores of psychiatric disturbance. However, males whose Mature scores increased over the 5-year period were also found to have subsequently lower disturbance scores.

As the authors point out, the interpretation of these findings is not entirely clear. It may well be that the defenses used in adolescence are precursors of later psychiatric disturbance. However, because the disturbance was only measured at the later date, there is no way to know whether the relation between earlier defense and disturbance might not also have existed at the earlier adolescent age—in which case it would be unclear whether there was a longitudinal causal relationship.

Two studies have investigated the relation between defense use in adolescence and later moral judgment. In the first (Hart & Chmiel, 1992), 42 boys (ages 13–14 and 16–18 years) were interviewed during adolescence and subsequently at 3–4 year intervals. The assessments included Kohlberg's Moral Judgment Interview (Colby & Kohlberg, 1987), which was subsequently coded to indicate the level of moral judgment attained. The interviews also provided additional information regarding life experiences, aspirations and family relationships. From these transcribed interviews, an independent coder used Haan's (1977) Q-sort to assess the use of defense and coping mechanisms. The results indicated that adolescent defense maturity (a summary measure based on both defense and coping mechanisms) was positively related to adolescent level of moral judgment; in addition, it significantly predicted *adult* moral maturity. Interestingly, the strength of this relationship increased as the men grew older. The correlation was positive but not significant at age 21; at ages 25 and 29, the correlation between *defense maturity* and level of *moral judgment* was significant. In contrast, adolescent use of immature defenses such as denial, regression, isolation and rationalization predicted lower levels of subsequent moral development. This relation between adolescent defense use and adult moral maturity held even when the initial level of adolescent moral maturity was controlled for (partialled out). Further, the use of cross-lagged correlations showed that the correlation from adolescent defense to adult moral level was always stronger than from adolescent moral level to adult defense, which is consistent with the assumption that adolescent defenses played a causal role in subsequent moral development.

A second study (Matsuba & Walker, 1998) also used Haan's Q-sort measure to assess defense use in 66 boys and girls who were in grade 5 or grade 10 (approximately ages 11 and 15 years). The Q-sort was based on a videotaped interview in which there was a discussion about moral conflicts. In addition, the Moral Judgment Interview was used to assess level of moral reasoning. Three years later the level of moral reasoning of these adolescents was assessed again. As in the Hart and Chmiel (1992) study, after controlling for initial level of moral reasoning, the results indicated that the use of immature defenses such as denial and projection in late childhood and adolescence was related to subsequent lower levels of moral reasoning. More mature defenses, such as intellectualization and sublimation, showed no relation with moral level assessed 3 years later (ages 14 and 18 years).

If earlier defense use does predict subsequent moral development, as these studies suggest, how might this linkage occur? The process of moral development from lower to higher moral stages involves a willingness to consider the inadequacies of one's current thinking for resolving moral conflicts, the capacity to consider new bases for moral judgments, and the ability to understand alternative perspectives. Immature defense mechanisms are likely to interfere with these processes—in which case progressive change, or development, will not occur (Hart & Chmiel, 1992).

Adult Studies

I reviewed, in detail, Vaillant's pioneering work on the longitudinal effects of defense mechanisms on adult development in my previous book (Cramer, 1991a). In summary, his work demonstrated, in two samples of men, that the use of mature defenses, assessed prior to age 50 years, predicted mental health, psychosocial maturity, job success and enjoyment, and marital stability. The participants in one of these samples had been studied since they were students at Harvard College. The other (the core city sample) had come from lower-class neighborhoods in Boston; the majority of these families were on welfare.[4]

More recent reports from Vaillant's work, based on these two quite different samples of men, have continued to show predictive relationships between earlier defense use and later functioning (Vaillant, 1993). In the college sample (for whom defense functioning was assessed from life information collected between ages 20 and 47 years), defense maturity predicted global mental health after age 50, psychosocial adjustment (including marital stability and job enjoyment) between ages 50 and 65, life satisfaction between ages 60 and 65, and self-reported physical functioning (ages 70–75). Also, earlier defense maturity predicted good physical health, as independently assessed by a physician at ages 50, 55, and 60. However, by age 65, and again at age 70, there was no relation between earlier defense maturity and independently assessed physical health.

Similar relations were found for the men of the core city sample. Defense maturity at age 47 predicted global mental health after age 50, joy in living at age 65, psychosocial adjustment at ages 50–65, and self-reported physical functioning (age 65). However, as in the college sample, independently assessed physical health at age 60 was not associated with earlier defense maturity (Vaillant, 1992, 1993, 2000).

Longitudinal study of a third group by Vaillant has demonstrated similar relations between defense maturity and psychological adaptation. In follow-up studies of Terman's (1959) sample of gifted children, the women in the group (n = 40) who were found to use more mature defenses between ages 20 and 70 were rated to have had greater job success at age 47, higher levels of psychosocial maturity and mental health, and higher levels of life satisfaction at ages 60–65 (Vaillant, 1993; Vaillant & Vaillant, 1990).

DEFENSES PREDICT PERSONALITY CHANGE: NARROW-BAND VARIABLES

In addition to the question of whether defense use in earlier life predicts standing on personality variables in subsequent years, there is the related question as to whether earlier defense use predicts subsequent *change* in personality. Although there is considerable evidence for personality consistency in adulthood, in the sense that the rank ordering of individuals on measures of personality traits remains quite similar across different ages, there is also repeated evidence of personality change, in the sense that the mean level of different traits changes as people grow older.[5]

The Berkeley Guidance study, discussed above, in addition to showing that childhood personality predicts later defense use, also demonstrated that defense use predicts personality change, which then predicts later adjustment (Cramer & Tracy, 2005). Using the statistical method of path analysis, we demonstrated that there was a significant pathway from early child personality through defense use to adult functioning. However, rather than finding a *direct* pathway from a particular childhood personality factor to the same adult personality factor (e.g., from childhood victimization to adult victimization), the results indicated that defense mechanisms intervened to "redirect" the pathway from child to adult personality. It was this redirected pathway, influenced by defense mechanisms, that then predicted change in personality, which in turn predicted psychological adjustment in early adulthood (see Figure 10.1).

Because Figure 10.1 is rather complex, it may be helpful to offer some explanation. At the far right of the figure, the three measures of adult psychological adjustment—psychological health, depression, and anxiety—are represented. Moving to the left in the figure, two measures of adult personality change (i.e., change from childhood to adulthood in self-confidence and outgoingness) are represented. As may be seen from the Figure, an increase in self-confidence is positively related to psychological health (beta = .50) and negatively related to depression (beta = −.41) and anxiety (beta = −.75). Likewise, an increase in outgoingness is positively related to

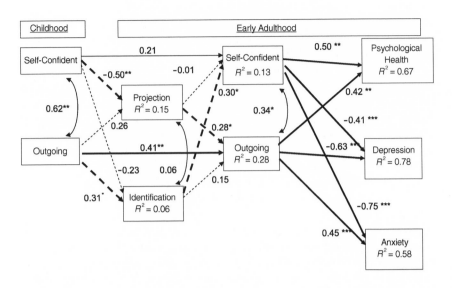

FIGURE 10.1. Standardized coefficients for regression effects in the path model from childhood personality to adult personality, as mediated through defense mechanisms to adult adjustment outcomes. Adapted from Cramer and Tracy (2005). Copyright 2005 by Elsevier. Adapted by permission. $^*p < .05$; $^{**}p < .01$; $^{***}p < .001$. ⎯⎯ = direct effect significant; ⎯ ⎯ ⎯ = mediated effect significant; ⎯⎯ = direct effect not significant; ⋯⋯⋯ = mediated effect not significant.

psychological health (beta = .42), negatively related to depression (beta = –.63), but positively related to anxiety (beta = .45).

Moving again to the left in the figure, we see that the change in self-confidence in adulthood is mediated by the use of the defense of identification (beta = .30), whereas the change in outgoingness is mediated by the use of projection (beta = .28). Finally, moving to the far left of the figure, we see that the use of projection was negatively predicted by childhood self-confidence (beta = –.50); in other words, children who were victimized (victimization is the opposite end of the self-confident factor) were more likely to use projection. Also, children who were outgoing were more likely to subsequently use identification (beta = .31).

Conceptually, these findings show that the *change* in victimization from childhood to adulthood was the strongest predictor of adult adjustment, and this change was significantly influenced by low use of the defense of identification. Those individuals who made little use of DMM Identification showed an increase in victimization at early adulthood. Importantly, the proclivity to use, or not use, this defense was determined not by childhood victimization but by the childhood characteristic of outgoingness: Children who were assessed as outgoing were more likely to use identification later.

A separate pathway showed that it was the change in the personality characteristic of outgoingness from childhood to adulthood that predicted all three of the adult adjustment measures; this change was influenced by the use of the defense of projection. In turn, the use of projection was related not to childhood outgoingness but to childhood victimization.

In sum, this study demonstrated that childhood personality predicts the subsequent use of defense mechanisms, and that these defense mechanisms then influence changes in personality from childhood to adulthood. In turn, it is these personality changes that are associated with adult psychological adjustment and maladjustment.

In Chapter 8 we saw that defense use is concurrently related to (1) the Big Five personality traits, (2) identity style, and (3) other personality variables. The study of Harvard men also demonstrated that a rating of the participants' defense maturity at ages 15–47 years was related to their subsequent Big Five scores at age 67. Maturity of defenses was a positive predictor of conscientiousness and a negative predictor of neuroticism (Soldz & Vaillant, 1999). Now we look at the question of whether earlier adult defense use might predict *change* in personality in later adulthood. The assumption here is that excessive reliance on immature defenses during adulthood would likely be associated with indications of personality problems. At the same time, theory leads us to expect that the unavailability of age-normative defenses might also have negative implications for adjustment (A. Freud, 1965). In other words, if either the defense used or the frequency of defense use (either too little or too much) deviates from the norm, this deviation may have negative consequences for the psychological well-being of the individual.

To investigate this issue, a longitudinal study of the relation between earlier defense use and subsequent adult personality development was carried out using information from the Berkeley Guidance Study and Oakland Growth Study at the Institute of Human Development. In this sample there were 155 men and women who had provided TAT stories at early adulthood (ages 30 or 37 years) and who also had been intensely studied by the institute staff at that age, at middle adulthood (ages 40 and 47 years) and at late-middle age (ages 54 and 61 years). Q-sorts were available for each participant at each of these adult ages. From these Q-sorts an assessment of the participants' standing on each of the Big Five personality dimensions and on each of the four identity styles could be determined. The concurrent relations between DMM defense use and Big Five personality and identity style at early adulthood were discussed in Chapter 8.

DEFENSE USE PREDICTS BIG
FIVE PERSONALITY CHANGE

Using this information, the DMM defense scores of these men and women, together with their IQ scores, were used to predict change in Big Five scores over a 24-year period, from early to middle adulthood, and from middle adulthood to late middle age (Cramer, 2003b). Because there is evidence that men and women may follow a somewhat different pathway of personality development (Helson et al., 1997; and see Chapter 9), the relation between defense use and subsequent personality change was studied separately for each gender. The inclusion of IQ as a possible predictive factor was done on the basis of earlier findings indicating that IQ moderated the relation between defenses and other personality variables (see Chapter 8).

The first step in this study was to determine whether there was change in the Big Five personality dimensions over the 24-year period of adulthood. The findings indicated that significant change did occur. Both men and women showed significant decrease in neuroticism and a significant increase in both extraversion and conscientiousness from early to middle adulthood. From middle adulthood to late-middle age, both men and women showed an increase in agreeableness, whereas women also showed a decrease in extraversion and conscientiousness. In addition, women showed an increase in openness from early to middle adulthood, whereas men showed a decrease on this dimension from middle adulthood to late-middle age.

Importantly, these changes in the Big Five personality traits during middle adulthood and late-middle age were predicted by the early-adult use of the DMM defenses of denial, projection, and identification, both separately and in interaction with IQ. Specifically, for females in middle adulthood, both strong and weak use of denial (curvilinear relation) predicted an increase in neuroticism, a decrease in agreeableness, and a decrease in conscientiousness. Strong use of projection predicted a decrease in extraversion. Both strong and weak use of identification (curvilinear relation) predicted a decrease in agreeableness. By late-middle age, females' earlier use of denial predicted an increase in conscientiousness and, at average and high levels of IQ, a decrease in openness.[6] Also for females at late-middle age, the earlier use of projection predicted an increase in extraversion, and, at low and average levels of IQ, an increase in conscientiousness.[7] Finally, the earlier use of identification predicted a decrease in neuroticism and an increase in conscientiousness.

Early-adult defenses were also significant predictors of personality change for the men in the group. At middle adulthood, earlier strong and weak use of denial (curvilinear relation) predicted a decrease in extraversion.

Strong use of projection predicted later increase in conscientiousness. At high levels of IQ, identification predicted an increase in both neuroticism and openness.[8] At late-middle age, defenses continued to predict personality change in men. Both strong and weak use of projection (curvilinear relation) in early adulthood predicted an increase in neuroticism and a decrease in both extraversion and agreeableness. Also, at low levels of IQ, projection predicted an increase in conscientiousness.[9] Finally, for men, the earlier use of identification predicted an increase in agreeableness at late-middle age. Overall, then, earlier defense use did predict personality change in adulthood.

The findings are also striking in demonstrating that, with increasing age, defenses become increasingly important for predicting personality trait change. For women in early adulthood, defenses alone (i.e., without a consideration of IQ) predicted two personality traits. By middle adulthood, defenses predicted change in four traits, and one of these trait changes was predicted by two defenses. By late-middle age, defenses predicted change in three traits, and one of these traits was predicted by two defenses. For men in early adulthood, defenses alone predicted one personality trait. In middle adulthood, defenses predicted changes in two traits. By late-middle age, defenses predicted changes in three traits, and one of those trait changes was predicted by two defenses.

In addition, during middle adulthood and late-middle age, there was increasing divergence between women and men in the relation of defenses to personality trait change. For women, all three defenses (denial, projection, and identification) were significant predictors of personality change. However, for men it was primarily the defense of projection that predicted personality change by late-middle age. This increasing importance of projection is consistent with the general finding that this defense is typically associated with males and masculinity (see Chapter 9 and Cramer, 1991a).

The findings of this longitudinal study also demonstrated that IQ and defense use interact in the prediction of change for all five personality traits, and the nature of that prediction is consistent across traits. As in the study showing that defenses and IQ predict level of ego development (Cramer, 1999b; see Chapter 8), strong defense use was related to a more positive personality picture for individuals with low IQs. In general, for both males and females with low IQs, the use of defenses—even immature defenses—may be seen as "compensatory," in that defense use is associated with an increase in positive personality traits and with a diminution of less desirable traits. At the same time, the use of these defenses by individuals with high IQs is a negative indicator for healthy personality development. [10]

DEFENSE USE PREDICTS IDENTITY CHANGE

This same group of 155 men and women were also studied to determine the relations between early adult defense use and subsequent identity development (Cramer, 2004). As in the previous study, DMM defense use was assessed from TAT stories told in early adulthood. Identity style was determined from the Q-sorts available for early adulthood (ages 30 and 37 years), middle adulthood (ages 40 and 47 years), and late-middle age (ages 54 and 61 years). These Q-sorts were matched (correlated) with prototype identity Q-sorts (Mallory, 1989) representing each of four identity styles—achieved, moratorium, foreclosure, and diffused.[11]

As described in Chapter 8, these styles can be differentiated in terms of two factors: (1) whether or not a commitment has been made to an ideological set of religious, political, and occupational values and goals, and to interpersonal concerns such as sex roles, sexual identity, and relationships; and (2) whether or not the individual has experienced some conflict or crisis in trying to establish these values, opinions, and goals. Individuals who have not made a commitment and who may or may not have experienced a crisis are considered to be in a state of identity diffusion. Those who have made a commitment, but not on the basis of having experienced a personal crisis (more likely on the basis of unquestioned acceptance of the values, opinions, and goals of their parents or other significant social group), are considered to be in a state of identity foreclosure. Those individuals who have not made a commitment but are currently in the process of exploration and/or experiencing a crisis are considered to be in a state of identity moratorium. Only those individuals who have both experienced a crisis and made a commitment are considered to be identity achieved.[12]

Previous research has shown that identity continues to change in adulthood in the direction of greater maturity (e.g., Pulkkinen & Kokko, 2000; Stewart, Ostrove, & Helson, 2001). Research has also shown that DMM defense mechanisms are related to identity status (see Chapter 5). Thus we might expect that identity change would be related to defense use. In particular, because the more mature defense of identification is both theoretically (Erikson, 1968) and empirically (Cramer, 1995, 1997a, 1998a, 1998b, 2001) related to the mature achieved identity style in late adolescents, it might be expected that the continued use of identification in early adulthood would predict subsequent change toward a more mature identity style. To investigate this possibility, the DMM defense scores of these 155 men and women from the Institute of Human Development study, together with their IQ scores, were used to predict change in identity style over a 24-year period, from early adulthood to middle adulthood, and from middle adulthood to late-middle age. [13]

The initial findings indicated that there was a significant increase in both the achieved and moratorium identity styles from early to middle adulthood. There was also a significant increase in the foreclosed style from early and middle adulthood to late-middle age.[14]

Having established that identity change does occur in adulthood, the next step was to determine whether defenses, along with IQ, would predict identity change. Regression analyses indicated that the increase in moratorium was predicted by the use of identification at early adulthood. However, the increase in the achieved style was primarily predicted by IQ—the higher the IQ, the greater the increase in achieved identity. Also, the use of projection by individuals at lower levels of IQ predicted a significant increase in the achieved style. In contrast to expectation, early-adult use of identification was a weak (marginally significant) predictor of a *decrease* in the achieved style. Together, these results suggest that the defense of identification is associated with a continuing search for identity—that is, with a continuation of the late-adolescent process.

Consistent with the assumption that the use of identification is associated with the process of identity exploration, we might expect that *not* relying on the defense of identification would hinder exploration and thus contribute to an identity style based on acceptance of the status quo—that is, to the foreclosed style. Thus it is notable that the *low* use of identification in early adulthood predicted an *increase* in foreclosure in middle adulthood. Further, at late-middle age, for higher levels of IQ, earlier low use of identification predicted further increase in foreclosure.

CONCLUDING REMARKS

I began this chapter with four questions that are interrelated but different. First, does the use of defenses change with age? There is considerable evidence that defense use does change in childhood and adolescence. (See also Chapter 2.) However, there is only one study that has investigated this question in adulthood. Vaillant (1976) reported that the Harvard men increased their use of mature defenses and decreased their use of immature defenses as they approached middle age. Further information on this question of defense change in adulthood, including data from women, is clearly needed.

Next, do early personality and experience affect later defense use? Our expectation here is that if early stress affects childhood personality and causes an age-appropriate defense to be overused at that time, the defense will likely become an ingrained part of the individual's personality and will continue to predominate beyond its age-appropriate period. This hypothesis was supported in three longitudinal studies. In one, psychological disturbance during ages 3–5 years predicted immature defense use at ages 8–10 years. In a second, psychological disturbance at age 3 predicted the use of the early childhood defense of denial at age 23. In the third, personality difficulties at ages 5–7 years predicted the use of the immature defenses of denial and projection at age 30.

The third question considered the other side of this issue: Does earlier defense use predict later personality? Studies with adolescents have shown that their use of immature defenses predicts psychological disturbance and lower levels of moral maturity in young adulthood. The many studies of Vaillant have shown, over a wide range of personality and life history variables, that men's use of mature defenses during earlier adulthood predicted myriad indications of later positive adjustment, whereas immature defenses were related to problems.

Finally, the fourth question asked whether earlier defense use predicts subsequent personality change. A study of both males and females from childhood to early adulthood demonstrated that defense use, influenced by childhood personality, predicted personality change in early adulthood, which in turn predicted psychological adjustment.

Studies with adults have also demonstrated that defense use predicts personality change. The study of Big Five personality traits showed clearly that trait change was predicted by defense, sometimes in interaction with IQ. It is also noteworthy that there is a change in the relation of defenses to personality over time. At middle adulthood, most women showed an increase in extraversion, but those who made strong use of projection at early adulthood showed a decrease in extraversion. However, by late-middle age, those who used projection showed an increase in extraversion, whereas most women showed a decrease. A similar change in the nature of the relationship between defenses and personality is seen for the trait of conscientiousness. Whereas most of the women increased in conscientiousnesss at middle adulthood, those who relied on denial at early adulthood showed a decrease. By late-middle age, when most women showed a decrease in conscientiousness, those who relied on denial showed an increase.

One question these research findings raise is why defenses should become increasingly important with age in the prediction of personality traits. Costa et al. (1991) have suggested that the use of mature defenses in adulthood reflects psychological adjustment rather than continuing development—the corollary being that those who use immature defenses will continue to function in a less well-adjusted manner. The present findings demonstrate that this maladjustment becomes increasingly evident with age. Adults who used immature defenses in early adulthood subsequently showed signs of maladjustment, whereas those who used a more mature defense subsequently showed an increase in positive traits. Although there are a few exceptions, the regression analyses generally indicated that high use of the more mature defense of identification in early adulthood subsequently predicted a more positive personality—low neuroticism, high agreeableness in males, and high conscientiousness in females—whereas use of the immature defenses of denial and projection subsequently predicted neuroticism and less of the favorable traits of extraversion and agreeableness. These results are consistent with those of Vaillant and Vaillant (1990), who found that maturity of defenses used prior to age 47 years was a significant predictor of the Harvard men's psychosocial adjustment and life satisfaction at age 65 years.

Although this description accounts for the subsequent relation between high defense use and personality traits, it does not accommodate the relation found between very low defense use in early adulthood and subsequent personality traits (i.e., the curvilinear relation of defense with personality). A. Freud (1965) discussed how normative deviation in defense use may be related to personality difficulties. She suggested that defenses that are used either too much or too little are likely to be indicators of psychological disturbance. Whereas defenses used at the normative level protect the individual from undue stress and anxiety, both inadequate defense availability (which leaves the individual open to emotional upset) and excessive defense use (which warps the individual's perception of reality) will negatively affect personality development. In our research, we found that those individuals who deviated in either direction from the normative level of defense use during early adulthood became more neurotic, less agreeable, less extraverted (men only) and less conscientious (women only) at subsequent ages than those individuals whose defense use during early adulthood fell within the normative range.

Although this second explanation overlaps with the first, the two explanations are based on different principles. In the first case, the negative effects of excessive use of an immature defense became more obvious with age, likely as a result of the cumulative distortions of reality testing in response to defense use. In the second case, the effects of the absence of defense protection became increasingly manifest as the individual grew older. However, in the absence of data on defense use during middle adulthood and late-middle age, both of these explanations are speculative.[15]

Our research also showed that adult change in identity status is predicted by earlier defense use. Whether or not identity continues to develop during adulthood, as well as the direction of that development, will be importantly affected by both defense mechanisms and intelligence.[16] In particular, the defense of identification, both singly and in interaction with IQ, is a strong determinant of identity development. As in previous investigations (Cramer, 1999c, 2004), this study again demonstrated the importance of the interaction between defense use and IQ for understanding adult development.

The results of this research also highlight the fact that there is specificity in the way in which defense mechanisms predict different aspects of adult development. In the study of Big Five personality change (Cramer, 2003b), the pattern of relations between defenses and personality traits was quite different from the relations between defenses and identity styles (Cramer, 2004). In the Big Five study, all three defenses—denial, projection, and identification—were found to be significant predictors of personality traits and of trait change across the 24-year span of adulthood. However, in the study in which the focus is on *identity* development, the defense of identification was the primary predictor of identity and identity change. In no case was denial found to be related to adult identity development, and projection was of minimal importance.

Finally, it should be emphasized again that in order to understand the relation between defenses, defense change, personality, and personality change, it is essential to carry out longitudinal studies. Only in this way can we discern the interrelationships among these factors. An important issue in this work is to ensure that the assessment of defenses is based on material that is independent from the information used to assess personality and life satisfaction (e.g., about job success and enjoyment, marital stability, and mental health). Otherwise, immaturity in one domain may well influence ratings in the other.

PART IV

Defenses and Psychopathology

There is increasing recognition in the mental health community that defense mechanisms constitute a critical component in the formulation of psychiatric diagnoses. This recognition is evidenced by the inclusion in the DSM-IV of a Defensive Rating Scale as a proposed new axis for the diagnosis of psychological disorders (see Skodol & Perry, 1993), and it is supported by a burgeoning number of research studies relating diagnosis to defense use.

In this part of the book I discuss research that shows how defense mechanisms are related to indications of pathology in both patients and in nonclinical individuals. Although these latter individuals are not diagnosed with a psychological disorder, they may harbor, to various degrees, indications of personality disorders, aggressive tendencies, depression, and other types of pathology and thus may be informative for our understanding of the role of defenses in pathological conditions.

In Chapter 11 I consider studies in which nonpatient groups of individuals are assessed for the presence of psychological disturbance and then see how this disturbance is related to the use of defenses. Although pathology in the participants of these studies is not great enough to require hospitalization, finding a relation with defense use even within this narrower range of disturbance would be a striking demonstration of the connection between pathology and defense use.

On the other hand, it could be argued that there is a qualitative difference between defenses associated with these lower-level indications of

221

pathology and the defenses associated with more extreme indicators. That is, at different degrees of intensity on the pathology dimension there may be qualitative differences in associated defense characteristics. For example, persons at the extreme of the dimension might, as a result of earlier experience or trauma, use different defensive strategies that are not found among persons in the moderate range. In this case, findings from research with nonclinical samples might not generalize to patient groups.[1] This possibility is addressed in Chapter 12, in which we consider the relation between defenses and pathology based on samples of patients who have been diagnosed with full-fledged psychiatric disorder. Chapter 13 focuses on how patients' defenses are affected by psychotherapy, and Chapter 14 presents in-depth case studies that illustrate how patients with different types of pathology make use of defense mechanisms.

CHAPTER 11

Defenses and Psychopathology in Adult Community and Student Samples

The idea that people might distort their perception of reality to protect themselves from anxiety and psychological distress was developed by Freud (1894) in the context of trying to understand the nature of psychopathology. Although the concept of defense mechanism has been considerably expanded and is now understood as a significant aspect of normal development and adaptive personality functioning, the idea that defenses, when used excessively, are related to psychopathology, continues to be important.[1] In a similar way, various adaptive mental capacities, such as the ability to ignore distracting stimuli, contribute to normal personality functioning, but when they are present in the extreme—for example, refusing to see the danger involved in a threatening situation—they are considered evidence of psychopathology. As another example, being alert and watchful in a situation known to be potentially dangerous is evidence of a resilient and adaptive personality, but hyperalertness and the expectation of danger and hostility at every turn, even in a placid situation, is evidence of pathology.

These modes of functioning—disregarding bothersome perceptions and hyperalertness to potential danger—may be understood as present in all of us to a greater or lesser degree. It is this issue of magnitude, or intensity, in these modes of functioning that differentiates the "normal" person from one who is considered to be psychologically disturbed.[2] This idea that the normal personality and the disordered personality represent different

223

points on the same continuum has received increasing prominence in recent years. Millon (1996) has stated that normal and abnormal are "relative concepts representing arbitrary points on a continuum or gradient" (p. 283), and Costa, Somerfield, and McCrae (1996) have noted that the "differences between normal and psychiatrically impaired individuals . . . are more quantitative than qualitative" (p. 47). Thus, although the extremes may appear to be qualitatively different, the presence of a personality disorder—the point at which normal personality becomes disordered personality—is defined by the degree to which selected personality features are manifest.

From this point of view, within any normal, nonclinical group we might expect to find individuals who possess more or fewer of the characteristics that define a psychological disorder. This dimensional approach to psychological disorders allows us to study nonclinical samples with an eye to enhancing our understanding of disordered psychological functioning. Thus we begin the chapter with a consideration of how indications of a personality disorder are related to defense use in a nonpatient sample.

DEFENSES AND PERSONALITY DISORDERS IN NONCLINICAL SAMPLES

Psychoanalytic theory provides a rationale for the grouping of the narcissistic, histrionic, and antisocial disorders into the same diagnostic cluster (DSM-IV, Cluster B)—namely, that they all derive from the same deviant personality structure: the borderline personality organization (Kernberg, 1975, 1994; Svrakic & McCallum, 1991). This underlying personality organization may be manifest in different ways, and it is these overt differences that distinguish the four personality disorders associated with the borderline personality organization. In turn, this shared origin suggests that there will be overlap but not identity among the prototypes for borderline, narcissistic, histrionic, and antisocial disorders. However, the borderline personality is generally considered to be more immature and more dysfunctional than the related personality disorders (Kernberg, 1975, 1994; Millon, 1996).

A review of the theoretical literature suggests that it is possible to differentiate among the antisocial, narcissistic, and histrionic personality disorders in terms of their relative developmental level, based on three criteria: (1) degree of self-focus, or egocentricity; (2) adaptational strategies used to satisfy needs; and (3) presence of conscience (Kernberg, 1975; Millon, 1996; Svrakic & McCallum, 1991). First, people who have an antisocial or narcissistic personality are similarly oriented toward meeting their own selfish wishes (Millon, 1996); they behave in ways that "benefit exclusively themselves" (Svrakic & McCallum, 1991, p. 187). In contrast, the person with a histrionic personality is oriented toward fulfilling the needs of others (Millon, 1996).

Second, although people with antisocial or narcissistic personalities show egocentricity, entitlement, and lack of empathy, they use different adaptive strategies to meet their needs. The person with a narcissistic personality tends to "seduce" the environment through superficial charm, exhibitionism, and "passive parasitic behavior," whereas the person with an antisocial personality tends to "destroy" the environment through actively aggressive acts (Svrakic & McCallum, 1991, p. 188). Following from this conceptualization, the frequency, nature, and severity of antisocial behaviors differ across the three personality disorders: for the person with an antisocial personality, these behaviors involve violence and property crimes; for the person with a narcissistic personality, they take the form of exploitation; for the person with a histrionic personality, *if* he or she engages in antisocial behavior, it is more likely to involve manipulation than overt aggression (Svrakic & McCallum, 1991).

A final basis for the differentiation among the three personality disorders is the level of conscience present. The person with an antisocial personality is characterized by little or no conscience, as seen in the absence of guilt about destructive acts; this is the critical differentiating feature between the antisocial and narcissistic disorders (Kernberg, 1989; Svrakic, McCallum, & Milan, 1991). The person with a narcissistic personality has "remnants of morality and honesty in some areas" (Svrakic & McCallum, 1991, p. 189); when confronted with the consequences of his or her antisocial acts, the person shows the ability to experience guilt. In contrast, "Histrionic persons manifest precise ethical norms" (Svrakic & McCallum, 1991, p. 190); in this group, there is clear development of conscience.

Considering these three criteria, the three personality disorders may be ordered in terms of developmental level reached:

• At the highest level is the histrionic personality: People with this diagnosis have the capacity to consider others; their strategies to meet their own needs may include the manipulation of others, but they have a clearly developed conscience and show concern for ethical behavior.

• At the next level is the narcissistic personality: People with this diagnosis are self-focused; their strategies include seduction and exploitation, but if confronted with the consequences of this behavior, they may experience guilt.

• At the lowest developmental level of the three is the antisocial personality: People with this diagnosis are self-focused; they use strategies of violence and active aggression and experience no guilt in connection with this behavior.

• Beneath this developmental hierarchy is the even earlier level of the borderline personality, which underlies each of the other personality disorders.

Just as the four personality disorders can be ranked in terms of their relative maturity, it is possible to order defense mechanisms in this way. At the lowest, most immature level are defenses such as splitting and denial; at a somewhat higher level of maturity is the defense of projection and, subsequently, identification. At the highest level of maturity are defenses such as sublimation and intellectualization (e.g., Bond, 1992; Cramer, 1991a; Vaillant, 1993).

According to theory, one of the major features of the borderline personality organization is the use of primitive defense mechanisms. These immature defenses include splitting, idealization, and neurotic denial/dissociation, among others (Kernberg, 1975; Masterson, 1985; Vaillant, 1994). The related personality disorders are also characterized by the use of low-level defenses, but there are also proposed theoretical differences in the defenses associated with these disorders:

- For people with an *antisocial* personality, the defense of projection is pervasive. These individuals disown their hostile impulses by attributing them to others and tend to blame their victims for their own harmful behavior. At the same time, they typically minimize, or are indifferent to, the harmful consequences of their actions—attitudes that represent aspects of the defense of denial.

- People with a *narcissistic* personality may rely on rationalization as a defense, but if this fails, they may revert to wishful fantasy or refuse to recognize disquieting information (i.e., denial); at times, people with narcissistic disorder "may be pushed to the point of employing projection as a defense" (Millon, 1996, p. 407).

- The present-day heir to hysteria, the *histrionic* personality disorder, is characterized by the use of the defenses of dissociation and neurotic denial; people with this disorder may also adopt a defensive stance of acting "as if" they were on stage—that is, assuming aspects of a borrowed identity (Millon, 1996; Vaillant, 1992).

Thus, although all four personality disorders (borderline, antisocial, narcissistic, and histrionic) are expected to be associated with the use of low-level defenses, there is again a suggested developmental ordering, with the borderline personality at the very lowest level, and the other three disorders showing some evidence of more advanced defenses.

These ideas were tested in a study carried out with the young-adult sample (Block & Block, 1980). Recall that these individuals were originally recruited for the study at age 3 years. By age 23, as young adults, they were functioning as members of the Bay Area community. Apart from having a higher than average IQ (mean = 114), they could otherwise be considered "normal." Nevertheless, as we would expect, they varied in degree of subclinical disturbance.

Using the Q-sort prototype approach, each of the study participants could be statistically described for the degree to which he or she demonstrated features of four DSM-IV personality disorders—the borderline, the antisocial, the narcissistic, and the histrionic personality disorders (Cramer, 1999b). The Q-sort prototypes were created by highly experienced clinical psychologists, who used the 100-items of the CAQ to describe each of the disorders, based on the DSM-IV criteria as well as their own clinical experience. Then the Q-sort of each participant was correlated with each of the prototypes. This correlation provided a measure indicating the degree to which the participant's personality was like that of the personality disorder. In this way, I assessed the borderline, narcissistic, histrionic, and antisocial personality syndromes (which are considered subclinical manifestations of their respective disorder), not for the purpose of diagnosis, but rather to determine how the different personality configurations related to the use of defense mechanisms. It was expected that persons who share the personality features that are associated with a personality disorder syndrome will also be likely to use the defenses that are characteristic of that syndrome.

In this study I investigated the relation of the three defenses of denial, projection, and identification, as assessed by the DMM, to the several personality disorder prototypes. Specifically, I expected that borderline personality syndrome (which represents the lowest level of psychological functioning) would be associated more strongly with denial (developmentally, the lowest level defense) than with the other two defenses. Because the other three syndromes theoretically have a borderline personality organization at their base, they too should be related to the use of denial. At the same time, because they represent different levels of ego development and are characterized by different adaptational strategies, they might be expected to show somewhat different patterns of defense use. The antisocial personality, next lowest in the developmental hierarchy, would also be expected to be associated with the use of projection, since the overriding propensity of this personality syndrome is to attribute hostility to others. For the narcissistic personality, which is developmentally more advanced than the antisocial, we would expect less use of denial and relatively greater use of projection. For the histrionic personality, which represents the highest developmental level of the three syndromes, we would expect some use of denial and projection, but also the possibility that aspects of the relatively higher level defense of identification might be used, consistent with both the higher developmental level and the strong other-person orientation of this syndrome (Millon, 1996).

The findings from the study supported these predictions, as seen in Table 11.1. The borderline prototype was associated significantly with the use of denial ($p < .008$), whereas the use of projection and identification were unrelated to this prototype. The antisocial, narcissistic, and histrionic prototypes were also significantly associated with the use of denial ($ps < .004$, .04, and .002, respectively). In addition, as predicted, they were also all associated significantly with the use of projection ($ps < .002$, .03, and .04, respectively). In contrast, none of the personality disorder prototypes was related to the use of identification.

Thus the DSM-IV Cluster B personality disorders were found to be associated with the lower level defenses of denial and projection, but not with the full-scale measure of the more mature defense of identification, in keeping with expectation. The findings also indicated that the theoretical ordering of the personality syndromes in terms of developmental level was related to the relative maturity of defense mechanisms used by each. Specifically, the lowest-level personality organization, borderline, was associated only with the lowest level of defense, denial. Syndromes linked with the borderline but representing somewhat higher levels of development—the narcissistic, antisocial, and histrionic prototypes—were characterized by the use of the relatively higher level defense of projection in addition to denial.

The DMM approach also allows for the coding of immature and mature forms of each defense. Within each defense the seven subcategories are arranged to represent a developmental continuum, from the earliest to more mature forms of the defense.[3] Thus, for each defense, it is possible to derive both immature and mature scores. Because the four personality disorders are hypothesized to be associated with immature levels of defense, it was of interest to determine the relation between these immature forms of the defenses and the four personality disorder prototypes.

To test this possible relation for each personality disorder, both the immature and mature levels of the three defenses were entered into a regression analysis to determine which defense(s) and level(s) would be the strongest predictors of each personality disorder prototype. The results indicated that the strongest predictor for the borderline prototype was the use of immature denial ($p < .009$); the addition of other defenses (both immature and mature levels) did not improve the prediction of the borderline prototype. For the antisocial prototype, the strongest predictor was immature projection, followed by immature denial ($p < .0005$). For the narcissistic prototype, the strongest predictor was immature projection ($p < .01$); the addition of other defenses did not improve the prediction. For the Histrionic prototype, the strongest predictor was immature denial, followed by immature identification ($p < .001$).

Thus, by examining the immature and mature forms of the defense

TABLE 11.1. Defense Mechanisms as Related to Personality
Disorder Prototypes

DSM-IV Cluster B	Denial	Projection	Identification
Borderline	.28**	.18	.03
Antisocial	.30**	.31**	.17
Narcissistic	.21*	.22*	.12
Histrionic	.31**	.21*	.16

Note. From Cramer (1999b); reprinted with permission from the *Journal of Personality.*
*p < .05; **p < .01.

mechanisms, further distinctions among the four personality disorders became apparent. First, it was the use of the *immature*, rather than the mature, forms of the defenses that characterized these personality syndromes. Second, the results indicated that the hierarchy of personality prototypes, from lowest (borderline) to highest (histrionic) level of functioning, was paralleled by a hierarchy in defense use. The borderline syndrome was associated only with the lowest level defense of immature denial. The antisocial syndrome is the next highest developmental level; in addition to the low-level immature denial, it was associated with the somewhat higher defense of immature projection. The narcissistic syndrome is the next highest developmental level; here immature denial was no longer associated with the syndrome—only the somewhat higher defense of immature projection was related. Finally, the histrionic personality syndrome, the most advanced developmentally, is the only syndrome to be associated with the more advanced defense of immature identification. However, contrary to expectation, the defense most strongly associated with this syndrome was immature denial, the least advanced of the defenses studied. This finding is consistent with the "*belle indifférence*" quality of the histrionic disorder but does not fit the developmental explanation.

An additional study with a nonpatient group also found a relation between defense use (DMM) and a measure of borderline personality disorder. In a study of college students, Hibbard and Porcerelli (1998) found that use of immature denial was positively related to scores on the Borderline Syndrome Index (Conte, Plutchik, Karasu, & Jerrett, 1980), whereas mature identification was negatively related.

The relation between DSM categories of personality disorder and defense maturity has also been assessed using the DSQ. Johnson, Bornstein, and Krutonis (1992), in a study of college students, related scores from the four factor scales of the DSQ-88 to scores on a self-report DSM-III-R personality disorder questionnaire (the Personality Diagnostic Questionnaire—Revised [PDQ-R]; Hyler, Skokol, Kellman, Oldham, & Rosnick, 1990).

Results indicated that the Maladaptive defense scale was positively related to scores on 9 of the 11 Personality Disorder scales. The Image Distorting scale was positively related to four of the Personality Disorder scales: Narcissistic, Antisocial, Passive–Aggressive, and Schizotypal. These two defense scales (Maladaptive and Image Distorting) correspond to Vaillant's (1977) "Immature" defenses. The Self-Sacrificing scale, which corresponds to Vaillant's "Neurotic" level, was positively related to scores on the Dependent Personality scale. The Adaptive scale, which corresponds to Vaillant's "Mature" level, was negatively related to scores on the Histrionic, Passive–Aggressive, and Dependent Personality scales; interestingly, it was positively related to the Schizoid scale.

Another nonclinical sample of 300 college students was studied for the relation between the three factor scales of the DSQ-40 and several measures to assess DSM-III-R personality disorders (Sinha & Watson, 1999). The eleven personality disorders were assessed using three alternative measures of the same disorders. The results indicated that the Immature scale predicted standing on all three measures for the avoidant, antisocial, passive–aggressive, borderline, and paranoid personality disorders, and on two of the three measures for the dependent, narcissistic, obsessive–compulsive, and schizotypal personality disorders. The Neurotic defense scale predicted standing on all three measures of dependent personality disorder. The Mature scale (negatively) predicted standing on all three measures of borderline and passive–aggressive personality disorders, and on two of the dependent personality measures.[4] As in the previous study, there was an unexpected positive relation between the Mature defense scale and one of the measures of schizoid personality. No information was provided regarding the relation of individual defenses to specific disorders. Overall, the findings from these two studies show that defense use, as assessed by the DSQ, is differentially related to indications of various personality disorders, but also that there is considerable overlap in the relation between defenses and type of personality disorder.

In the preceding studies, the assessment of personality disorders was based on continuous measures. Maffei et al. (1995) have argued that these results, in which the various personality disorder scales are treated as continuous measures, demonstrate the relation of defenses with personality dimensions, or traits, rather than with psychiatric diagnoses, which are made in terms of categories. To determine if defenses would differentially predict membership in categories of psychological disorder, Maffei et al. (1995) studied the responses of 256 Italian medical students to the PDQ-R (Hyler et al., 1990), using the technique of cluster analysis. This procedure identified three clusters, or categories, of students based on the degree of personality impairment: (1) those for whom there was no evidence of impairment (28%), (2) those for whom there was moderate impairment

(47%), and (3) those for whom there was high impairment and a probable personality disorder (25%). Membership in these three categories was then related to defense use, as assessed by the DSQ-36. Significant differences in scores on the Immature defense scale were found: the high-impairment group used more immature defenses than the moderately impaired, who in turn used more than the unimpaired. The three groups did not differ in the use of neurotic or mature defenses.

The separate categories of personality disorders have also been shown to be related to defense mechanisms, as assessed from interview ratings, in a large group of nonpatient men (Vaillant, 1994; Vaillant & McCullough, 1998). This "core city" sample of men was originally selected during junior high school as a contrast group to a sample of juvenile delinquents (Glueck & Glueck, 1966). These nondelinquent boys were subsequently followed for a period of 35 years by Vaillant (1983), who interviewed them periodically. From these interviews, vignettes were selected that illustrated the participants' responses at times of conflict and crises. One set of raters assessed the use of defenses from these vignettes; another set evaluated the men for the presence of a personality disorder at age 47, using DSM-III (American Psychiatric Association, 1980) criteria.

Of this nonpatient sample, 24% (74 men) were diagnosed as having a personality disorder. Of these, 66% were rated as relying on immature defenses (including schizoid fantasy, projection, passive–aggression, hypochondriasis, acting out, and dissociation/denial). Further analysis indicated that specific diagnoses were associated with the use of specific defenses. For example, as predicted, projection was associated with the diagnosis of paranoia; in fact, 100% of the men with this diagnosis were rated as using projection. The diagnosis of antisocial personality disorder was highly associated with the use of the acting out defense; 75% of the men with this diagnosis used this defense; in addition, 63% were rated as using dissociation/denial.[5] The diagnosis of narcissistic personality disorder was primarily associated with the use of dissociation/denial (83%), with a lesser percentage of this group using projection. In general, these findings agree with those using the DMM approach to assess defenses (described above; Cramer, 1999b). Together, these studies using non-self-report measures indicate that specific defenses are integrally associated with different diagnostic entities. It is for this reason that Vaillant concluded that defense mechanisms are "a valuable diagnostic axis for understanding psychopathology" (1994, p. 49).

DEFENSES AND PATHOLOGICAL AGGRESSION

The DMM has been used to study the relation between defense use and pathological aggression. In one study (Kim, 2001), male college students were asked "Have you hit, kicked, punched or otherwise hurt someone within the past year?" They were further queried if this aggressive act had occurred with a stranger, friend, partner, or family member. From the larger group of students, 30 who reported having been involved in violent behavior toward a stranger were selected and compared with 30 students who reported no violent behavior. Each of these groups were individually administered the TAT; the stories were coded with the DMM for the use of defenses. As in the earlier findings regarding antisocial personality (Cramer, 1999b; Vaillant, 1994) and conduct disorder (Cramer & Kelly, 2004), the use of denial was stronger in the violent group than in the nonviolent group. The two groups did not differ in the use of projection. Notably, the nonviolent group scored higher on the defense of identification, although the difference was not statistically significant (due to considerable variability in both groups). Interestingly, none of the three self-report DSQ scales (Immature, Neurotic, Mature) differentiated the two groups. Again, it is a non-self-report measure that revealed a significant difference in defense use between the violent and nonviolent groups—a difference not found when defenses are assessed by self-report. Additional results indicated that the DMM Projection scale was positively related to the MMPI-2 Psychopathic Deviate scores, and to the DSQ Immature scale ($r = .60$).

Similar findings were obtained in a study by Porcerellli, Cogan, Kamoo, and Leitman (2004). DMM defense use by male college students was studied in relation to self-reported use of violence in reaction to conflict with strangers or partners. As in the previous study, the use of denial was related to the report of violence toward strangers. Also consistent with the earlier study, the use of identification was negatively related to the report of violence toward strangers and partners. In addition, the use of projection was positively related to the report of violence toward partners.

In a third study of pathological aggression, parents who had been convicted of child abuse ($n = 32$) were compared with patients who had anxiety disorders ($n = 119$) and with a normal population reference group ($n = 204$) (Brennan, Andrews, Morris-Yates, & Pollock, 1990). Although the abusive parents did not differ from the patients with anxiety for symptoms reported on the SCL-90, they had significantly higher scores on the Immature defense factor of the DSQ-88, as compared to either the patient or the normal reference group. The predominant defense of the abusive parents was projection, which they reported more frequently than either of the other two groups; they also reported using more denial. It seems likely that these defenses contribute to the parents' abusive behavior in that the defenses produce a distorted view of the child's behavior. As a result of using projection, hostile intentions are attributed to the child and then retaliated against by the parent, and the negative consequences of this retaliatory behavior are then denied.

DEFENSES AND DEPRESSION

In addition to demonstrating the relation of defenses to DSM personality disorders and aggressive psychopathology, other research has focused on the role of defenses in dysphoria and depression. In three studies using the DSQ-88 to assess defense use, the Immature defense scale was found to predict level of depression, as assessed by the Beck Depression Inventory (BDI). The Mature defense scale was negatively related to depression, and the Neurotic scale was unrelated to depression (Kwon, 2000, 2002; Kwon & Lemon, 2000). Similar findings were obtained from a group of adult college students (mean age = 31 years; Flannery & Perry, 1990). The Immature (Maladaptive) scales of the DSQ (both DSQ-88 and DSQ-67) were positively related to scores on the BDI as well as to scores on the Taylor Manifest Anxiety Scale (Taylor, 1953).

In a large-scale population study of Canadians (*n* = 667), depression, as assessed by the self-report Center for Epidemiologic Studies—Depression scale (CES-D) (Radloff, 1977), has also been found to be related to immature defense use as assessed by the Q-sort Adaptive Defense Profile (ADP; MacGregor, Davidson, Rowan, et al., 2003). A similar result was found in a study of Canadian university students (*n* = 133). Immature defense use, as assessed by the ADP, was related to higher scores on the BDI (Davidson et al., 2004).

Finally, in two studies with the DMI as the defense measure, TAS was a positive predictor of depression (BDI) and PRN was a negative predictor (Kwon, 1999, 2000b).

DEFENSES AND OTHER INDICATIONS OF PATHOLOGY

In another study with a nonclinical sample of 350 people from the community (Muris & Merkelbach, 1996), the DSQ-36 was related to the SCL-90-R pathological symptom scales (Derogatis & O'Cleary, 1977) and to Eysenck's neuroticism scale (Eysenck 1998). The results indicated that the individual immature defenses of undoing, projection, acting out, devaluation, passive–aggression, and somatization were positively related to the total score on the SCL-90-R. With the exception of undoing, these relations were significant even when the contribution of neuroticism was partialled out. Among the mature defenses, only humor was (negatively) related to the measures of pathology.

Another study related measures of the Japanese translation of the DSQ-88 to measures of psychiatric symptoms on the Cornell Medical Index Questionnaire in a group of 270 Japanese university students: The Immature defense factor was positively related to symptoms of anxiety, depression, and impulsive anger; the neurotic factor was related to anxiety; and the mature defense factor was unrelated to any of these symptoms (Nishimura, 1998).

A further study of college students related their DSQ-36 responses to self-reported phobic tendencies (social phobia, agoraphobia, blood injury phobia; Muris & Merkelbach, 1996). The five immature defenses (projection, devaluation, undoing, acting out, and somatization) were positively related to social phobia, agoraphobia, and the total fear score. Two of the mature defenses (suppression, sublimation) were negatively related to these indications of pathology.

The relation between defense use and psychological pathology was also investigated in the core city sample of men (Soldz & Vaillant, 1998). In this study, rather than relating defense use to categories of personality disorder, as discussed earlier in this chapter (Vaillant, 1994; Vaillant & McCullough, 1998), the men were grouped into categories in terms of their defense use, and this grouping was related to life functioning. Two coders were given an extensive summary of interviews conducted with the men at age 47 years; each rated the use of 15 nonpsychotic defenses on a 3-point scale (defense absent; defense noted one or two times; defense noted three or more times or was most frequent). The ratings of the two coders were then combined. Subsequently, based on cluster analysis, five clusters of men were identified. One of these clusters included men who used mature defenses. Two clusters included men who used neurotic defenses; one of these was characterized by high use of all defenses, especially the use of "obsessive defenses of Isolation and Reaction formation" (Soldz & Vaillant, 1998, p. 107), as well as dissociation, displacement, and suppression. Men in the other neurotic cluster were characterized by low use of most defenses, with the exception of repression, displacement, and isolation. Two further clusters were characterized by men who used immature defenses. The first included men who relied on projection, fantasy, displacement, isolation, and reaction formation. The second consisted of men who used passive–aggression, acting out, dissociation/denial, and hypochondriasis.

Membership in the five clusters was found to be differentially related to a group of life variables that were also assessed from the interviews of the men at age 47. In general, the men in the mature defense cluster seemed to be functioning well in a broad range of domains, including positive mental health. Men in the two neurotic defense clusters functioned better than men in the immature clusters but not as well as those in the mature defense cluster. Men in the immature defense clusters evidenced a number of life problems; those in the second immature defense cluster were functioning the worst of all. This latter group exhibited the poorest global mental health, the greatest number of antisocial responses to stressful situations, were more likely to have a problem with alcohol, and occupied a lower social class at age 47 than men in the other clusters. At the time of interview, the men in both of the immature clusters had spent more time unemployed, indicated less job satisfaction, and were less likely to be in a lasting marriage than the men in the other three clusters. By age 60 years, men in the second immature defense cluster were medically evaluated as having the poorest physical health.

CONCLUDING REMARKS

Although the research reviewed in this chapter is based on nonclinical samples of students and community members, such samples provide clear indications that defense use is related to symptoms of psychopathology. Taking the view that psychopathology exists on a continuum from very little (normal) to extreme (psychiatric diagnosis), these findings demonstrate that both the degree and the type of defense used are related to the degree of pathology, at least within the normal to subclinical range. Whether this relation is also true at the more extreme levels of psychological disturbance (clinical psychopathology) is considered in the next chapter.

In any case, there is consistent evidence that defense use is concurrently associated with subclinical pathology. Number of psychopathological symptoms, depressive tendencies, and phobias are all correlated with the use of immature defenses; depression and phobias are also negatively related to the use of mature defenses. Further, there is evidence that different types of personality disorder are related to different types of defenses, and that there is a congruence between developmental level of pathology and developmental level of defense.

Defense use has also been found to be related to pathological aggression; this relation depends on the object of the violent behavior. As compared to nonviolent men, male college students who reported engaging in violence toward strangers were more likely to use denial. In contrast, the use of projection was associated with violence toward partners. Use of the more mature defense of identification was negatively related to both stranger and partner violence. Consistent with these results are the findings that child-abusing parents are more likely to use the defenses of projection and denial. One way to understand these connections between defense use and violent behavior is to assume that the use of these immature defenses distorts the aggressor's view of the victim, first, by mistakenly attributing hostile intentions to the victim through projection, especially when the victim is known to the aggressor, and second, by not recognizing (denying) the pain and suffering caused to the victim. The effect of the combination of these defenses then "justifies" the aggressor's violent behavior.

In all of these studies demonstrating the relation between defense use and pathology, an important, but unanswered question remains: Is it the presence of pathology that results in the use of particular defenses, or is it the continuing use of maladaptive defenses that eventually results in the occurrence of pathological symptoms (cf. Maffei et al., 1995)? An understanding of the relation between pathology and defense use requires longitudinal research.

CHAPTER 12

Defenses and Psychopathology in Adult Psychiatric Patients[1]

*I*n the previous chapter we saw that indications of psychopathology in nonpatients were related to their use of defense mechanisms. In this chapter I consider three related questions:

1. Does defense use by psychiatric patients differ from that of non-patients?
2. Can defense use differentiate among different diagnostic groups?
3. Are specific defenses associated with specific diagnoses?

The answers to these questions may depend, to some extent, on the defense measures used. We begin by considering studies in which defenses were assessed using the DMM.

PSYCHOPATHOLOGY AND THE DMM

One of the first investigations using the DMM to study defense mechanisms was conducted with a group of seriously disturbed hospitalized psychiatric patients from the Austen Riggs Center in Stockbridge, Massachusetts. As part of an intensive study of the effects of psychoanalytically oriented psychotherapy (Blatt & Ford, 1994), TAT protocols were available from the time the patients entered the hospital and again after 15 months of treatment. This information was available for 90 patients, most of whom were diagnosed as having either psychotic or borderline personality disorder (BPD).

The "before" and "after" stories were DMM coded for the use of the three defenses of denial, projection, and identification, making it possible to relate defense use to diagnosis and to other aspects of the patients' functioning (Cramer, Blatt, & Ford, 1988). In addition, as is discussed in Chapter 13, change in defense use was determined after a period of treatment.

The results showed that, on admission to the hospital, patients with a diagnosis of psychosis were higher in total defense use than were the patients with BPD ($p < .005$). In particular, the patients with psychosis made greater use of the defense of denial; they also tended to use more projection and identification (Cramer, 1999a) (see Figure 12.1). What is striking here is that severity of pathology is related to intensity of defense use, especially the use of the immature defense of denial.

The 90 patients in the Riggs study were also clinically assessed for their characteristic personality organization to determine if they were primarily anaclitic or introjective (Blatt, 1990).[2] The anaclitic personality is characterized by a concern with interpersonal relatedness, dependency, and communion with others. In contrast, the introjective personality is characterized by a concern with self-definition, separateness, and agency. When the anaclitic and introjective groups were compared for the use of DMM denial, projection, and identification, they did not differ significantly. Contrary to expectation,[3] there was a tendency for anaclitic patients to use identification to a greater degree than the introjective patients.

The most interesting finding, however, was that the relation between defense use and pathology differed for the two groups. For the anaclitic group, the use of defenses was significantly associated with a number of clinical symptoms, as assessed by the Strauss–Harder Clinical Symptom Scales (Strauss & Harder, 1981). Anaclitic patients who used denial had more bizarre–disorganized symptoms, more bizarre–retarded symptoms and poorer interpersonal relations, although their perception of others was more likely to be benevolent. Their high scores on projection were also related to poor interpersonal relations but not to bizarre symptoms or benevolent perception of others. In contrast, the use of identification by anaclitic patients predicted fewer interpersonal problems and fewer psychotic symptoms. For the introjective group, the use of identification was positively associated with perceptions of others as malevolent and destructive (Cramer et al., 1988). Thus the use of defenses by these two groups had different implications for their psychological functioning.

Initially, we were surprised that the anaclitic and introjective groups did not differ in their use of the three defenses, as we had expected from theory. Further consideration raised the possibility that some factor other than diagnosis (such as gender) may have clouded the differences. Concep-

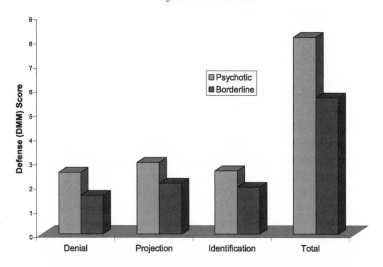

FIGURE 12.1. Defense use by psychotic and borderline patients.

tually, many of the features defining the anaclitic personality are similar to cultural conceptions of femininity—and, indeed, the largest number of individuals meeting the anaclitic criteria are females. Likewise, the features defining the introjective personality are similar to the cultural conception of masculinity—and the largest number of individuals meeting the introjective criteria are males. There is, then, a gender congruency, both theoretically and empirically, between *anaclitic* and *female*, on the one hand, and *introjective* and *male*, on the other.

In the clinical population of the Riggs study, as expected, the majority of the females were assessed as anaclitic, and the majority of the males were assessed as introjective. However, there were also patients who might be described as gender incongruent—anaclitic males, and introjective females (Cramer & Blatt, 1993). For these individuals, their central identification—that is, their identity—was culturally incongruent with their biological gender. We expected that this incongruence might be a source of inner conflict and, as such, would intensify the use of defense mechanisms.

We know from other research that defense use is related to gender and gender orientation (see Chapter 9). Denial is more characteristic of women and is associated with a feminine orientation, whereas projection is more characteristic of men and is associated with a masculine orientation, at least in men. In this case, the gender-congruent anaclitic women should use the expected defense of denial, and the introjective men the expected defense of projection. However, the gender-incongruent patients (anaclitic men and introjective women) might not show the expected use of defenses.

That is, an interaction between gender and personality organization might cloud the defense results when only personality organization is considered.

To investigate this possibility, the four patient groups (male/female × anaclitic/introjective) were compared for defense use at the time they entered the hospital (see Figure 12.2). Looking first at the gender-incongruent patients, we see that anaclitic males had a significantly higher level of defense use than the (gender-congruent) introjective males ($p < .06$); likewise, the introjective females had a significantly higher level of defense use than the (gender-congruent) anaclitic females ($p < .02$). This higher level of defense use in the gender-incongruent patients was due both to their higher scores for projection and to their greater use of the defense of identification— that is, the defense that is closely linked to the development of identity. These results demonstrate that in this patient group, it is not personality organization, per se, that is related to defense use; rather, it is an incongruent match between personality and gender that accounts for the greater use of defenses. Further, the results suggest that the use of the defense of identification by highly disturbed patients was associated with their psychological conflict around gender identity.

The Riggs study was important for two reasons: (1) it demonstrated the usefulness of the DMM approach for studying clinical patients, and (2) it supported the idea of a developmental hierarchy of defenses. As has been shown in previous studies of children with different levels of chronological maturity (see Chapter 2), this hospital study demonstrated that those pa-

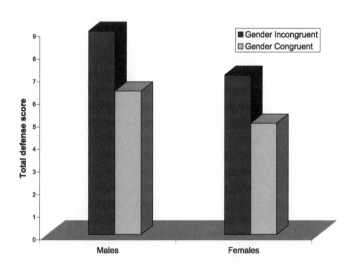

FIGURE 12.2. Total defense use on entrance to hospital. From Cramer (1999a); reprinted with permission from Lawrence Erlbaum Associates, Inc.

tients at the lowest level of psychological functioning—the psychotic patients—made greater use of the immature defense of denial. Further, this study demonstrated a relation between the level of defense use and the level of pathological symptoms. Use of the lowest-level defense of denial predicted the presence of bizarre pathological symptoms and problematic interpersonal behavior. The somewhat more mature defense of projection predicted interpersonal problems but not low-level, bizarre symptoms. The most mature defense, identification, was predictive of fewer psychological symptoms, but was found to be especially associated with problems of gender-incongruent personality organization.

A second investigation of hospitalized psychiatric patients with a variety of diagnoses (including schizophrenia, major depression, posttraumatic stress disorder, and personality disorders) used the DMM to assess defense use and yielded results highly similar to those of the Riggs study (Hibbard et al., 1994). In this research, VA patients' use of defenses was contrasted with that of college students from Tennessee (Hibbard et al., 1994). It was expected that the patients would make greater use of the lower-level defenses of denial and projection, whereas the college students would show greater use of the more mature defense of identification. In fact, as can be seen in Figure 12.3, the psychiatric patients (Patients-2) did score higher on denial and projection than the students (College-2), although the differences were not statistically significant. However, the patients' scores on identification were significantly lower than the college students' $(p < .02)$.

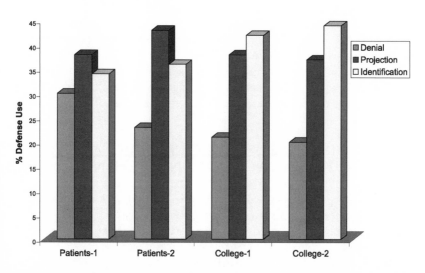

FIGURE 12.3. Defense use in two studies of psychiatric patients and college students.

Subsequently, I compared Hibbard et al.'s (1994) data with my own from the Riggs patients (Patients-1) and from Massachusetts college students (College-1). As may be seen in Figure 12.3, the results are highly similar. In both studies the psychiatric patients score relatively higher on denial, whereas the college students score higher on the mature defense of identification. The somewhat higher score on denial for the Riggs patients may reflect the fact that this sample included *all* patients admitted to the hospital, whereas the Hibbard study relied on patients who agreed to volunteer for the study; these patients may have been less psychologically disturbed and, in turn, less prone to use such a primitive defense as denial. Despite this difference, the overall similarity between the two sets of data—based on different patients and different college samples and collected and coded by two different examiners—is quite striking.

An additional study demonstrating the relation between DMM defense use and the diagnosis of paranoia is discussed below.

FURTHER STUDIES OF DEFENSE USE
BY PSYCHIATRIC PATIENTS

In addition to the two studies using the DMM just described, there have been numerous other investigations of the use of defense mechanisms by psychiatric patients. Most of these studies rely either on the DSQ or the DMRS to assess defense use. Some of these studies focus on the question of whether patients from broad diagnostic categories (e.g., neurotic, personality disorder) differ in defense use from nonpatients. Others focus on differences in defense use by patients in discrete diagnostic categories (e.g., panic disorder, BPD). Although some studies contain both types of comparisons, the report below first examines the comparison of patients (various diagnostic categories) with nonpatients. This is followed by investigations that focus on specific diagnostic categories, including paranoia, personality disorders, anxiety disorders, mood disorders, and others.

DOES DEFENSE USE BY PSYCHIATRIC PATIENTS
DIFFER FROM THAT OF NONPATIENTS?

To answer this question, we consider a series of studies that compared psychiatric patients with nonpatient controls. The assessment of defense use in these studies has been based on various versions of the DSQ (DSQ-88, DSQ-81, DSQ-72, DSQ-40, DSQ-36), with different versions sometimes yielding different defense factor scales, especially when patient characteristics differ. Nevertheless, there are consistent findings showing differences between patients and controls.

Patients scored higher on the Immature defense scale and lower on the Mature scale, as compared to controls (Bond, 1992; Bond & Vaillant, 1986; Sammallahti & Aalberg, 1995; Sammallahti, Aalberg, & Pentinsaari, 1994; Simeon, Guralnik, Knutelska, & Schmeidler, 2002). Findings for the Neurotic scale differ. Some studies find no difference between patients and controls (Sammallahti & Aalberg, 1995; Sammallahti et al., 1994), whereas others report that patients have higher scores on the Neurotic scale (Andrews, Pollock, & Stewart, 1989; Simeon et al., 2002). This difference may be due to the different composition of the patient groups in the various studies. In the Simeon et al. (2002) study, all patients were diagnosed with depersonalization disorder, and in the Andrews et al. (1989) investigation, only patients in certain subcategories of anxiety disorders differed from those in the control group.

A comparison of the patients with panic disorder, agoraphobia, social phobia, and obsessive–compulsive disorder (OCD) with individuals in the control group indicated that patients in the panic disorder group did not differ from those in the control group for DSQ-36 defense use. Patients with agoraphobia or OCD scored significantly higher on the "Neurotic" factor then did the controls. Patients with social phobia or OCD scored significantly higher on the "Immature" factor and lower on the "Mature" factor than those in the control group (Andrews et al., 1989).

Further study of the Andrews et al. (1989) defense data examined scores on the individual defense scales and contrasted the separate categories of anxiety disorders—panic disorder (with or without agoraphobia; $n = 78$), social phobia ($n = 23$), and OCD ($n = 18$)—with 204 individuals of similar age from the general population (Pollock & Andrews, 1989). As compared to those in the control group, patients with panic disorder used more displacement, somatization, reaction formation, and idealization; patients with social phobia used more displacement and devaluation and less humor; patients with OCD used more undoing, projection, and acting out, and less humor.

In a subsequent study the DSQ-72 responses of these patients were used, along with others, to construct a shortened DSQ-40 (Andrews et al., 1993; see Chapter 16). As with the DSQ-72, the new version indicated that the group of patients with anxiety disorders ($n = 200$), as compared to those in the control group ($n = 388$), were more likely to endorse the neurotic defense of reaction formation and the immature defenses of projection, displacement, somatization, and devaluation. They were also less likely to endorse the mature defenses of humor, suppression, and sublimation.

CAN DEFENSE USE DIFFERENTIATE
AMONG DIAGNOSTIC GROUPS?

Several studies have investigated the use of defenses by people in specific diagnostic groups to determine whether specific defenses are associated with specific diagnostic entities. The question being asked in these studies is not how patients differ from controls but how patients from different diagnostic groups differ in their use of defenses.

Why might defense use and diagnosis be related? Different explanations with alternative orderings of causal events are possible. In one explanation the psychological disturbance develops first, and the defense is then brought into play to compensate for, or reduce, the upset caused by it. In this case, the nature of the psychological disturbance is responsible for the type of defense that is engaged to protect the self against that disturbance. This explanation fits well with theories that focus on disorders as products of biological factors.

A different explanation focuses on the defense as primary and the disorder—that is, the symptoms that are used to diagnose the disorder—as the result of using the maladaptive defense. This idea has been a part of psychoanalytic theory for a long time. For example, A. Freud wrote that neurotic symptoms are the result of an "unvarying use of a special form of defense" (1936, p. 34). In the psychoanalytic model the functioning of a particular defense produces the symptoms that define the diagnosis.

Yet a third explanation derives from self psychology (Kohut, 1977). Here the problems or weaknesses in the underlying self-structure are seen as responsible for the psychological disturbance. At the same time, and as a parallel development, defense mechanisms function both to conceal this disturbance and to protect the self. Consistent with this theory is the idea that the defense mechanisms used would be those available at the period of development during which the psychological disturbance began. Thus disturbances hypothesized to begin very early in life (BPD, narcissistic personality disorder) would be associated with very primitive defenses (e.g., splitting, primitive idealization), whereas those beginning later—for example, paranoia—would be associated with more advanced defenses such as projection.

In any case, whatever the causal relationship between defense use and type of psychological disorder, the theories agree that different defenses can be expected to be related to different disorders. As expressed by Laplanche and Pontalis, "Which of the [defense] mechanisms predominate in a given case depends on the type of illness [diagnosis] under consideration" (1973, p. 109).

In this section of the chapter I consider the empirical evidence for the association between specific defenses and specific diagnoses. I am not suggesting that diagnosis could be made solely on the basis of knowledge of defenses. Yet it is possible that differential defense use should be a critical component of diagnostic decision making.

Paranoia

The use of projection is associated with the diagnosis of paranoia both theoretically and diagnostically. The paranoid patient's unrealistic expectation of danger and harm from the environment is understood to be a result of the attribution of his or her own hostility or other personally unacceptable impulses onto others, who are then feared. To test this formulation, Worth (1998) used the DMM to assess the use of projection by paranoid and nonparanoid psychiatric patients. In a carefully controlled study, the archival records of a large inner-city hospital provided MMPI scores from male in- and outpatients. Men with Minnesota Multiphasic Personality Inventory (MMPI) Scale 6 *T*-scores of 70 or above constituted the paranoid patient group (*n* = 26); those with *T*-scores of 69 or below formed the nonparanoid patient group (*n* = 27). The two groups were highly similar for age, education, and IQ. They were also determined to adequately represent the larger population of patients from which they were drawn.

Existing TAT stories for these patients were coded for projection (DMM) by two raters who were unaware of the patients' diagnoses or other information. The results indicated that projection was significantly more frequent in the paranoid than in the nonparanoid group (*p* < .01). Further, the paranoid patients had higher scores for all seven subcategories of DMM projection, and they were especially likely to use the immature forms of the defense.

Personality Disorders

A Finnish study (Sammallahti et al., 1994) compared patients with personality disorder (*n* = 59) with patients with neurosis (*n* = 42) for their scores on the four defense factors of the DSQ-88. Testing the parallelism of the profiles of the two patient groups revealed significant differences. Notably, patients with personality disorders had higher scores on the Immature (Borderline) scale.

In another Finnish study (Sammallahti & Aalberg, 1995), a comparison of people with personality disorders (*n* = 31) and those with neurosis (*n* = 42) also indicated that the two clinical groups differed only on the Borderline factor scale; patients with personality disorders scored higher than patients with neurosis (Sammallahti & Aalberg, 1995). Looking more closely at the Borderline factor scale, it was the Omnipotence/ Devaluation and Projective Identification subscales that were responsible for the difference between the patient groups. The two groups did not differ on the Mature, Neurotic, or Immature defense scales.

In contrast, other early attempts to differentiate among diagnoses, and especially to differentiate patients with BPD from other patients on the basis of defense use (DSQ), were largely unsuccessful (Bond, 1990; Bond & Vaillant, 1986; Bond et al., 1989; Perry & Cooper, 1986).

In an early study by Perry and Cooper (1986) of 81 patients with BPD, antisocial personality disorder, or bipolar Type II affective disorder, the DMRS was used to assess five summary defense scales: Action, Borderline, Disavowal, Narcissistic, and Obsessional. These summary defense scales did not significantly discriminate among the three diagnostic groups. However, the defenses did show a differential pattern of relations with the different diagnostic scale scores. There was a marginally significant correlation between the borderline personality disorder scale and the Action and Borderline defense scales (Immature: DMRS levels 1 and 2). Also, the number of antisocial personality disorder symptoms was found to correlate with the Disavowal and Narcissistic defense scales (Immature: DMRS levels 3 and 4), whereas the bipolar II symptom scores were found to correlate with the Obsessional (Neurotic: DMRS level 5)[4] defenses.

A study by Bond and Vaillant (1986) using the DSQ-81 also attempted to demonstrate different defense use by the different diagnostic groups of personality disorder, psychosis, major affective disorder, and anxiety. However, there was no definitive relationship between diagnosis and defense use, nor could defense use predict diagnostic category. The exception to these findings was with the affective disorder group, who, like the control group, used "adaptive" defenses more than the other three defense styles.

Another attempt to relate diagnosis to a revised DSQ-88 measure of defenses, which may have included some of the previous study's patients, was equally unsuccessful (Bond, Perry, Gautier et al., 1989). Defense use did not differentiate among diagnoses of personality disorder ($n = 27$), psychosis ($n = 8$), major affective disorder ($n = 25$), dysthymia ($n = 22$), anxiety ($n = 27$), or adjustment disorder ($n = 32$). Further, the DMRS measure of defenses also did not differentiate among these diagnostic groups.

An additional investigation of the patients with personality disorders from these two studies (i.e., Bond & Vaillant, 1986; Bond et al., 1989) was conducted to determine if those with a BPD could be distinguished from the other personality disorders by the defenses that they use (Bond, 1990). From theory (Kernberg, 1967), it would be predicted that the patients with BPD would use image-distorting defenses (splitting, projective identification, omnipotence/devaluation, and primitive idealization) more often than would people with the other personality disorders. However, a comparison of the two groups indicated no difference in DSQ-88 defense use. Indeed, if a BPD underlies the other personality disorders (see Chapter 11), then we would expect to find similarities in the defense use of all people with personality disorders.

Nevertheless, in the second study (Bond et al., 1989), when the DMRS was used to assess defense use, the six patients with BPD scored higher on the Immature and Image-Distorting defense scales, as compared to patients with other personality disorders. In another very small sample of patients with personality disorders, a DMRS assessment of defenses used during five consecutive sessions at the initial stage of therapy revealed differences between six patients with BPD and five patients without BPD (Perry, 2001). The patients with BPD had a greater percentage of low-level "action" defenses and, to a lesser extent, "major image-distorting" defenses (the two lowest levels of defense in the DMRS hierarchy).

The only study that showed the DSQ to differentiate between BPD and other psychiatric diagnoses was conducted with a larger sample from outpatient clinics, using a diagnostic interview especially devised for the diagnosis of BPD (Bond, Paris, & Zweig-Frank, 1994). Seventy-nine women with BPD were compared with 72 women who were patients but did not have BPD. Using the DSQ-88, the patients with BPD were found to use more "maladaptive" and more "image-distorting" defenses than the patients without BPD. In contrast, the latter group used more "adaptive" defenses. The authors suggested that their success in differentiating patients with BPD from other patients, in contrast to the earlier studies, resulted from using a larger patient sample and a better method of assessing BPD.

A different approach for determining the relation between DSQ defenses and diagnosis was used by Soldz et al. (1995) with a group of psychiatric outpatients. Rather than asking if the different diagnostic groups use different defenses, the investigators determined if different defense use predicted different disorders. Using the DSQ-88, the three scales resulting from a factor analysis of this group (Mature, Immature, and Withdrawal defenses) were entered into a regression analysis to predict each of 13 personality disorder diagnoses, as determined from a structured clinical interview. The results indicated that the Immature defense scale predicted borderline, paranoid, narcissistic, histrionic, dependent, passive–aggressive, and self-defeating personality disorders. The Withdrawal scale scores positively predicted schizoid, schizotypal, avoidant, and obsessive–compulsive personality disorders and were a negative predictor of histrionic personality disorder. The mature defenses did not predict any of the individual personality disorders.

The authors noted that because defenses are also related to the Big Five personality traits (see Chapter 8), and these Big Five traits are related to pathology, the defense–pathology connection might be due to standing on these traits. To investigate this possibility, the effect of the Big Five variables was statistically controlled; the results indicated that the relations between defense and diagnosis were generally unchanged. Thus, despite the overlap between defense style and Big Five personality traits, the authors concluded that defense style makes a unique contribution to understanding psychopathology, beyond that provided by the Big Five model.

Two further studies focused on the question of whether defense use predicts personality disorders. In one, 55 psychiatric inpatients with mixed DSM-IV Axis I disorders were assessed for the presence of an Axis II personality disorder on the basis of the Structured Interview for the DSM-IV (Pfohl, Blum, & Zimmerman, 1994). Diagnostic criteria were rated on a 4-point scale and then added together to give a score for each personality disorder. Of the group, 66% satisfied at least one criterion for at least one personality disorder. Defense use was assessed with the DSQ-40. Subsequent analyses indicated that the Immature defense scale predicted the BPD diagnosis on the basis of the defenses of displacement and acting out (Devens & Erickson, 1998).

The second study, with 50 outpatients who were seeking treatment, used the same method to assess the presence of a personality disorder (Lingiardi et al., 1999). Personality disorder diagnosis was then related to defense use, as assessed by the DMRS. The histrionic diagnosis was related to the narcissistic defense level (especially to the defenses of idealization and omnipotence) and to the borderline level (especially splitting), as well as to the individual defenses of acting out and affiliation. The antisocial diagnosis was related to the action level (especially acting out) and to the individual defenses of projection and intellectualization. The borderline diagnosis was related to the action level (especially acting out). The narcissistic diagnosis was related to the individual defense of acting out.

Although both of these two studies show correlations between personality disorder diagnoses and differential defense use, it is important to note that the correlations are driven by the inclusion of individuals with no personality disorder diagnosis—that is, by what might be considered a nondisorder control group. For this reason, the results primarily show that persons with a disorder have higher defense scores than those without a disorder.

In one final study showing the relation of personality disorder and defense use, a large sample of patients with eating disorders ($n = 114$) was studied by Bulik, Sullivan, Carter, and Joyce (1997). Half of these women, ages 17–45, were also alcohol dependent, and those who were alcohol dependent were more likely to be diagnosed with a comorbid personality disorder. This latter group had higher scores on the DSQ-88 Immature scale than did the nonalcohol-dependent patients with bulimia. The two groups did not differ on the Neurotic and Mature scales.

Anxiety Disorders

Several other investigations have focused on the relation between anxiety disorders and defense use. One question is whether the different types of anxiety disorders can be differentiated from each other on the basis of the use of different defenses.

For example, patients with (DSM-III-R) anxiety disorders (panic disorder, social phobia, or OCD) were compared for defense use (Pollock & Andrews, 1989). Profile analyses of DSQ-88 defense use by the different anxiety groups significantly differentiated the patients with panic disorder from patients with social phobia or OCD and also differentiated between patients with a social phobia and those with OCD. Patients with panic disorder were more likely to use displacement, reaction formation, and somatization; patients with social phobia used devaluation and displacement; and those with OCD used undoing, acting out, and projection.

However, in a subsequent study (Andrews et al., 1993), using either the new DSQ-40 or the new DSQ-72 (in which two items specifically focused on anxiety symptoms were removed), the different anxiety disorders (panic/agoraphobia, social phobia, and obsessive–compulsive) did not differ significantly from each other.

Patients with panic disorder have also been contrasted with patients diagnosed with dysthymia. In one study using the DSQ-36 to assess defense use, the patients with panic disorder were found to use different defenses than patients with dysthymia and to differ from patients without a psychiatric diagnosis (Spinhoven & Kooiman, 1997). Specifically, the patients with panic disorder ($n = 47$) had higher scores on the Immature and Neurotic scales and higher scores on the individual defense scale of Idealization.

The use of defenses by patients with panic disorder ($n = 22$) and patients with (DSM-III-R) dysthymia ($n = 22$) was also studied using the DMRS (Bloch, Shear, Markowitz, Leon, & Perry, 1993; Busch et al., 1995). The two patient groups were comparable for age, gender distribution, race, and education. The authors reported that patients with panic disorder did not score higher than patients with dysthymia on any of the seven defense levels of the DMRS (Busch et al., 1995). However, as reported in Bloch et al. (1993; see below), they did score significantly lower on several scales. Also, patients with panic disorder made greater use of reaction formation and undoing.

Mood Disorders and Depression

A further comparison of DMRS defense use of the Dysthymic and Panic Disorder patients (Bloch et al., 1993; Busch et al., 1995) indicated that patients with dysthymia had higher DMRS scores on the Action, Disavowal, and Narcissistic defense scales (levels 1, 3, and 4). Specifically, they used more projection, projective identification, devaluation, acting out, passive–aggression, and hypochondriasis. Bloch et al. (1993) also reported that a post-hoc analysis of the data from Perry and Cooper (1986) indicated that patients diagnosed with chronic depression were characterized by the DMRS use of devaluation, passive–aggression, and hypochondriasis.

DSQ-40 defense use has been related to number of depressive episodes and number of suicide attempts in a group of hospitalized patients with a diagnosis of major depressive disorder (n = 77; Corruble et al., 2003). Patients with recurrent episodes had higher scores on the Immature defense scale, as compared to those with single episodes. Although the number of suicide attempts was not significantly different between the personality-disorder and no-personality-disorder groups, the relation of defense use to number of suicide attempts depended on the presence of a comorbid personality disorder. For patients with a personality disorder, the number of lifetime suicide attempts was correlated with the Neurotic scale scores, especially the defense of undoing; scores on the Immature and Mature defense scales were unrelated to number of suicide attempts. For patients without a personality disorder, the number of suicide attempts was correlated with scores on the Immature scale, especially projection, passive–aggression, somatization, acting out, and splitting; scores on the Neurotic and Mature scales were unrelated to suicide attempts. In addition, patients who were diagnosed with a personality disorder had lower scores on the Mature defense scale than those without a personality disorder (Corruble et al., 2003).

Suicidal patients' use of defenses has also been contrasted with that of nonsuicidal patients (Apter et al., 1989). Thirty patients who had been admitted to the hospital following a suicide attempt were compared to 30 nonsuicidal patients hospitalized for other psychiatric reasons. The suicidal patients represented a variety of diagnostic categories; the nonsuicidal patients were matched with them for sex, age, and diagnosis, including affective disorder, personality disorder, or schizophrenic spectrum disorder. Defense use was assessed from the eight defense scales of the Life Style Index (Plutchik, Kellerman, & Conte, 1979). The results indicated that the suicidal patients scored significantly higher on the defense of regression. All patients were also assessed for suicidal risk using a self-report scale; this measure was found to be positively related to the use of regression and displacement and negatively related to denial.

Continuing study of these 60 patients while they were in the hospital indicated that 20 became violent toward a staff member or fellow patient. A comparison of this violent group with the remaining nonviolent patients indicated that the former scored higher on displacement and lower on reaction formation. All patients were also assessed for risk of violence using a self-report scale. Risk of violence was found to be positively related to the defenses of regression, displacement, and compensation and negatively related to repression.

An interesting question was raised in a study of hospitalized adults (ages 18–45) with a diagnosis of major depressive disorder; the DMI was used to assess defense use. The central question the investigators examined was whether depressed patients are more pessimistic and thus more likely to use the defense of turning against the self (TAS), or whether nondepressed normals are more likely to be overly optimistic, which the investigators believed would be demonstrated by their greater use of reversal (REV) and principalization (PRN) (Margo, Greenberg, Fisher, & Dewan, 1993). Patient scores were compared with the mean scores of contrast groups constructed from previous studies. For females, the contrast mean was based on the original DMI publication (Gleser & Ihilevich, 1969); for males, the contrast mean came from an unpublished dissertation (Gladstone, 1976). As compared to the previous DMI mean scores, both men and women in the depressed patient group had lower scores for REV and PRN. Also, within the patient group, scores on the Beck Depression Inventory (BDI) were negatively related to REV and PRN. On the other hand, the choice of TAS by the male patients with depression and of turning against the object (TAO) by the female patients with depression was greater than that of the contrast group male or female mean. The choice of TAS by patients was also positively related to BDI scores.

Apart from the rather serious problem of the choice of contrast groups, there is also an interesting issue to consider regarding the meaning of lower PRN and REV scores among patients with depression. Although the authors concluded from these findings that nondepressed people maintain their psychological health by being overly optimistic (REV, PRN), similar to the idea that denial promotes mental health (cf. Taylor & Armor, 1996), an equally plausible interpretation is that patients with depression are unduly pessimistic. Indeed, looking at the reported means for the depressed group, this latter interpretation seems likely. The mean REV score for patients with depression (both men and women) ranks fifth (i.e., the lowest) of their five defense scores. However, the mean REV scores of the contrast groups are not noticeably high; out of the five defenses, REV ranks third (women) or fourth (men) as a defense choice. This analysis does not suggest that the contrast groups rely excessively on REV as a defense.

ARE SPECIFIC DEFENSES ASSOCIATED WITH SPECIFIC DIAGNOSES?

A final question to be raised in this chapter, which focuses on the use of defenses by patients with diagnosed psychopathology, is whether defense use is related to different pathological symptoms. At the beginning of the chapter, I presented evidence that the use of denial, projection, and identification was differentially related to the presence of particular clinical symptoms (see p. 238). Distinct relations between particular DMRS defense styles and symptoms have also been reported for a group of psychiatric patients with a diagnosis of BPD, antisocial personality disorder, or bipolar type II affective disorder (Perry & Cooper, 1989). The patients were rated over a period of 1 year by observers for the presence of depressive, anxious, and antisocial symptoms; they also provided self-ratings for depression and anxiety. Action and Borderline defense scales (Immature: levels 1 and 2) were found to be positively related to observer- and self-rated symptom scales of depression and anxiety. The relations between the Disavowal defense scale (level 3) and symptoms differed depending on whether the symptoms were observer- or self-rated. When symptoms of depression and anxiety were rated by observers, there was a positive correlation between symptom scores and Disavowal scores. In contrast, when the symptom scores were based on self-ratings, there was no correlation with the Disavowal scale. The Narcissistic defense scale (level 4) was correlated only with the observer-rated antisocial symptoms. Finally, the Obsessional defense scale (level 5) was negatively correlated with observer- and self-reported measures of depression and anxiety.

In another study of this group of patients, 52 individuals diagnosed with BPD, antisocial personality disorder, or bipolar type II affective disorder were followed for 1 year, during which time they were periodically assessed for defense use (DMRS), life stresses, psychotic symptoms, and depression (Perry, 1988). Examining the relation between defense use and pathology, the results indicated that the Action defense scale (Immature: level 1) and the Borderline scale (Immature: level 2) were correlated with an increase in depressive symptoms but not with a major depressive episode. The use of borderline defenses was also related to the occurrence of psychotic symptoms, as was the individual defense of "bland denial." In contrast, the use of narcissistic defenses (level 4) was *negatively* related to the occurrence of a major depressive episode. The author suggested that both borderline and action defenses may make an individual vulnerable to an increase in chronically existing depressive symptoms, but these defenses are not associated with higher rates of acute major depressive episodes. Narcissistic defenses, on the other hand, may provide a protective effect against such episodes.

Another group of 50 outpatients with mixed DSM-IV Axis II personality disorder diagnoses were assessed for defense use with the DMRS and for psychiatric symptoms with the SCL-40 (Lingiardi et al., 1999) prior to the beginning of therapy. The action defenses correlated with nearly all of the symptom scales. The borderline defenses, and especially splitting, correlated with the scales for depression, anxiety, paranoid ideation, and psychoticism.

Defense use, as assessed by the DMRS, was also related to adequacy of psychological functioning, as clinically rated by the Global Assessment Scale (GAS), in a patient group that included individuals who were diagnosed with BPD, antisocial personality disorder, or bipolar type II affective disorder (n = 76; Perry & Cooper, 1989). All diagnostic categories were combined into a single group. This analysis indicated that the action defenses (Immature: level 1) and the borderline defenses (Immature: level 2) of the patient group predicted low scores on the GAS, whereas the obsessional (DMRS level 6) defenses predicted high GAS scores.

This finding was repeated with the group of 50 outpatients mentioned above (Lingiardi et al., 1999). Scores on the GAF were negatively related to action defense scores and positively related to obsessional defense scores.

CONCLUDING REMARKS

The research evidence is consistent in showing that patients differ from nonpatients in their use of defense mechanisms. Regardless of the method used to assess defenses, patients as a group show greater use of immature defenses and less use of mature defenses. Patients in individual diagnostic categories, however, may differ from nonpatients at only one level of defense (i.e., immature, neurotic, or mature). These findings, showing that the presence of pathology is related to greater use of immature defenses and less use of mature defenses, are consistent with the results obtained from nonpatient samples (see Chapter 11).

The findings are less clear, however, as to whether diagnostic categories can be differentiated by patients' use of defenses. Although there are theoretical reasons to expect such differentiations to occur, the research findings are inconsistent. Attempts to demonstrate differences in DSQ defense use by BPD patients, as compared to patients with other personality disorders, have generally been unsuccessful. This outcome may reflect the salient position of BPD at the basis of all personality disorders (see Chapter 11). Alternatively, the inconsistent results may be a function of the method used to assess defenses; two studies with the DMRS, although based on very small numbers of patients with BPD, have shown that they used more of the lowest-level defenses, as compared to patients with other personality disorders. However, it is also possible that the use of videotaped interviews to assess the DMRS defenses may produce a "halo" effect, such that the evidence of borderline pathology in the interview influences the rater to code defenses known to be characteristic of the borderline personality. Similarly, viewing a nonborderline patient may increase the coding of nonborderline defenses. As noted by Bond et al. (1989), this confounding of clinical information does not occur with the DSQ.

The method used to assess defenses has also been shown to produce different results in studies of patients with varying types of anxiety disorders. For example, the older version of the DSQ (DSQ-88) differentiated among subcategories of anxiety disorder, whereas the newer versions (DSQ-72, DSQ-40) did not. Similarly, the DSQ-36 showed that patients with panic disorder scored higher than patients with dysthymia on the Immature and Neurotic scales, whereas the DMRS did not show patients with panic disorder to score higher on any of its seven defense levels.

Finally, there is evidence that different types of defenses are related to different types of symptoms. Also, lower-level defenses are associated with a greater number of pathological indicators, whereas more mature defenses are associated with fewer symptoms. Significantly, these relations differ somewhat depending on whether it is an observer or the patient who reports on symptom presence.

Overall, then, although the use of defense mechanisms does differentiate between patients and nonpatients and does relate to symptom presence, there is no compelling evidence that diagnostic groups can be clearly differentiated by the use of defenses. In a positive light, this finding of virtually no relation between defense style and diagnosis has been taken as an indication that, because the two factors are independent, there is need for a new, separate DSM axis for defense mechanisms in addition to the diagnostic axis (Bond & Vaillant, 1986). In this case, defense assessment would not contribute to diagnosis but would facilitate therapeutic approach.

CHAPTER 13

Defenses and Psychotherapy

In the previous two chapters we have seen that indications of pathology and pathological symptoms are related to the use of several defense mechanisms or defense styles. The explanation of this relation is open to different interpretations, as discussed in Chapter 12. It may be, for example, that the use of immature defenses contributes to the development of pathology. On the other hand, it could be that the presence of psychopathology results in the use of immature defenses. Or, the use of particular defenses and the presence of pathology may both be the result of some third factor that is responsible for their covariation. Correlational studies cannot differentiate among these possibilities.

Nevertheless, given the defense–pathology relation, we might wonder how the experience of psychotherapy affects the use of defense mechanisms. If therapy reduces psychopathology, does it also change the use of defenses? If so, are these changes dependent on the type of pathology being treated? In this chapter, I review research studies that have focused on changes in defense use by psychiatric patients in conjunction with the experience of psychotherapy. The studies are grouped in terms of the method used to assess defense use. In the next chapter I consider individual case studies to examine in greater detail how defenses change.

RESEARCH WITH PSYCHIATRIC PATIENT GROUPS

As described in Chapter 12, one of the earliest studies using the DMM approach was conducted with 90 psychiatric patients from the Austen Riggs

Center. During their stay at the hospital, these seriously disturbed patients received psychoanalytically oriented psychotherapy. Most patients were diagnosed with psychosis ($n = 29$) or BPD ($n = 50$). There were extensive clinical case records, nursing reports, and other data available for the duration of patients' stay in the hospital. In addition, TAT stories and other projective test data were available for the patients as they entered the hospital and again after they had received 15 months of treatment. The TAT stories of each patient were coded for defense use at the time of entry to the hospital and after the 15 months of treatment. In addition, the presence of psychiatric symptoms and the capacity for interpersonal relatedness were assessed at both times.

As discussed in Chapter 12, on entrance to the hospital, the patients with psychosis made greater use of defenses, especially the defense of denial (see Figure 12.1). Strikingly, after 15 months of treatment, these patients showed a sharp decrease in total defense use.[1] As can be seen in Figure 13.1, this decrease was greatest for the defense of denial ($p < .02$); the use of projection and identification also decreased, but the difference was not statistically significant. A similar comparison for the patients with BPD indicated a slight decrease in projection and identification, but the differences were not significant.

Further, for the total group of patients ($n = 90$), the decrease in all three defenses following treatment was significantly associated with a re-

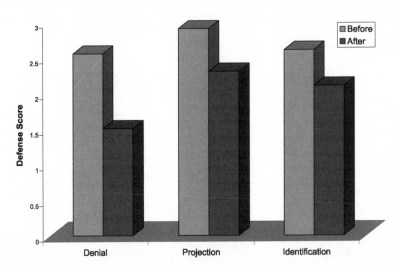

FIGURE 13.1. Defense use by psychotic patients before and after 15 months of treatment. From Cramer (1999a); reprinted with permission from Lawrence Erlbaum Associates, Inc.

duction in the occurrence of bizarre–disorganized pathological symptoms, as assessed by clinicians using the Straus–Harder Case Record Rating Scale (Strauss & Harder, 1981). This was true for both groups (psychosis and BPD) as well as for the remaining patients with other diagnoses. Notably, within each of these patient groups, the decrease in bizarre–disorganized symptoms was primarily due to a decrease in the use of denial. In addition, for patients with psychosis, a decrease in projection was associated with better interpersonal relationships.

The relation between defense use and change in the WAIS-IQ was also determined. At admission to the hospital, the use of identification among the patients with psychosis was negatively related to WAIS-IQ ($p < .05$). After 15 months of treatment, a decrease in the use of identification by these patients was associated with an increase in IQ.

Because previous studies of personality had demonstrated that defenses and IQ interact in predicting personality change (see Chapter 8), further study of the Riggs patients was undertaken to determine how IQ might interact with the use of defense mechanisms to predict change in pathology following treatment. This study focused on the 70 most seriously disturbed patients (diagnosed with psychosis or severe personality disorder), in whom clinical change was seen most clearly (Cramer, 2005). Regression analyses indicated that the interaction between defense change and IQ was a significant predictor of clinical change. For patients with lower IQs, a decrease in the use of defenses after 15 months of treatment predicted a decrease in symptom level and an increase in interpersonal functioning. Thus, for these patients, (1) a decrease in the use of identification predicted a decrease in neurotic symptoms, (2) a decrease in the use of projection predicted a decrease in bizarre–retarded symptoms, and (3) a decrease in denial predicted a decrease in impulsivity. Likewise, a decrease in identification and in projection both predicted an improvement in interpersonal functioning.

The corollary of this finding, however, is that an increase in defense use by patients with lower IQs predicted increased symptom manifestation. In turn, this finding suggests that for seriously disturbed individuals who have lower IQs, defenses function to support their pathological symptoms. This finding stands in contrast to the earlier studies of psychologically healthy individuals with lower IQs, for whom defenses functioned to support favorable personality characteristics (see Chapter 8). Taken together, these findings suggest that, for individuals with lower IQs, defenses function to maintain or strengthen the existing personality organization—an adaptive, positive organization in psychologically healthy individuals or a pathological organization in psychologically disturbed individuals. A decrease in the use of defenses among individuals with lower IQs will result in a decrease of positive traits in healthy individuals and a decrease of pathological symptoms in disturbed individuals.

For individuals with higher IQs, the reverse association between defense and symptom change was found. Midway through their treatment, an increase in defense use predicted decreased symptoms and more adequate interpersonal functioning. Thus (1) an increase in the use of identification predicted a decrease in neurotic symptoms and more adequate interpersonal functioning, (2) an increase in the use of projection predicted a decrease in bizarre–retarded symptoms and improved interpersonal functioning, and (3) an increase in denial predicted a decrease in impulsivity. This pattern suggested that for patients with higher IQs, defenses function to control or suppress manifestations of pathology.

COMPARISON OF MOST IMPROVED
AND LEAST IMPROVED PATIENTS

Another way of examining the data from this clinical sample is to compare those patients who were determined by clinical ratings to be most improved after 15 months of treatment ($n = 18$) with those determined to be least improved ($n = 13$). It was expected that the most improved patients would show the greatest decrease in defense use, especially primitive defense use. The results supported this prediction (see Figure 13.2). After treatment, the most improved patients showed the greatest decrease in their use of

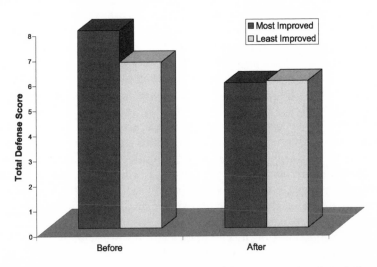

FIGURE 13.2. Defense use by most improved and least improved patients before and after treatment.

defenses, again due primarily to the significant decrease in the use of denial ($p < .05$).

COMPARISON OF ANACLITIC
AND INTROJECTIVE PATIENTS

It is also possible to examine these data through a different lens in order to investigate more complex aspects of personality and pathology. Here we consider the relation of defense use to two types of personality organization (Blatt, 1990). As described in Chapter 12, the anaclitic personality is characterized by a concern with interpersonal relatedness, dependence, and communion with others. In contrast, the introjective personality is characterized by a concern for self-definition, separateness, and agency. Accordingly, there is a gender congruence, both theoretically and empirically, between being female and the anaclitic personality organization, on the one hand, and between being male and the introjective personality organization, on the other. However, some patients were gender incongruent—anaclitic males, introjective females. For these individuals, their central identification— that is, their identity—is culturally incongruent with their biological gender.

As we saw in Chapter 12, this potential conflict intensified the use of defense mechanisms. On entrance to the hospital, both the male and female gender-incongruent patients ($n = 31$) showed a higher level of defense use than the gender-congruent patients ($n = 59$; $p < .007$). Strikingly, at this time, gender-incongruent patients used defenses that were consistent with the opposite gender. That is, anaclitic men tended to use more denial (statistically found to be more frequent among women), whereas introjective women used more projection (statistically found to be more frequent among men). However, after 15 months of treatment, the gender-incongruent patients shifted from gender-incongruent to gender-congruent defenses— that is, anaclitic men used more projection, and introjective women used more denial.

Also as discussed in Chapter 12, at admission to the hospital, gender-incongruent patients made greater use of identification—the defense that is closely linked to the development of identity (see Figure 13.3). It is interesting to see what happened with the defense of identification after 15 months of treatment. In the usual course of development, a growing boy will identify with other boys and men who are significant in his life, acquiring their masculine characteristics, and a girl will identify with girls and women and thus acquire feminine characteristics. However, the anaclitic boy or man has adopted defenses and other personality characteristics usually found in women, and the introjective girl or woman has adopted defenses and characteristics usually found in men. In these gender-incongruent patients there

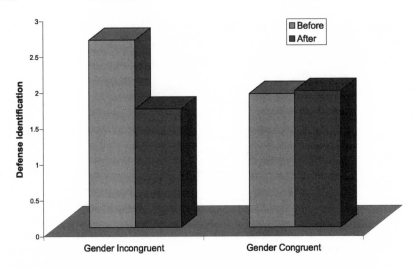

FIGURE 13.3. Gender-incongruent and gender-congruent patients before and after treatment.

is a tension or conflict between the nature of their personality organization and their biological sex. Under these circumstances, to maintain the conflicted identity and to manage attendant anxiety and protect self-esteem, identification is used as a defense. We expected that as the identity conflict was resolved, the use of identification would decrease. This prediction was confirmed. Using identification scores derived from stories told in response to the same TAT cards, Figure 13.3 shows that after treatment there is a highly significant ($p < .005$) decrease in the use of identification by the gender-incongruent patients, but no change for the congruent patients, with the result that now the two groups do not differ in the use of this defense. We may interpret the decrease in the defense of identification—the defense that had been closely associated with the gender-incongruent identity—to indicate that the conflict around the gender-incongruent personality organization was modified through treatment, so there was less need for the functioning of the defense.

Use of the other two defenses, denial and projection, also decreased in both patient groups after treatment, but only one change was statistically significant: There was a significant decrease in the use of denial among the gender-congruent patients ($p < .05$). Interestingly, the use of projection continued to be greater for the gender-incongruent patients than for the gender-congruent patients.

Further study of these patients demonstrated that their changes in defense use during treatment were related to changes in clinical symptomatology, interpersonal relations, and investment in object relationships. To summarize these results for gender-incongruent patients: (1) an *increase* in gender-congruent defenses was related to psychological improvement, and (2) a *decrease* in the defense of identification was related to better psychological functioning. Again, the implication of the use of the defense of identification by gender-incongruent patients was highlighted. As discussed above, in these patients strong use of identification appears indicative of psychological disturbance, or conflict, rather than an indication of psychological strength. In contrast, for gender-congruent patients a decrease in gender-congruent defenses of denial and projection and an increase in the use of identification were related to psychological improvement. For these patients, better functioning was linked to less use of immature defenses and greater use of a more mature defense.

In another study of a group of 30 well-educated middle-class professional patients (mean age = 45 years) with a DSM-III-R diagnosis of dysthymic disorder, the DMM was used to assess defense change after treatment (Little, 1998). Scores of these patients on scales representing the anaclitic (dependent) and introjective (self-focused) personality types, based on the Depressive Experiences Questionnaire (Blatt, D'Affitti, & Quinlan, 1976), were also obtained, as was their tendency toward depression (based on both self-report BDI and clinical ratings). After the initial assessment, patients were assigned to one of two treatment groups: medication only, or medication plus group therapy. The group therapy began after 8 weeks of medication treatment and continued once a week for 16 additional weeks.

At intake, the two treatment groups did not differ in DMM defense use, nor did they differ on the depression measures. After the 24 weeks of treatment, the use of denial had decreased for the patients in both treatment groups. Defenses were then related to clinical assessment scores. At intake, identification was negatively correlated with BDI scores; denial and projection were unrelated to BDI. However, neither initial level of defense use nor change in defense use predicted change in either the BDI or the clinical rating of depression after treatment.

Also, at intake, scores on both the anaclitic and introjective dimensions were positively correlated with the use of projection and negatively related to the use of identification. High scores on both personality dimensions also predicted a decrease in the use of identification at the end of treatment, and high scores on the introjective dimension predicted a decrease in the use of denial.

DSQ STUDIES

Change in defense use following treatment has also been studied using the DSQ to assess defenses. In one study the effects of short-term treatment were investigated in 31 patients admitted to a psychiatric hospital with a diagnosis of major depressive disorder (Kneepkens & Oakley, 1996). The treatment, which averaged 7 days in length, consisted of counseling, therapeutic milieu, and (in some cases) antidepressant medication. At admission and again at discharge, patients completed the self-report DSQ-40 and the Center for Epidemiologic Studies—Depression scale (CES-D) measure of depressive symptom level (Radloff, 1977). The results indicated a significant decrease in immature defenses at discharge, a significant increase in mature defenses, and no change in neurotic level defenses. There was also a decrease in depressive symptoms, but the relation between defense change and symptom change was not reported. As a cautionary note, the authors point out that the changes in self-report of defenses may also have been prompted by symptom change, by medication change, or by participant selection factors (half of the patients tested at admission did not complete the questionnaires at discharge).

A similar study attempted to compare patient defense scores with those of a control group (Akkerman, Carr, & Lewin, 1992). Patients with a diagnosis of major depressive disorder ($n = 37$), who received either in- or outpatient treatment (psychotherapy and antidepressant medication) were given the DSQ-36 at admission and again 2 months after therapy had begun. At the latter time, the patients were no longer diagnosable as depressed, according to the DSM-III-R criteria for depression, due to symptom remission. A comparison of self-reported DSQ-36 defense use at the two time periods indicated a decrease in immature, neurotic, and mature defenses, but only the immature decrease was statistically significant ($p < .05$). These patient scores were then compared with those of nonpatients from an earlier study by Andrews et al. (1989). This comparison indicated that the patients with depressive disorder used more immature defenses at admission but did not differ from those in the control group 2 months later. In contrast, they used fewer mature and more neurotic defenses both at admission and 2 months later. Thus the primary change in defense use over this 2-month period was a decrease in self-reported immature defenses. This decrease was paralleled by a decrease in self-reported depressive symptoms. Again, the actual relation between defense change and symptom change was not provided.

A further study examined the use of DSQ-88 defenses in a group of outpatients diagnosed with (DSM-III-R) OCD ($n = 17$), both before and after a 7-week period of group behavioral psychotherapy. The findings showed that scores on the (mature) Adaptive scale increased, and this increase was correlated with decreased depression (BDI) and decreased OCD symptoms. However, there was no change on the (immature) Maladaptive, Image-Distorting, or Self-Sacrificing scales. The only individual defense to show change was that of undoing, which decreased over the period of treatment (Albucher, Abelson, & Nesse, 1998).

A group of patients suffering from panic disorder with agoraphobia

(n = 29), who had previously been treated unsuccessfully with drug therapy, participated in cognitive-behavioral group therapy for 12 sessions over a period of 4 months (Heldt et al., 2003). All patients completed the DSQ-40 at the beginning of the therapy. This pretherapy defense use was related to therapy outcome—that is, to remission of symptoms. The results showed that initial low Neurotic and low Immature defense scale scores predicted symptom remission. However, when a comorbid diagnosis of depression/dysthymia was controlled for, only the low neurotic defense score predicted symptom remission. Notably, there was no association between symptom remission and reaction formation, undoing, or denial.[2]

DMRS STUDIES

The DMRS measure of defense mechanisms has also been used to determine if defenses predict patients' reactions to treatment, with varying results. In one study both the DMRS and the DSQ-88 were used to assess defense functioning prior to and following 40 sessions of outpatient psychodynamically oriented therapy (Hersoug et al., 2002). The most frequent diagnoses of the 43 patients were anxiety disorder and personality disorder. For both the DMRS and the DSQ-88, a single measure of Overall Defense Functioning (ODF) was determined.[3] In addition to the defense assessments, patients completed the SCL-90-R, from which the Global Severity Index (GSI; Derogatis, 1983) was determined.[4] Patients also provided a rating of their alliance with the therapist.[5]

The results of this study indicated that scores on the DMRS-ODF were at a significantly more mature level after therapy ($p < .001$), with most of the change occurring after session 16. However, scores on the DSQ-ODF were essentially unchanged. Further, although the GSI indicated improvement after therapy, and the alliance with the therapist had increased, neither of these changes were predicted by either of the defense measures.

In contrast, a study by Hoglend and Perry (1998) found that initial level of defense mechanisms did predict therapy outcome. Patients included those with a primary diagnosis of major depression (n = 16) and those with a nondepression diagnosis (primarily anxiety disorder: n = 18). They received either in- or outpatient weekly therapy and antidepressant medication when appropriate. At intake, patients were assessed for defense use with the DMRS and again 6 months later, following treatment. Clinicians also assessed DSM-III-R Axis I GAF at both times. In addition, most patients completed the DSQ-88 and the self-report GSI at both time periods.

The focus of this study was to determine the best predictors of patient functioning after 6 months of treatment; the two groups of patients (with and without depression) were studied separately, likely because the importance of defense functioning was different for the two groups. For the patients with depression, overall defense maturity (DMRS-ODF) at intake predicted higher GAF and lower GSI after 6 months of treatment. In a subsequent regression analysis of the patients with depression, defense functioning at intake was a better predictor of these outcome variables than was initial GAF, although the small number of patients available for this analysis (n = 15) raises questions regarding the reliability of this result. For the patients without depression, intake DMRS-ODF did not predict either of the outcome measures (GAF, GSI). However, initial defense maturity for patients without depression, based on the self-report DSQ, predicted the 6-month outcome GAF. This result was not found for the patients with depression.

Subsequently, the patients with depression were divided into two groups: Those who were more improved, and those who were less improved, than predicted by their original GAF score. Comparing the two groups, it was found that the more improved group had a higher ODF score at intake. On closer inspection, this result reflected the finding that only one individual defense—self-observation—from the highest ODF level was more frequent in the more improved group. In contrast, for the less improved group, scores on eight of the lower-level defenses that had previously been found to be associated with depression were more frequent at admission, as compared to the more improved group. Overall, these findings may be interpreted in two ways: Either the use of higher-level defenses is a positive prognostic sign of therapeutic outcome for patients with depression, or, more likely, the use of lower-level defenses is a negative prognosticator.

A study that raises questions about the meaning of defense change over the course of therapy was carried out with 61 patients who were given four psychodynamic therapy sessions, using the Brief Psychodynamic Investigation method (BPI; Gillieron, 1989) (Drapeau, De Roten, Perry, & Despland, 2003). Most of these patients were seeking help for mood (62%) or anxiety (36%) disorders. Using the DMRS, patients' defenses were assessed at each of the four sessions. Results showed that the number of defenses used decreased from the first to the middle two sessions, and again from the middle to the last session. At the same time, the maturity level of defenses used (ODF) increased at the fourth session. This increase in ODF was due to an increase in the "obsessional" defenses (level 6), especially intellectualization, and a decrease in the "narcissistic" (level 4) defenses, especially devaluation and idealization.

The authors noted that such change in defense functioning over a very short period of time is different from the results of other studies (e.g., Hersoug et al., 2002). They suggest that in the initial interview, the stress, unfamiliarity, and/or the more nondirective, open-ended nature of the interaction may have resulted in an unusually high rate of low-level defenses, thus artificially inflating the baseline data. In contrast, the fourth session was more structured. Overall, the findings raise the important issue of how the frame and style of the therapy may influence the patient's use of defenses.

An earlier report of this BPI study (Despland, de Roten, Despars, Stigler, & Perry, 2001) investigated the relation between defense use and therapist's style of intervention in determining the patient's alliance with the therapist. Twelve patients (11 women, 1 man) were selected to represent three different styles of alliance, as this occurred over the four therapy sessions: alliance high and stable (n = 7); alliance continually improving (n = 10); alliance low and stable (n = 4). Using the DMRS, level of ODF and scores for the seven defense levels were determined for the first therapy session. Interestingly, the three alliance groups did not differ on these defense measures. However, when each patient's average ODF (from 1 [low-level action defenses] to 7 [high-level adaptive defenses]) was compared with the therapist's average style of intervention (from 1 [supportive] to 7 [exploratory]) during the initial therapy session, greater similarity between ODF and intervention level predicted greater therapeutic alliance in the third and fourth sessions.

Further investigation of defense change over a longer (40 weekly sessions) psychotherapy, using two different manualized treatment approaches (both psychodynamically oriented, but one more confrontational, the other more insight-oriented) was conducted with 28 outpatients (Winston, Winston, Samstag, & Muran, 1994). The majority (75%) of the patients were well-educated women with diagnoses of depression or anxiety disorder, along with DSM-III-R Cluster C personality disorders. The defense coding system used was based on Vaillant's (1977) four-level hierarchy and was thus similar to the DMRS. Both patient defense use and "therapist intervention addressing the defense" (TAD) were coded on a minute-by-minute basis for four therapy sessions: one session from each of the first, second, third, and fourth groups of 10 visits. For each of the sessions, the average number of defenses used from each level was determined, as was the average number of therapist TADs.

Analyses of these data indicated that level 4 defenses (mature) were used very infrequently. Also, because there were no patients with psychosis in the group, level 1 defenses (psychotic) were not included. Thus only level 3 (intermediate)[6] and level 2 (immature) defenses were studied. The results indicated that there were significant correlations between the frequency of patients' use of both intermediate and immature defenses and the frequency of TADs. In terms of defense change, across the four quartiles of treatment, the insight therapy patients showed a significant decrease in the use of intermediate defenses (e.g., intellectualization, verbal denial, undoing, displacement, minimization, sarcasm) but no significant change in the use of immature defenses. The confrontational therapy patients showed no changes in the use of either level of defense, even though the confrontational therapists addressed the patients' defenses significantly more often than did the insight therapists. Further, although outcome measures (SCL-90-R and others) indicated general pre- to posttherapy improvement, there was no relation between change in defense level and outcome.

Defense functioning has also been used in an attempt to predict patients' continuance or discontinuance of psychotherapy (Perry, 2001). Fourteen outpatients diagnosed as having personality disorder and/or depressive disorder were audiotaped during five therapy sessions at the beginning of treatment; defenses were coded using the DMRS. Patients were subsequently divided into those who remained in the treatment after 1 year (n = 8) and those who had dropped out (n = 6). The latter group had significantly lower ODF scores at the beginning of therapy.[7] Those who remained in therapy showed a tendency toward using more "mature" (level 7) and more "obsessional" (level 6) defenses at the beginning of treatment. However, dropout status was also related to frequency of therapy sessions offered. All of the dropout patients were seen once weekly, whereas there were no dropouts among those seen twice weekly. Thus the possible relation of defense maturity to therapy continuation is confounded in this study with frequency of treatment.

In another study 50 patients seeking outpatient twice-weekly therapy were assessed for defense use with the DMRS prior to the beginning of treatment (Lingiardi et al., 1999). Of this group 30% dropped out of treatment within the first 2 months. Although diagnosis did not differentiate between the dropouts and those who remained in therapy, the use of the defense of disavowal was found to be more characteristic of the dropout group.

There is little information available regarding defense change in adolescents undergoing psychotherapy. A study of 37 hospitalized adolescents (mean age = 13 years), primarily diagnosed as having conduct or affective disorder, used the DMI to assess defense choice at admission and again after 9 months of treatment (Noam et al., 1991). On the basis of their change in level of ego development (Loevinger, 1976) over the 9-month period, some of these adolescents were described as "progressors" (those who had advanced at least one half stage in their level of ego development) and others as "nonprogressors" (those who had not advanced one half stage in their level of ego development). The two groups did not differ in defense choice at admission. However, the progressors were found to have increased their choice of REV and decreased their choice of projection after treatment, whereas the nonprogressors showed no change. Notably, these findings were not due to differences between the two groups in initial ego level, IQ, age, gender, or socioeconomic status.

CONCLUDING REMARKS

The findings from studies of defense mechanisms and psychotherapy can be related to three general questions:

1. Do defenses change after therapy?
2. If defenses do change, does this change relate to symptom change?
3. Does the initial level of defense use predict symptom change?

Comparisons of defense use before and after therapy generally show that the use of immature defenses decreases and the use of mature defenses increases. However, this shift varies somewhat by defense measure and diagnostic group. For example, using the DSQ, mature defenses were found to increase in a group of patients with OCD, but there was no change in the use of immature defenses. As another example, in a group of patients with anxiety and personality disorders, mature defenses increased when assessed by the DMRS, but no change was found when they were assessed by the DSQ.

Again, findings regarding the question of whether defense change is related to symptom change vary for different diagnoses and different defense measures. On the positive side, study of hospitalized patients with psychosis or BPD showed that a decrease in DMM immature defense use was related to a decrease in pathological symptoms. Also, outpatients with OCD showed that an increase in DSQ mature defenses was related to a decrease in symptoms, and adolescent inpatients demonstrated that an increase in DMI mature defense use was related to an increase in level of ego development. However, for patients with dysthymia, there was no relation between DMM defense change and change in measures of depression. Nor did women outpatients with diagnoses of depression or anxiety disorder show a relation between change in defense level, as assessed from interviews, and change in pathological symptoms.

Finally, the findings again vary by diagnosis and defense measure for the question of whether pretherapy level of defense use predicts posttherapy outcome. On the one hand, DSQ defenses initially assessed at a mature level did predict more favorable outcome for patients with agoraphobia. On the other hand, defenses initially assessed with the DMM did not predict therapy outcome for patients with dysthymia, and defenses initially assessed with the DSQ and DMRS did not predict outcome for patients with anxiety and personality disorders. Even more complicated, initial defense maturity, as assessed by the DMRS, predicted better outcome for patients with depression, but not for patients without depression, whereas in the same study, initial defense maturity, as assessed by the DSQ, predicted better outcome for patients without depression, but not for patients with depression.

Finally, there is some evidence that the relation between patients' defense level and therapists' type of intervention predicts therapeutic alliance, and that change in patients' defense use is related to type of intervention. In this regard, Vaillant (1994) has cautioned that therapists should proceed with care and sensitivity in the treatment of patients' defense mechanisms: "By thoughtlessly challenging irritating, but partly adaptive, immature defenses, a clinician can evoke enormous anxiety and depression in a patient and rupture the [therapeutic] alliance" (p. 49).

CHAPTER 14

Case Studies

In this chapter we look more closely at the use of defense mechanisms by several individuals who are experiencing a serious psychological disorder. For each of these cases, the DMM is used to assess defenses. Examples of each patient's TAT stories and defense coding are provided.

The first case is that of a convicted serial killer. An examination of his use of defenses illustrates how they may contribute to pathological behavior. A second case contrasts the defenses of a 10-year-old boy prior and subsequent to 4 years of psychological treatment; here we see significant maturation in defense use. A third set of cases again contrasts defense use prior and subsequent to therapy, demonstrating how both diagnosis and age are important factors in understanding changes in defense use. The final case tracks defense change in a 10-year-old boy during 2 years of intensive treatment.

"BEN": A SERIAL KILLER

The use of defenses by an extremely violent individual was studied by Porcerelli, Abramsky, Hibbard, and Kamoo (2001). This man, a 24-year-old African American named Ben,[1] was a serial sexual homicide perpetrator, having murdered 13 women over a period of 9 months. From his TAT stories, both his typical use of defense mechanisms (DMM) and his characteristic mode of perceiving others (Social Cognition and Object Relations Scale; SCORS; Westen, Lohr, Silk, Gold, & Kerber, 1989) were coded. Together, these two measures suggested that this was a man who relied on immature forms of denial and projection as a way to rid himself of aggressive and sadistic impulses. In conjunction with a difficulty in differentiating between self and others, these defenses contributed to his perceiving his victims as threatening objects, against whom he must protect himself.

Aspects of these defenses and the blurring of boundaries between self and others can be seen in the following extracts from two of the TAT stories he told. To Card 1 (picture of a young boy seated in front of a violin), he responded:

> *Okay, here we have a little boy, and he is being pressured into taking violin lessons. He do not want to be taking them because they are so boring. . . . So they spend hours and hours studying, as boring as it is. Now from the look of it, I would say this one got upset with him making too much noise of not doing something and hit him. [Who would that be? Who is upset?] This father. His father is mad at him because he considered the instrument to be sissyish, you know. Women play violins, you know, cellos and shit like that. Anyway, he was yelling back and forth, you know, just yelling back and forth, and the father struck him. The little boy was in his room looking at this and wondering why. [Wondering why?] Why can such an instrument cause him so much trouble. . . . I see nothing but sorrow in the whole future. Like I say, he is going to spend the rest of his life trying to please his father. His father is never going to be pleased.*

To TAT Card 2 (farm scene; man plowing fields, pregnant woman looking on, a young woman with books in the foreground), he responded:

> *Here we have the mother and son working on the farm, you know. The woman there, she likes the son. The mother won't let her get next to her son because she is scared that the daughter is going to take her son away. . . . I believe the mother is going to take the girl away. The son has been with the mother for so long, you know, listening to her, her guidance and everything. Until the mother dies, he is going to be there on that farm working. . . . His mother is the only protection, the only love he will ever have. When she dies, he is going to be all alone. He is going to be resentful towards any woman, anyone because his mother is dead. That is the same thing.[2]*

In these two stories, the projection of hostility onto the characters is clear. The father, mad at the young boy for being involved with womanly activities, hits him and rejects him. Notably, the cause for this aggression is attributed to the (feminized) violin rather than to either of the merged characters. The mother in Card 2 fears the girl will interfere with her relationship with the son and so "takes the girl away"—but then the mother dies. Both stories also demonstrate the blurring of boundaries between characters. Card 1 depicts a single figure, the boy, seated in front of the violin. But the storyteller quickly moves to merging the boy with another (unexplained) figure: "They spend hour and hour studying . . . , " and then one of the merged-figure combinations aggresses on the other: "this one (unexplained—there is only *one* figure in the picture) . . . got upset . . . and hit him." Ben's description of this merging creates confusion in the examiner, who must ask "Who would that be? Who is upset?"

In Card 2 this merging is seen in the idea, first, that the woman/daughter and mother are both competing for the son, and the mother is scared that "the daughter is going to take her son away." This merging is continued in the later repeated phrase "the mother is going to take the girl away." The boundaries are thus blurred as to who is going to remove whom from the scene. Further blurring of boundaries between mother and other women is seen in the closing statement "he is going to be resentful towards any woman, anyone because his mother is dead. That is the same thing."

Let us look now more closely at the case and at Ben's use of defense mechanisms, as assessed with the DMM from his TAT stories. Ben was an illegitimate child. His mother was addicted to cocaine, which she obtained by earning money as a prostitute. His father was unknown to Ben, and his mother was jailed when he was 2 years old. He and his younger brother then had a very disturbed, deprived, and disrupted childhood. Nevertheless, he and his brother maintained a "reunion fantasy" in which they could create the perfect family by getting back together with their idealized mother. Ben experienced a multitude of placements in foster homes and institutions; in the latter, he experienced a homosexual relationship with a male staff member.

By 10th grade Ben had left school and become involved in heavy drug use; he hustled as a homosexual prostitute. His only meaningful attachment was to his brother, who managed to live a relatively stable life and would allow Ben to live with him as long as he was drug free. When Ben reverted to drug use, his brother ordered him to leave his home. Two weeks later, the killings began. Over a period of 9 months, Ben murdered 13 women, all of whom had records of prostitution and crack cocaine use. All were murdered in the same way: they were bound, beaten, raped, sodomized, and finally strangled to death.

While in custody, Ben was evaluated; this evaluation included telling stories in response to nine cards from the TAT. Formal analyses of his stories were used to assess his capacity for forming relationships with others (SCORS: Westen et al., 1989) and his use of defenses (DMM). Results from the SCORS indicated that people were seen in complex ways but were easily confused or merged—there was difficulty maintaining the separateness, or boundaries, between different individuals. Further, there was evidence of a desire to be loved but deficits in the capacity to experience pleasure from mutual relatedness. These factors, in combination with themes of sadistic aggression, resulted in a picture in which the protagonist was left feeling empty and unloved. His orientation toward others was basically narcissistic: His primary concern was gratification of his needs (Porcerelli et al., 2001).

The stories were also coded independently by two raters, using the DMM, for the use of defenses. These stories provided adequate material to code 52 instances of defense use. Fifteen percent of these reflected the use of denial; notably, all of these were instances of immature denial. Projection responses made up 51% of the defense scores, with 59% of these at the immature level. In fact, 52% of the projection score was comprised of responses to the single, immature category titled "attribution of hostile or normatively unusual feelings or intentions to a character." This result is consistent with the prior observation that Ben has difficulty in differentiating among people, including himself and others, so that his own rage and malevolence are perceived as residing in others. Overall, the frequent use of denial and projection are highly similar to that found in the community sample study showing the relation between defense use and antisocial personality (Cramer, 1999b).

Unexpectedly, 34% of Ben's defenses were coded as identification. Whereas in normal samples identification generally represents a mature defense, previous studies of pathological patient groups have suggested that the use of identification in these groups may be indicative of a conflicted or pathological identification that interferes with, rather than promotes, normal development (Cramer & Blatt, 1990; see Chapters 12 and 13). When the authors examined Ben's identification responses, it appeared that this was the case. These responses displayed a frustrated wish for contact with a sadistic father as well as an inability to separate, psychologically, from a controlling mother, with whom he identified both as a way to prevent abandonment and to contain his rage toward her. These and other aspects of the identification responses suggest that the type of identification being manifest is pathological in nature.

"MARTIN": A 10-YEAR-OLD BOY

The following case was assessed by Dr. Francis Kelly at a community mental health center (Kelly, 2003). Dr. Kelly did the psychological evaluation and has generously provided the case history and diagnostic information. He is, however, not responsible for my interpretation of the material.

As a child grows older, we expect to see developmental changes in the use of defense mechanisms. The TAT stories from a boy named Martin illustrate these changes. However, in Martin's case, early trauma had contributed to a delay in his psychological development, so that when he was first evaluated at age 10 years, his defense mechanisms were more like those of a 5-year-old. With treatment, a subsequent evaluation at age 14 showed developmental progress, although he still lagged behind the expected defense profile for his age group.

Martin's earliest years were characterized by severe attachment problems. Unpredictable in his behavior, Martin alternated between clinging and rageful outbursts—both of which occurred in the context of neglect and physical abuse. An elderly, sickly father who was his caretaker died when he was 4 years old. When he began school and continuing until he was evaluated at age 10, Martin was unable to connect with peers, seemingly unaware of how to negotiate social interactions. He also had learning problems related to his psychological difficulties. To ensure his attendance, his mother frequently remained at the school during the first several years. When not at school, Martin spent his time alone, watching television. At age 10, Dr. Kelly noted a clinical impression of a schizoid–depressive disorder, with DSM-IV-TR diagnoses of dysthymic disorder, early onset; disruptive behavior disorder; and separation anxiety disorder, early onset.

Following the initial evaluation, Martin began long-term individual psychotherapy that continued for 4 years. By age 14, his overall functioning had improved; he showed greater self-control, better academic functioning at school, and improved ability to get along with family members. However, he still lacked the ability to relate to peers, with whom he demonstrated a hostile–avoidant pattern.

After 4 years of treatment, his therapist left the agency, and his mother did not keep his appointments with a newly assigned therapist. However, as Martin became more withdrawn, with suicidal and homicidal thoughts, his mother renewed contact with the agency, and Martin was seen for a second evaluation.

As part of this assessment, Martin was given the TAT, as had occurred during the initial assessment at age 10. It is thus possible to compare his stories and defense use at the two ages, both prior and subsequent to treatment. Although chronological development is confounded with possible treatment effects, such a comparison is interesting in its demonstration of the change in defense predominance.

To illustrate these changes, Martin's stories in response to three TAT cards are given, first for age 10 and then for age 14. Following each story, phrases that indicate the use of defenses are highlighted, and the particular DMM defense score that applies is given in parentheses; *D*, *P*, and *I* indicate the defenses of denial, projection, and identification, and the numbers following each letter refer to the subcategory of the defense that is scored.

(See Chapter 15 for a description of the seven subcategories of each defense.)

Here are Martin's TAT stories:

Card 1: A young boy seated in front of a violin.

Age 10: A kid learning how to play one of these things. . . . I hate these [TAT cards]. I did these last year. I don't know what happens. He's sighing. I don't know what happens. He goes to the bathroom and tells time.

Faced with a task he is unable or unwilling to complete, Martin has his character escape from the situation ("he goes to the bathroom") (avoiding reality; D4); he then adds a peculiar outcome ("tells time"; P7). These two components of his story are in no way suggested by the picture and do not represent reality as it is generally understood (we do not go to the bathroom to tell time). In my experience, this peculiar ending is unique to this boy. His use of denial to avoid anxiety results in this peculiar ideation.

Age 14: Boy maybe 4 or 5 looking at a violin. Wondering how to play it. Just got done practicing it, thinking what he should do. Definitely thinking. Hard to tell . . . puts it away or could pick it up and play. I'd put it away and take out the guitar. Looks a little bit upset or not satisfied with his work. Some scratches he overlooked . . . or string could have broke.

Now, Martin is able to create a story. Although there is still some tendency to avoid the situation ("I'd put it away and take out the guitar"), he manages to keep focused on the task ("Definitely thinking"). There is some evidence of projected dissatisfaction ("upset, or not satisfied"; P1), which is then attributed to the violin ("some scratches"; P2).

Card 2: Farm scene: a young woman in the foreground with books in her hand; a man in the background, working in the fields; an older pregnant woman looking on.

Age 10: Harvesting for the winter . . . and they . . . one guy gots [sic] no pants . . . these are underwear. Nothing else. I don't know.

In this more complex picture, Martin is unable to integrate the various characters. To deal with this complexity, he ignores the presence of (fails to see: D1) the pregnant woman and the girl holding books (D1) and focuses only on the man. The use of denial continues in his misperception (D2) of the man when Martin claims that the trousers the man is wearing are underwear.

Age 14: Guy digging up crops. Pregnant lady leaning against a tree, hoping he'll get through the day alive. Young lady holding books. Bunch of houses and rocky land. Go in the house and start eating. The young girl looks worried. . . . The guy no telling, can't see his face. Pregnant lady looks happy probably cause she's pregnant. Nope, nothing else here.

On this occasion, all three characters are recognized and described with some attempt at a story line. The use of denial has been replaced by projection, beginning with the unusual attribution that the pregnant woman hopes the man will "get through the day alive" (P1). There is nothing in the picture that would explain this concern, nor is any reason given by the storyteller. This statement is followed by an example of circumstantial thinking (P3); the storyteller says he cannot imagine what the man's feelings might be *because* he can't see his face.

Card 6BM: An elderly woman stands looking out the window; a tall young man stands in the middle of the room, looking down.

Age 10: I can't say. A girl looking out the window and a man wondering what she's doing. Then she jumps off the United States Building. I'm just saying she does.

The response begins with Martin's saying he "can't" say what is going on (D4). This is followed by a misperception of the age of the female character (D2), which is followed by further denial of the reality of the picture (the "United States Building"; D5)—there is nothing in the picture to suggest the presence of a large building. (Perhaps he is referring to the equally nonpresent Empire State building?) This statement is then followed with another denial of reality—"I'm just saying she does" (D5)—that is, it didn't really happen.

Age 14: Son who came home to give bad news to mother. The way he's dressed looks like someone died. Or the mother could have asked him over to tell him his father died. Then he goes home . . . and hard to tell. No telling, just a picture.

This time the characters are correctly recognized as an elderly woman and younger man. The use of projection becomes evident in the circumstantial thinking—"The way he's dressed looks like someone died" (P3)—that is, using dress as a justification for the projected idea of death, which is further amplified in the idea that "his father died" (P5). At the end of the story, the use of denial reappears—"No telling, just a picture"—that is, it isn't real (D5).

I used stories told to the same seven TAT cards at both ages to compare Martin's use of defenses at ages 10 and 14. As might be expected, he told somewhat longer stories at the older age. Because longer stories provide more opportunities for coding defense use, to compare scores at the two ages, it is a good idea to transform the absolute defense scores into relative scores, in which the relative use of each defense is expressed as a percentage of the total defense score. For example, the relative use of denial is determined from the ratio: denial / denial + projection + identification. In this way, we have an estimate of defense use that is not influenced by story length.

The relative scores for Martin's use of defenses at ages 10 and 14 are presented in Figure 14.1. Martin's defense pattern at age 10 is clearly immature. Denial is his predominant defense (60%), with the use of projection considerably less frequent (33%). Normatively, we would expect projection to be the predominant defense in a 10-year-old boy, with relatively little use of denial. By age 14, Martin shows the age-appropriate predominance of projection (88%), with little use of denial (4%). However, he still lags behind developmentally in his minimal use of identification (8%), which should have increased by this age.

It is difficult to determine whether the developmental advance in Martin's use of defenses has occurred as a result of the therapeutic endeavor or from advancing age. However, it appears that his use of defenses at the beginning of treatment had been delayed by social–psychological experiences rather than by some intellectual deficit, because his intellectual functioning

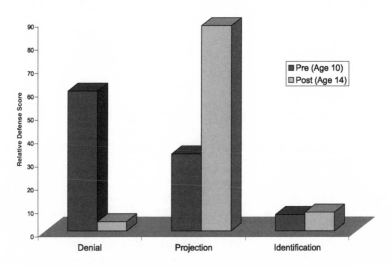

FIGURE 14.1. Martin: Defense use pre- and posttreatment.

was determined to be in the normal range (Wechsler Intelligence Scale for Children–III [WISC-III] Full-Scale IQ = 90). Subsequent advance in defense maturity may then also be attributed to social–psychological experiences.

THREE FEMALES: BEFORE AND AFTER TREATMENT

Thus far we have considered defense use in an adult man and a preadolescent boy. In this section we consider three females who were assessed both prior and subsequent to experiencing psychotherapy. The discussion of these three cases is based on material provided by Drs. Stephen Hibbard, Francis Kelly, and John Porcerelli,[3] each of whom supervised the assessment of one of the patients. The follow-up assessment of these three patients after a period of treatment provides an opportunity to examine not only changes after therapy but also how age and diagnosis may contribute to these changes.

The first patient, Karen, was assessed at ages 10 and 12 years. At the initial evaluation she was characterized as being at a borderline level of personality organization. Her DSM-III-R diagnoses, provided by a multidisciplinary assessment team, were posttraumatic stress disorder, chronic; disruptive behavior disorder, NOS; dysthymic disorder, early onset. The second case, Jennifer, a 31-year-old single woman, was assessed prior to treatment and again after time-limited therapy of 12 sessions. She was described as functioning at a neurotic level of personality organization, with no clear DSM diagnosis but indications of a personality disorder with histrionic, anxious, and depressive features. The final case, Mrs. S, was assessed at age 38 when she was admitted to a psychiatric hospital subsequent to auditory and visual hallucinations. She was described as functioning at a psychotic level of personality organization, with paranoid and histrionic features. The consensus diagnosis given by her treatment team was DSM-III-R brief reactive psychosis.

"Karen"[4]

At age 10 years Karen was first seen for psychological assessment following discharge from a psychiatric facility where she had been hospitalized twice within a 6-month period because of depression, self-abusive behavior (scratching and cutting herself), and psychotic ideation. Both at home and in school she demonstrated significant mood instability, oppositional and defiant behavior, along with periods of intermittent verbal and physical aggression as well as explosive outbursts. She was unable to initiate or maintain consistent, positive ties to peers, teachers, or family members.

Her developmental history included longstanding affect, mood, and behavior regulation problems that were first noted in the preschool years and occurred within the context of intrafamilial chaos and discord. Her parents divorced when Karen was 4 years old; this termination of the marriage was prompted by her father's intermittent sexual and physical abuse of the mother and his two daughters. Following the dissolution of the marriage, Karen and her sister remained in the custody of their mother. The family subsequently has had no contact with the father. The mother described an array of early-onset (age 4 years) and enduring functional concerns about Karen: temper tantrums, sleep difficulties, nightmares, somatic complaints, and shyness with strangers. Prior to her hospitalizations, Karen was depicted as increasingly contrary, defiant, distractible, labile, anxious, and fearful; she did not want her mother to leave her alone at home for even a brief period of time.

Upon discharge from her second psychiatric hospitalization at age 10, Karen returned home and began weekly individual and family psychotherapy; in addition, she was placed on Ritalin, Paxil, and Risperidal. She began to attend a therapeutic day school and was also involved with a structured after-school day treatment program that emphasized therapeutic activities and socialization skill enhancement. As an additional support, the family had access to stabilization emergency services.

Two years of concerted multimodal therapeutic interventions served to stabilize Karen and ultimately resulted in significant amelioration of behavioral, mood, affect, and interpersonal problems. When seen for follow-up psychological evaluation at age 12, she was continuing to function well in her therapeutic day school, and plans were being formulated for her to return to a public school setting. Her explosive and volatile outbursts had ceased at home and in school; she was making friends and spoke positively about the changes in her life.

The DMM was used to code stories given in response to the same eight TAT cards at the beginning (age 10 years) and after 2 years of treatment (age 12 years). A comparison of Karen's use of defense mechanisms at these two ages indicated that the total defense scores remained the same at the two ages (total scores of 26); however, the relative use of the three defenses changed markedly (see Figure 14.2). At age 10, pretreatment, the relative use of defenses was denial, 35%; projection, 44%; identification, 30%; at posttreatment the relative percentages were denial, 15%; projection, 44%; identification, 41%.

Although not as extreme as found with Martin, Karen's use of defenses at age 10 again demonstrates immature psychological development. Her use of denial reaches 35%, whereas normative expectation for her age is around 12%. Different from Martin, she shows the age-expected increase in the use of identification. These results are discussed further after considering the other two cases.

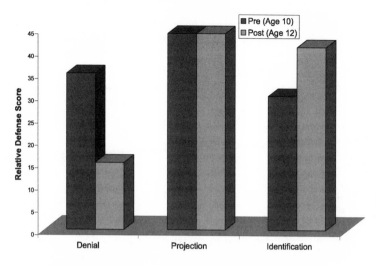

FIGURE 14.2. Karen: Defense use pre- and posttreatment.

Examples of Karen's Pre- and Posttreatment TAT Stories

To illustrate changes in defensive mechanisms from admission to discharge, TAT responses from Card 6GF (a young woman sitting on a sofa, looking over her shoulder at an older man) are reported along with DMM scores.

> *Pretreatment, age 10 years, 2 months, Card 6 GF: I don't know. I don't have any story for this one . . . nothing there. [Tell me what you see.] They really love one another . . . maybe . . . I don't know. She is a famous movie star . . . but she doesn't like him, they broke up I guess. [What happens?] He broke up with her because he saw another woman—they really weren't made for one another. [How does he feel?] Happy, I guess . . . I don't know. Maybe upset . . . don't know.*

DMM—DEFENSES

Denial (3): Reversal ("they really love one another . . . . they broke up")

Denial (3): Reversal ("she doesn't like him . . . he broke up with her")

Denial (4): Negation ("nothing there")

Projection (1): Attribution of negative emotion, unexplained ("she doesn't like him")

Identification (6): Role differentiation ("movie star")

Total: Denial = 3; Projection = 1; Identification = 1.

Posttreatment, age 12 years, 5 months, Card 6 GF: They're at a movie and she gets spoken to by the manager because she's talking. "Pipe down you or you'll leave!" And when the movie is over she stays . . . works there for the rest of her life. She was with her dad because she wanted to spend quality time with him. [How does she feel?] She feels all funny because she doesn't know it was the manager . . . but likes him. [What happens in the future?] I told you . . . she works there.

DMM—DEFENSES

Identification (3): Regulation of behavior ("Pipe down or you'll leave")
Identification (5): Working ("works there for the rest of her life")
Identification (6): Role differentiation ("manager")
Total: Denial = 0; Projection = 0; Identification = 3

Whereas the initial story is a romance fantasy filled with emotional ambivalence, the second story is about real people engaging in real-world activities. This advance in ego functioning is also seen in the decreased use of denial. Suggestions of male idealization in her second story may contribute to the increased use of identification at age 12.

"Jennifer"[5]

At age 31 Jennifer applied for services at a psychological training clinic. On entry into treatment, she indicated two areas of concern: lack of energy, with inability to focus on cognitive work, and difficulty in romantic relationships.

Jennifer was the younger of two daughters. She had a highly conflicted relationship with her father, who was alcoholic and hostile when drinking. When Jennifer was 16, at her urging, her mother asked her father to leave the household. The parents were divorced soon thereafter. Jennifer subsequently provided some emotional caretaking for her father, about which she was highly ambivalent.

Jennifer reported having had several boyfriends from her late teen years through her 20s, but none of these had lasted over a year. Eight months prior to coming into treatment, she had been let go from a highly desirable position as a graphic artist/designer. Her description of being let go implied that she was not able to get along with her boss.

Jennifer was seen in weekly psychotherapy; she was not given psychotropic medications. The therapy consisted largely of supportive, client-centered interventions. Defense mechanisms were assessed using the DMM from stories told in response to 14 TAT cards, both before and after therapy. The results indicated a decrease in the overall use of defenses, from a pretreatment total score of 44 to a posttreatment score of 25, which was likely related to her self-reported decrease in anxiety and other psychiatric symptoms. Equally informative, the relative use of the three defenses changed after treatment (see Figure 14.3). Denial decreased from 52 to 32%, projection increased from 27 to 36%, and identification increased from 21 to 32%. Each of these changes indicates a movement toward defense maturity, although the use of denial continues at a rather high level. Based on a large sample ($n = 120$) of community women in their 30s, we would expect the relative use of denial to be 26%, projection to be 46%, and identification to be 28%.[6]

Examples of Jennifer's Pre- and Posttreatment TAT Stories

Changes in defense use are illustrated in the following stories in response to TAT Card 4 (woman holding the shoulders of a man, who is turned away) pre- and posttreatment.

Pretreatment, Card 4: Um, well, this kinda looks like um . . . [Make up a story.] Okay, well, he's . . . they're in a movie, he's the actor, she's the actress, and uh, I guess it's sort of . . . he's obviously turning away, but not necessarily from her. I think he's actually more interested in something else, or going somewhere else but she doesn't look like she's

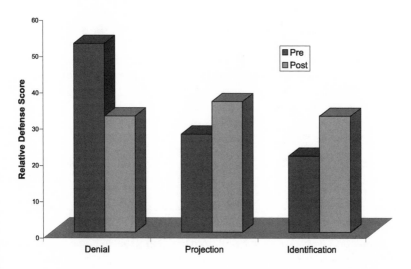

FIGURE 14.3. Jennifer: Defense use pre- and posttreatment.

tormented either, like "Oh my God, you're leaving me." It's more like she's kinda concerned. He's just sort of interested in something else, but she's not like terribly concerned about herself. She's not like, "Oh, you're leaving me," you know, it's more like, "Oh, what's wrong. Tell me what's going on." And I don't really know . . . maybe he's catching a bus. Or, you know, they . . . but I don't really see it as, like, they're not having, you know, they're not having problems between themselves. It's just, whatever. [What led up to it?] They were talking to one another. [How does it turn out?] Um, well, it's a movie, so, uh, I guess it turns out okay, in the end, but, I don't know, she probably follows him. . . . [That's it?] Yeah.

DMM—DEFENSES

Denial (4): Negation (scored 5 times) ("He's turning away, but not necessarily from her"; "she doesn't look like she's tormented"; "she's not like terribly concerned about herself"; "she's not like, Oh, you're leaving *me*"; "they're not having problems between themselves")

Denial (5): Denial of reality ("It's a movie")

Projection (1): Attribution of unusual intention ("Maybe he's catching a bus")

Identification (6): Role differentiation (scored twice) ("actor"; "actress")

Total: Denial = 5; Projection = 1; Identification = 2

Postreatment, Card 4: He just has a crazed, wild look in his eyes. He's ready to bolt. She has this "kiss me" look on her face. I don't know what exactly is going on. He looks like he's ready to get up, but she has this, "Okay, he's just going away. I just want to get your attention." [Feel?] He feels anxious. She feels the need to distance herself from his anxiety, but he will, regardless of how good she is, he will go his own way.

DMM—DEFENSES

Denial (4): Negation ("I don't know exactly what is going on")

Projection (1): Attribution of unusual emotion to eyes ("crazed, wild look in his eyes")

Projection (1): Attribution of unusual emotion to face ("this 'kiss me' " look on her face")

Projection (1): Attribution of unusual emotion ("I just want to get your attention")

Identification (3): (Self) regulation of behavior ("he will go his own way")

These two stories are striking in their demonstration of the recurring strong use of denial pretreatment and its near absence posttreatment. Rather than the repetitive denial of feelings seen in the first story, the second story presents the characters as filled with projected emotion.

"Mrs. S"[7]

At age 38, suffering from hallucinations and threatening to kill her parents, Mrs. S was admitted to a psychiatric hospital on a petition by her parents. She believed her body had been invaded by an evil spirit, which later was described as the husband who had recently left her. It was at this time that her functioning began to deteriorate. She began locking all the doors in the house, fearing that a man who looked like her husband would come to the house and harm her. She also began to deny ever having been married (massive denial). On several occasions she failed to turn off the gas stove. Due to her increasing withdrawal and confusion, she could no longer function at work and eventually had to leave her job. Whenever her parents tried to reason with her, she became more confused or enraged.

Mrs. S was seen three times a week in individual psychoanalytic/ supportive psychotherapy. Her treatment included antipsychotic medication, group (milieu) therapy, and art therapy. She eventually began to talk about the "evil spirit" that had invaded her, saying it was hard for her to sleep because he rapes her at night. Other boundary disturbances were noted early in her treatment. For example, just after a patient had yelled at her, Mrs. S said to her therapist, "You are so angry with me today." On another occasion, when asked about her separation from her husband, Mrs. S remarked that the therapist looked "so sad."

In time, her reports of the evil spirit began to vacillate between an evil spirit that wanted to rape and kill her and one that was getting to know her and love her. During the latter half of the second month of treatment, Mrs. S told the therapist that the evil spirit inside of her looked just like her husband. The therapist said that she must miss him and wish that she could keep him with her. She responded by saying that she thought she just saw a cross in the window and that "it must mean that there are a lot of sad people in the world."

During her third month of treatment, Mrs. S's thinking became less concrete; she began describing experiences and memories in more complex and less distorted ways. She could express anger toward her husband for leaving her. Mrs. S also reported that the "evil spirit" was "shrinking" inside of her and was confined to her abdominal region. In subsequent sessions Mrs. S revealed having intense sadness over not having a baby. She spoke directly of her anger toward her husband for making her wait to have a child and how a hysterectomy had ended all her hopes.

After 4 months of intensive treatment, Mrs. S had made significant improvement. She was no longer a threat to herself or others. She demonstrated positive interactions with her parents during family meetings with the social worker as well as a greater capacity to verbalize painful feelings of loss and anger, and she expressed an eagerness to "get back to life." Prior to discharge, Mrs. S was, at times, able to talk about and feel the losses that she had suffered (husband, job, independence, hysterectomy). As for the delusion of an evil spirit, Mrs. S told the therapist that it still existed but that she was not crazy enough to keep telling people about it.

At a 6-month follow-up to her hospital discharge, she spoke with pride about moving into her own apartment and getting her "old job back" as a florist. She asked the social worker to say hello to some of the members of her treatment team and to thank them for helping her "during my crazy spell."

A comparison of the DMM defense scores for Mrs. S, pre- and posttreatment, shows this improvement in functioning. Her total defense score of 56 prior to treatment decreased to 43 after treatment. In terms of the individual defenses, denial decreased from 26 to 16%, projection decreased from 41 to 23%, and identification increased from 33 to 60% (see Figure 14.4).

Examples of Mrs. S's Pre- and Posttreatment TAT Stories

To illustrate changes in defensive mechanisms from admission to discharge, TAT responses to Card 5 (woman looking into a room) are reported along with DMM scores.

> *Pretreatment, Card 5: There is a question on the lady's face pertaining to what she sees in the room. She's looking for an individual who came from the same area. The room appears homey and comfortable. I see astonishment in her eyes. [Astonishment?] And she appears to see . . . or something that's not there. Maybe she walked into the room and something's missing. Seems to be coming out from the dark, like coming out of a galaxy (?) I pick it up by the swirling stars (points to a tiny spot on the card).*

DMM—DEFENSE SCORES

Denial (2): Misperception ("swirling stars")
Projection (1): Attribution of emotion to face ("a question on the lady's face")
Projection (1): Attribution of emotion to eyes ("astonishment in her eyes")
Projection (7): Bizarre, very unusual story
Total: Denial = 1; Projection = 3; Identification = 0

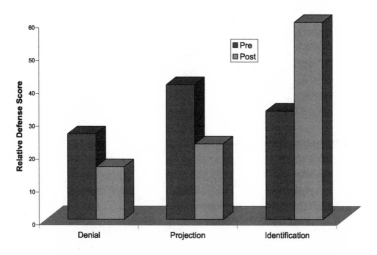

FIGURE 14.4. Mrs. S: Defense use pre- and posttreatment.

Posttreatment, Card 5: I see a woman who doesn't think she's going to enter, just opened to see what's going on inside the room. She was coming up from the cellar or basement. The picture looks like it's from the 30s or 40s. Whatever was in the room took her by surprise and disbelief. But she doesn't seem to be in a hurry to move away. She's just staring. I don't know what else to say. Maybe someone was in the house that she didn't intend on seeing. I think the outcome is going to be utter surprise or disbelief because that's the look showing on her face. [Who was in the room?] Maybe a husband. Maybe he came home from the day at work and maybe she's questioning him as to why he left the business at an early time. He didn't call first.

DMM—DEFENSE SCORES

Denial (4): Negation ("she doesn't seem to be in a hurry")
Projection (1): Attribution of emotion to face ("the look showing on her face")
Projection (2): Ominous additions ("whatever was in the room took her by surprise and disbelief")
Identification (5): Work, delay of gratification ("day at work")
Identification (6): Role differentiation ("husband")
Total: Denial = 1; Projection = 1; Identification = 2

The first story conveys a sense of considerable cognitive disarray. Things are not as they appear to be, and there is a swirling sense of general confusion. In the second story, a lesser sense of confusion continues, and the attempt to distance herself from the situation is not successful. The major difference in this second story is that the delusional galaxy is replaced with a real-life confrontation with the husband. It may be that the extreme increase in the defense of identification on this second occasion is a result of her experience with her therapist, and supports her capacity to confront feelings about her husband.

Karen, Jennifer, and Mrs. S: Changes in Defenses after Treatment

Relative defense scores are again used so that in a comparison of the defenses used by these three patients differences in age and/or diagnosis do not affect the length of stories told. In this way we have a picture of defense use that is not influenced by story length or number of stories told. Using these relative scores, some interesting results emerge (see Figure 14.5). Considering the patients' defense use profiles side by side, we see that in each case the relative use of the immature defense of denial decreased after treatment (denial-pre vs. denial-post), and in each case the relative use of the defense of identification increased. The picture is somewhat different for the defense of projection. Here Karen remains about the same pre- and posttherapy, Jennifer shows an increase, and Mrs. S shows a large decrease in the use of projection.

Two factors can be considered regarding the changes in projection. First, for Karen, an early adolescent, projection is the normative defense, so we should expect to see prominent use of the defense throughout this period of development, as found. Second, it is important to note that the *relative* increase in Jennifer's use of projection is a function of the decrease in the *absolute* use of denial. The absolute number of projection responses actually decreased from 12 pretreatment to 9 posttreatment, whereas the absolute number of denial responses pretreatment (23) decreased to an absolute number of 8 denial responses posttreatment.

The very high identification score of Mrs. S (60%) is noteworthy. Although such high scores often occur with students of college age, they are rare in older adults from the general population. Mrs. S's score, coupled with her hospitalization for psychosis, is reminiscent of findings from hospitalized adults at the Austen Riggs Center (Cramer & Blatt, 1990). Those findings demonstrated that very high identification scores were often associated with a "false" identity rather than with healthy, mature ego integration (see Chapter 12). One wonders, then, about Mrs. S's posttreatment personality and whether there is some aspect of a "false self" being manifest, perhaps hinted at in her comment that she is no longer "crazy enough to keep telling people about her pathology"—that is, the surface self she presents to others differs from what lies underneath. Perhaps this presentation reflects a currently strong identification with her therapist, as sug-

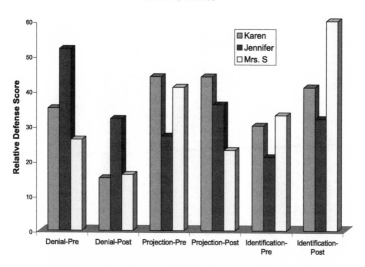

FIGURE 14.5. Defense use for Karen, Jennifer, and Mrs. S pre- and posttreatment.

gested in the posttherapy TAT story discussed above. In any case, we see that structural change in the use of defense mechanisms has occurred for all three patients; they are all functioning at a higher defense level after treatment.

Another finding becomes clear when we consider these patients in terms of *age* rather than diagnosis. Developmental differences are important to keep in mind, especially when working with children. Here we must always be aware that some change in defenses can be expected as a result of maturation. Research studies have shown that there are certain ages at which this is most likely to happen; for example, there is a significant decrease in the use of denial between 6½ and 7 years; there is a significant increase in projection between 8 and 9 years; and there is an increase in identification between 14 and 16 years (Cramer, 1997b; see Chapter 2).

Using normative data for girls helps us to more clearly understand the change that occurred in Karen's use of defenses (see Figure 14.6). The solid gray bars represent normative expectations at age 10 years; the striped gray bars represent Karen at age 10 years, 2 months. The solid black bars represent normative expectations at age 12; the striped black bars represent Karen at age 12 years, 5 months. As we can see, pretreatment Karen uses denial much more than would be expected for a child of her age; posttreatment, however, she is approximately at a normative level for denial. For projection, Karen is approximately at normative level both at pre- and posttreatment. For identification, she is below normative level pretreatment but at normative level posttreatment. Thus the immaturity in de-

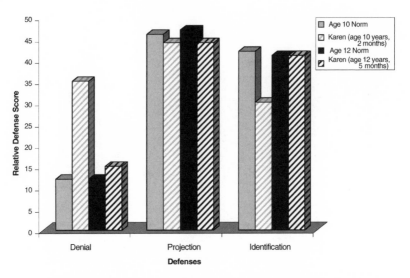

FIGURE 14.6. DMM normative expectations in relation to Karen.

fense functioning at age 10 years, 2 months has developed into a normative level at posttreatment.

As these findings demonstrate, when evaluating children's use of defenses, we should keep in mind some general developmental expectations and interpret findings not only in terms of individual change due to treatment but also in terms of change that might be expected as a result of maturation.

"JIM": A PSYCHOANALYTIC PATIENT[8]

In the previous cases, we compared the use of defenses before and after therapy. In the case of Jim, we trace the use of three defenses, as assessed with the DMM, as these occurred during the course of a 2-year psychoanalytic treatment. Here the DMM is used not only to assess the use of defenses in the patient's TAT stories but also to assess defense use that occurs during the therapy sessions that are reported. A full description of the content of the treatment sessions is available in Colarusso (1991, 2000).

At the beginning of treatment, Jim was nearly 10 years old. He was good looking, intelligent, and outgoing. However, he had difficulty making friends, was willful, had temper tantrums, and acknowledged that he was unhappy. He also described a phobia: He feared snakes in his bed. On the basis of diagnostic interviews with parents and child, as well as psychological testing, he was diagnosed as suffering from an anxiety neurosis with phobic and obsessional features.[9]

For a 10-year-old boy, both clinical observation and empirical research provides us with clear expectations regarding the use of denial, projection, and identification. From psychological testing (cf. Schwartz & Eagle, 1986) we would expect to find that the defense of denial, although characteristic of the 5-year-old and still used to some degree by the 7-year-old, has been largely relinquished by age 10. Empirical research also shows that 10-year-old boys no longer rely on denial as a prominent defense (see Chapter 2). Instead, the typical 10-year-old shows a greater use of projection.

Research findings with the DMM (see Chapter 2) led to the following expectations: A nearly 10-year-old boy would be assumed to show a relatively low use of denial (11%), with the prominent use of projection (52%) and some indication of the early components of identification (37%). When Jim's six TAT stories from the beginning of treatment were systematically evaluated for the use of these three defenses, the results indicated a pattern that is more characteristic of younger children: denial = 50%; projection = 33%; identification = 17%. Thus, at the beginning of his childhood therapy, rather than showing a predominant and age-appropriate use of projection, Jim relied heavily on the use of denial. The defense of identification, which should be increasing at this age, is notable by its near absence. At this point, Jim's use of defense mechanisms was developmentally immature.

Examples of his use of denial on the TAT are seen in the story given in response to Card 1 (a young boy seated in front of a violin).

Once upon a time a boy was playing his violin and he kept on practicing for a couple of years. Then he just got mad at his violin— no one knows why, but he did. His violin broke for some reason but nobody knew it—but he was glad it was broken because he didn't want to play it anymore . . .

Here Jim, the storyteller, twice denies that anyone knew the reason why the boy was mad and why his violin broke ("he got mad . . . no one knows why"; "his violin broke for some reason but nobody knew it"). This condition of "not knowing" also occurs in his story given in response to Card 3BM, where "nobody knew what to do," and to Card 15, "he didn't know what names [he] should call them."

His story in response to Card 2 (a farm scene, with a man plowing the fields, a pregnant woman looking on, and a younger woman standing with books in her hand) also demonstrates his use of denial.

Once upon a time, a man was exploring a cave and he saw some cave drawings and he started to draw—to copy—the cave drawings down and when he got to the museum he took a photo of it—but when he got there—there was a picture of it in the newspaper that saw him photographing the cave drawing—and he became one of the best known cheaters in the world. So when he got home everybody started shouting at him, "What did you do that for?" And then—the end.

This story is striking in its complete omission of (i.e., "not seeing") the three characters depicted in the picture: the woman in the foreground, the pregnant woman leaning against a tree, and the man plowing the field. When the examiner asked Jim directly who these people are, he again used denial, saying, "I don't know." With further pressure from the examiner, it becomes clear that Jim has "seen" the issue of pregnancy, but he quickly adds another denial that the man and woman could have a baby. Further examples of denial occur on other TAT cards, on the Rorschach, and in the diagnostic interviews with Dr. Colarusso. Such prevalence of denial in a 10-year-old boy is age inappropriate, and the occurrence of projection is noticeably less than would be expected at 10 years of age.

When we turn to the material describing the early therapy interactions between Jim and his therapist, we again see the predominance of denial and the relative absence of the age-appropriate defense of projection. In the following material, I trace systematically the occurrence of denial and projection, as these are described at different points in the therapy. If defense development is to get back "on track," the use of denial should markedly decrease, with a corresponding rise in projection.

In the early sessions denial occurred around the possibility that Jim harbored aggressive impulses; this possibility was consistently denied. For example, during his play in Session 25, Jim stated that he was going to bomb the Empire State Building, but he denied that anyone would get hurt (he says, "no one" is inside); he also denied that the analyst might be angry about a mark he made on the wall. In the next reported session (35), Jim denied the wish to oppose the analyst and, in his play, denied that he and the analyst were harmed by bombs dropped, despite the enormous power used to destroy the house they were in. In a subsequent session (37), the analyst began to interpret Jim's defenses, calling attention to the defensive behavior and its possible function.

At this point in the therapy, the defense of projection began to emerge. By Session 85, Jim stated that his parents "don't want me to be big and strong because they don't want me to order them around." This projection was immediately interpreted ("I guess you feel that's what you would like to do"). The interpretation met with resistance and was then followed by Jim withdrawing from the discussion, a regression to the earlier defense of denial. But he recovered, and the therapist then called attention to another projection ("I guess you feel that I was playing a trick on you"), to which Jim agreed.

In Session 86 the therapist returned to Jim's projection ("they don't want me to boss them around"). In contrast to the resistance following the interpretation of this statement in Session 85, this time Jim accepted the interpretation: "It's true. I would [like to boss them]." In this same session, an early form of identification occurred, when Jim decided to play a game of solitaire *with* the analyst, who commented on this identification process: "We're going to combine our power." Jim was then described as "basking in the warmth of identification with the analyst-father" (p. 211). At this point in the treatment, all three defenses—denial, projection and identification—are seen in the interaction between Jim and his analyst.

After this time, Jim's behavior and analytic material were noted to be age appropriate. He has a healthy romantic interest in girls, has made friends, is successful in team sports, and has distanced himself from overinvolvement with his parents, insisting on more autonomy. In his analyst's assessment, he has returned to the developmental mainstream. Termination was now seriously discussed between patient and analyst. During this time, Jim's use of identification as a defense against the impending loss was seen in his putting on the analyst's jacket; the defense was interpreted. The importance of maintaining the bond between them was also expressed in Jim's crafting of a ring for his analyst. At 12 years of age, the analysis was terminated.

If we had complete transcripts of all the analytic sessions, it would be possible to provide a very accurate description of Jim's use and change of defenses as the analysis progressed. Lacking this, it is still possible to divide the analysis into the seven phases indicated by the analyst in his report and then make a rough estimate of the occurrence of the three defenses during each phase. Obviously, this is not an "accurate" account; it is meant only as an indication of how we might proceed in using the present approach to study defense change in analysis, where some interesting trends can be observed.

In the opening phase (Sessions 24–99), based on a count of defense use, denial appears as the most frequent defense (67% of all defenses mentioned); projection (13%) and identification (20%) are used noticeably less often. In the next phase (Sessions 100–125), there is evidence of Jim interpreting his own use of denial. In the third phase (Sessions 133–179), the relative use of the three defenses has shifted to a more age-appropriate distribution: denial (28%), projection (43%), identification (28%). There is also evidence during this phase of Jim's interpreting his own use of projection.

However, following this phase, according to the analyst, "the most painful part of the analysis" began. This painful part was accompanied by a regressive shift in defense use. During this fourth phase (Sessions 196–203), denial again is most prominent (62%), followed by projection (26%)

and identification (12%). Also, during this phase, Jim provided his own interpretation of his use of denial. During the next phase (Sessions 211–235),
the use of denial continues to predominate (71%), with projection following (28%) and no evidence of identification from the material provided.
The last two phases (Sessions 272–282 and 314–356) provide no mention
of defense use, with the exception of the two examples, given above, of
identification with the analyst during termination.

If we take an overall view of this material from the perspective of the
use of age-appropriate defense mechanisms, the general impression is that, at
the beginning of the analysis, there was excessive use of the age-inappropriate
defense of denial and inadequate use of the defense of projection. As the
analysis progressed, there was more evidence of projection, and then of
identification, as would be expected in a boy approaching adolescence.

These interesting "results" raise certain questions. They are interesting
in that they show, during the first half of the analysis, a shift in the use of
defenses from an age-inappropriate to an age-appropriate pattern, suggesting a healthy developmental progression. However, as the analysis moves
into the "most painful" part, there is a reversion to the age-inappropriate
defense of denial. Nevertheless, the use of age-appropriate projection is
maintained at a somewhat higher level than was found in the initial stages.
Unfortunately, we do not have sufficient information about the content of
the last two phases to know whether, having worked through these painful
issues, there was again a shift to the more age-appropriate pattern of
defense use, as had occurred earlier. Certainly the absence of presenting
symptoms and the evidence for developmentally appropriate concerns and
behaviors would suggest this to be the case. It would have been very interesting, at this point, to have independent information from psychological
testing to assess the relative use of the three defenses—that is, to determine
to what degree Jim had returned to the "mainstream" of defense mechanism development.

CONCLUDING REMARKS

In this chapter we have seen how an assessment of defense use can comple-
ment and add to our understanding of a patient's pathology. As we have
noted in other cases of pathological aggression (see Chapter 11), the defense combination of denial and projection in a serial killer can be seen to
contribute to the manifestation of violent behavior. The study of individual
cases also demonstrates the change in defense use associated with the experience of psychotherapy that has been reported from larger group studies
(see Chapter 13). In each of the individual cases discussed, the use of immature defenses decreased after therapy, whereas the use of mature defenses

increased. In fact, when transcripts from therapy sessions at different points in the treatment are available, it is possible to assess defense change as it occurs over the course of the therapy.

Finally, in the study of defense change in children who are in treatment, we must be mindful of the relation between maturational level and defense expectations. Whereas an adult's decrease in the defense of projection may be a sign of better functioning, this may not be the case for an early adolescent, for whom the use of projection is age appropriate.

PART V

Assessment of Defenses

*I*n my own work I have found that the use of narrative stories is a particularly successful means for studying defense mechanisms. Whereas *reading* stories provides a view of the material world and the social environment outside of the self, the *creation* of stories reflects the inner environment of the storymaker—his or her wishes, hopes, fears, and quirks. As Dan McAdams (1993) has phrased it, "Storytelling appears to be a fundamental way of expressing ourselves and our worlds to others" (p. 27). In this expression of self, the storyteller's typical defenses will be manifest.

In the approach to storytelling known as the Thematic Apperception Test (TAT), we do not ask people to tell stories about themselves—we do not ask explicitly for a description of the "personal myth" (McAdams, 1993, p. 12). Rather, we present a pictorial rendition of what might be described as "life moments"—scenes that depict life experiences that are more or less familiar to the storymaker—and ask for a story about that situation. What is interesting about this procedure is the myriad reactions that occur to the same black-and-white picture. For example, consider the TAT picture of a scantily dressed man clinging to a rope. What is clearly, to one storyteller, an athletic man climbing up a rope in a sports competition is, to another, a man escaping from a fire in the bedroom of his mistress, climbing down the rope to save his life. Assuming that the two storytellers are telling their stories under similar circumstances, to the extent that both of them are reacting to the same picture, the differences in their reactions must come from inner differences in wishes, motives, and fears. In this sense, the story each composes tells us something about each person's personal myth, even though this information was not explicitly requested.

295

In many ways, stories are particularly well suited to provide information about defense mechanisms. The open-ended nature of stories allows for a relatively free expression of thought processes. This unhampered verbal production gives us a window into discovering the thought processes of the individual, including the working of defense mechanisms.

Based on the theoretical description of denial, projection, and identification provided in Part II, the rationale for using narrative materials to assess these defenses is discussed in Chapter 15. The revised Defense Mechanism Manual provides the explicit coding rules to assess each of the three defenses. The Manual is available at www.williams.edu/Faculty/Cramer/cramer.html.

Chapter 16 describes several other methods of assessing defense mechanisms, including the DMRS and the DSQ.

CHAPTER 15

Explaining the Defense Mechanism Manual[1]

*I*n this chapter a narrative approach to the assessment of defense mechanisms is described. The choice of this approach was based on several considerations. A defense mechanism is a thought process that may take different forms and be expressed through a variety of content. For these reasons, the assessment method should allow for thought processes to be revealed in an unhampered and undirected fashion, in an open-ended format where no stereotyped response is readily available. Although these thought processes may not be observed directly, they can be inferred from verbal behavior. Because defense mechanisms are rather complex mental processes, they are more likely to be revealed in relatively extensive samples of verbal behavior than in single-word responses. Finally, some means must be available for two or more independent observers to decide whether or not a defense was used. The method that most closely approximates these various requirements is the TAT, for which the DMM was especially developed to score defenses. The manual may also be used with the Children's Apperception Test (CAT), or with any other narrative material. The manual itself may be freely downloaded from www.williams.edu/Psychology/Faculty/Cramer/cramer.html (select Defense Mechanism Manual).

Why should we expect to find defense mechanisms used in this kind of storytelling or narrative material? First, recall that our definition of a defense mechanism is a cognitive operation that functions to protect the individual from anxiety or loss of self-esteem. In the storytelling procedure, the person is placed in a situation with an unknown examiner who, by virtue of being the examiner, is in a position of authority. For many persons, this is a situation that will increase anxiety, especially if the examiner is seen as someone who is judging the storyteller. Second, the storyteller is requested, on the spot (i.e., without preparation), to create an imaginative story about a somewhat ambiguous picture. Such a request may be experienced as a demand to demonstrate intelligence, creativity, quickness, or other positively valued aspects of the self. The feeling of being "examined" may be especially strong if the storytelling occurs in an institutional setting. But even in a more benign setting, the storyteller's self-esteem may be challenged, and this challenge will contribute to some anxiety associated with the storytelling process.

Thus the request to tell a story may be expected to arouse some anxiety and some self-esteem concern in many people; in turn, this arousal will activate the use of defense mechanisms. Then we may expect that the stories they produce will reflect the activation of these defenses. That is, the way in which the story is told will be influenced by the operation of defenses.

In earlier chapters the components of the defenses of denial, projection, and identification were discussed from theoretical and developmental points of view (see Chapters 3, 4, and 5). In this chapter I use the components of the defenses as the basis for assessing defense mechanisms in TAT stories, and I formulate the components in a way that they may be identified in the thematic productions of children and adults. These formulations provide the basis for the Defense Mechanism Manual (DMM).

For each defense the components have been arranged into seven scoring categories. Each of these categories is discussed and illustrated in the remainder of the chapter. An attempt is made to provide the reader with the kind of thinking and rationale that formed the basis for the development of the scoring categories. In the DMM numerous examples from various TAT and CAT cards are given. Also, specific rules for scoring or not scoring a category, and for differentiating between similar categories, are provided.

ASSESSMENT OF DENIAL WITH THE DMM

In Chapter 3 we saw that the defense of denial can be manifest in different components. Some of these components (e.g., failure to perceive, avoidance of perception, perceptual errors, reversal, and negation) are closely tied to perception and were grouped together in the previous discussion as constituting aspects of perceptual denial. Other components (e.g., unfounded optimism, idealized goodness, maximization and minimization of an idealized object's qualities, and daydreams [fantasied or enacted]) were discussed as contributing to the establishment of an alternative reality—that is, the imposition of a personal fantasy onto experience.

In this section we examine these components as they may appear in stories told in response to the TAT. Seven scoring categories have been developed to help locate them. In most cases, a single component is represented by a single category. However, the components of avoidance of perception and of daydreams have been combined into a single category called *denial of reality*.

Scoring Categories of Denial

The seven categories for scoring denial are as follows:

1. Omission of major characters or objects
2. Misperception
3. Reversal
4. Negation
5. Denial of reality
6. Overly maximizing the positive or minimizing the negative
7. Unexpected goodness, optimism, positiveness, gentleness

Using the Scoring Categories for Denial

For each of the scoring categories of denial, an example is given from stories told in response to TAT Card 1, which depicts a young boy seated in front of a table, on which a violin lies.[2]

1. *Omission of major characters or objects.* This category represents the most primitive component of denial: the failure to perceive what is there to be seen. Scores in this category refer to the failure to perceive salient stimuli that are seen by nearly all one's peers. The category applies only to the major or obvious objects; these are specified for each card. Omission of any of these objects in the story told is scored according to a prescribed plan.

For example, in TAT Card 1, the omission of either the boy or the violin from the story is given a score of 1. However, if perception of the object is implied in the story by including a reference to the function of the critical object, an omission is not scored.

The following story, told in response to TAT Card 1 by an adolescent boy, illustrates the category of omission:

> *This boy is one of many children in a classroom. He is unsure of many of the answers for the questions which have been given him on the test*

he is taking. He'll casually glance over at the answers the other children have on their papers. He won't get caught and will probably do very well. . . .

In this boy's story there is no mention of the violin, nor is there any reference to music or to practicing. The presence of the violin in the picture is not acknowledged.

Occasionally, especially with young children, the storyteller may perceive the critical object but not know what it is or what to call it. Different reactions are possible to this problem situation. If the storyteller makes no reference to the unknown object and thus acts as though there is nothing there to be explained, the category of omission is scored, as previously described. However, if the storyteller acknowledges that something is there but that it is unknown to him, then he has made an accurate assessment of reality. This nondefensive reaction is illustrated in the following story in response to TAT Card 1:

That's a little boy. He's down on his workbench and he's looking this over and he's wondering what it is. And he's wondering if he'll ever find out. He can't wait till his father comes home so he can ask his father. And he's kind of sitting there wondering when his father will come home.

In this creative, adaptive solution to the problem of seeing something but not knowing what it is, the storyteller incorporates the problem he faces into the story itself. He openly discusses his lack of knowledge, rather than denying it. In such a case, omission is not scored.

2. *Misperception.* There is a third way in which "not knowing" the meaning of an object may be handled. Rather than blotting it out completely or acknowledging her ignorance, the storyteller may change the object into something it is not. In such a case, a misperception has occurred.

This category also represents a primitive component of denial. Misperception may be used defensively against "not knowing," as previously described. It may also occur because the perceptual process is pathologically distorted. In either case, the disturbing external stimulus is handled by changing it into something it is not.

Misperception, as a component of denial, is scored for any unusual or distorted perception of a figure, object, or action in the TAT picture that is without sufficient support for the observation—but only if the projected image is not of ominous quality. (Misperceptions that are ominous are scored under projection.)

The following story, told in response to TAT Card 1 by a kindergarten girl, illustrates the category of misperception, in which the violin is misperceived as a mirror:

The boy is looking in the mirror at himself. And, he is wondering about how he is going to look for the party, and he doesn't know what to wear.

3. *Reversal.* As a component of denial, reversal modifies the disturbing aspects of reality by changing them into their opposite. On the TAT, reversal can be seen when the usual perception of the card is changed into its opposite, when the story itself involves a reversal of theme or details, or when a character takes on qualities that were previously stated to be the opposite, including a change of sex. The concept of reversal involves both ends of a continuum (e.g., happy–sad; strong–weak; honest–dishonest).

The following story by a 12-year-old boy, told in response to TAT Card 6BM (see Chapter 14, p. 275), illustrates the component of reversal:

This looks like a man that was a gunman for his gang. The mother found out and disowned him, though she didn't want to. Then the son goes out and makes good. He gets a good job after helping the police round up a gang of gamblers or crooks.

4. *Negation.* Although negation is sometimes considered to be a separate defense, it can be considered a component of denial as well, for it changes the real to the not-real, the truth to the untruth. Negation is accomplished by assigning a negative value, a minus sign, to an experience that if acknowledged, would produce pain. As such, it refers to only one end of a continuum that either *is* or *is not* (i.e., is negated). Negation stands in contrast to reversal, which involves both ends of the continuum. Not all negative statements, of course, are defensive. Sometimes the defensive aspect of a negative statement can be determined from its unusual or unexpected nature. In this case, the action or event that is negated would not be expected to happen, so the need to point out that it did not happen is felt as unnecessary (e.g., "He wasn't thinking about killing his mother"). Other times, the defensive nature of the negation is more straightforward; for example, "He fell from the top of the building, but he didn't get hurt."

Negation is scored if a character in the story "does not . . . " any action, wish, or intention that, if acknowledged, would cause displeasure, pain, or humiliation. It is also scored if the storyteller negates or denies a fact or feeling. Also, references to doubt as to what the stimulus card is are scored. Such comments are based on the assumption that the stimulus card *is* something, and the defense is seen in the expression of doubt that the card may *not* be that thing. The following story in response to TAT Card 1 illustrates the category of negation:

> *Johnny is staring at the violin. . . . He has thought about breaking the violin but won't. . . . He will soon forget his problems.*

Negation is also illustrated in the following story of an 11-year-old boy, told in response to TAT Card 12M (young man lying on couch, older man leaning over him, hand outstretched): "Here is a sick woman . . . the woman doesn't feel anything; she's just sleeping." As in the previous story, the negation—the sick woman "doesn't feel anything"—is accompanied by another component of denial, namely, the avoidance of reality ("she's just sleeping"), which is discussed in Category 5.

Negation also occurred in the story discussed under category 1, omission. In that story, the boy who is looking at the answers of other children "won't get caught."

5. *Denial of reality.* This category includes two of the components of denial discussed in Chapter 3: avoidance of a situation and daydreaming. They are grouped together because they share a characteristic of denial through the *avoidance* of reality rather than through rejection (omission), distortion, or change. This avoidance is accomplished either through a physical action or through a mental fantasy that allows an escape from the real into the unreal.

Physical avoidance may occur by refusing to (1) look at something that would be unpleasant to see, (2) think something that would be unpleasant to think, or (3) hear something that would be unpleasant to hear (e.g., "He doesn't listen to what his mother has to say because he knows she is angry at him").[3] In a more extreme form, this kind of avoidance of reality is accomplished through falling asleep, fainting, or dreaming—all of which remove the individual from the possibility of perceiving reality.

Avoidance of reality through the use of fantasy (e.g., daydreaming) occurs in two ways. First, the fantasy, which is clearly false with regard to reality, may be used to avoid thinking about what is really happening. Or the knowledge that fantasy exists may be used to deny the reality of a painful situation, by attributing to it the unreal status of being "only a dream" or "just make-believe."

The following story, told in response to TAT Card 1 (the boy and the violin) by an 11-year-old girl, is an example of the denial of reality through physical avoidance:

> *There's a boy looking at his violin, looking like he does not want to practice. So . . . he's plugging his ears so he won't have to play it to his teacher for the concert.*

Avoidance or denial of reality through the use of fantasy is illustrated in the following story, also told in response to TAT Card 1 by an adolescent girl:

> *The little kid is in a school. . . . Possibly he has just been scolded by the supervisor and has realized it is useless to try to fight back, so he returns to his own thoughts.*

The use of fantasy to deny reality may be very straightforward, as in the following story of an 11-year-old boy told in response to TAT Card 7GF. (Older woman sitting on a sofa, alongside a girl who holds a doll.)

> *The girl doesn't have any brothers or sisters, she's just daydreaming about having a little baby sister or brother—she wants one real bad. . . .*

6. *Overly maximizing the positive or minimizing the negative.* This category represents one of the components of Pollyannish denial. It may occur as an aspect of idealization and may be accompanied by a note of unfounded optimism. Its purpose is to magnify positive experiences and reduce or eliminate the impact of events that are painful. On the TAT it is seen in any gross exaggeration or underestimation of a character's qualities, including power, size, beauty, or possessions. The following story, told in response to TAT Card 1 (the boy and the violin) by an adolescent girl, illustrates the use of maximization:

> *This boy, John, is a very talented young musician. . . . He has played at such renowned places as Carnegie Hall and Denver Atheneum. Even though he's only four. . . .*

7. *Unexpected goodness, optimism, positiveness, gentleness.* Again, this component is a part of Pollyannish denial. It represents the continuing need to see the world as only a positive, pleasure-giving place, despite evidence to the contrary. It involves an imposition onto reality of variants of the inner defensive fantasy that this is the best (sweetest, kindest, gentlest, etc.) of all possible worlds. It includes instances in which the developing story leads one to expect a negative outcome, but then, without adequate explanation, everything works out for the best. It also includes instances in which negative experiences are treated as unimportant, reacted to with a "sour grapes" "I didn't want it anyway" attitude, or willingly accepted as part of one's "fate." Often a saccharine "life is beautiful" flavor is present in these stories. Occasionally, this component is expressed through a stance of naive wonder or awefulness.

The following story, told in response to TAT Card 1 by a college freshman, illustrates this category, as well as the component of maximization discussed in the previous category:

> *Jeremy was alone. The tinseled tree and paper wrappings had been put away for another year. . . . The violin . . . began to make the most beautiful music this world has ever heard. And that music led Jeremy away into another world filled with smiles that didn't fade and tinseled trees that grew all year long.*

ASSESSMENT OF PROJECTION WITH THE DMM

We turn now to the second defense, projection. As with denial, the various components of projection, which were discussed in Chapter 4, are used to establish scoring categories. Although some of these components involve the attribution of feelings or affective states to people or things, other components are concerned with the attribution of responsibility to external causes. When hostile feelings are projected onto others and the source of responsibility for events is felt to be external, then the world is perceived as a frightening place wherein one may expect to be attacked or trapped, and it is necessary to protect oneself from such attack and plan for escape. In the extreme, this constellation may create a bizarre view of reality. Expression of these thoughts are also components of projection.

In this section we examine the components of projection as they appear in stories told in response to TAT cards. Although mindful of certain problems attendant on assessing projection in a projective test,[4] we nevertheless proceed to score projection based on the occurrence of certain themes or ideas in the stories. These themes are scored when they are attributed to any character in the story or when they occur as a justification for the story given by the storyteller. Although one might argue that only those attributions made to the hero of the story should be considered projections (based on the assumption that the hero represents the storyteller), we instead take the point of view that each character, object, and event in the story represents some facet of the storyteller's psyche. Because projection involves putting the "bad," negative, and unacceptable onto something outside of one's psyche, we therefore score all unexplained or unjustified negative feelings, intentions, and events that occur in the story as instances of projection.

Seven scoring categories have been developed to help locate the components of projection. The attribution of negative feelings or intentions is separated from the attribution, or addition, of negative objects or qualities of objects to the stories. Likewise, the attribution of responsibility to external causes forms a separate category. In addition, three categories include different expressions of the idea that the world is a dangerous place in which one must assume a protective stance. The final category covers instances in which projection contributes to the expression of bizarre thoughts.

Scoring Categories for Projection

The following is a summary of the seven scoring categories of projection:

1. Attribution of aggressive or hostile feelings, emotions, or intentions to a character, or the attribution of other feelings, emotions, or intentions that are normatively unusual
2. Addition of ominous people, ghosts, animals, objects, or qualities
3. Magical or circumstantial thinking
4. Concern for protection against external threat
5. Apprehensiveness about death, injury, or assault
6. Themes of pursuit, entrapment, and escape
7. Bizarre or very unusual story or theme

Using the Scoring Categories of Projection

1. *Attribution of aggressive or hostile feelings, emotions, or intentions to a character, or the attribution of any other feelings, emotions, or intentions that are normatively unusual.* This category includes instances in which negative feelings are attributed by the storyteller to a character in the story, as well as instances in which one character in the story attributes negative feelings or intentions to another character. However, the attribution of negative feelings is scored *only* if there is no justifiable reason for the attribution. Negative feelings that are clearly the result of something that has happened are not scored as projection.

Many stories include instances in which a negative feeling or intention is attributed to one character. In the following story (told in response to TAT Card 17BM [a partially clad man clinging to a rope] by an adolescent girl) it is made clear that a man is the victim of his uncle's bad intentions; there is no redeeming justification for these intentions:

> *This is a man who was in an insane asylum. He wasn't really insane, but a rich uncle wanted all his money, thus had him committed. . . .*

Occurring less often is the instance in which one character in the story attributes a negative intention to another character in the story. For example, in the following story told in response to TAT Card 1 (the boy and the violin) by an adolescent girl, the boy in the story attributes negative intentions to his father:

The boy has just gotten an expensive violin for his birthday. His father
. . . gave it to him for something to do. The boy cannot play football
like his friends, because he is a hemophiliac. . . . The boy is upset. . . .
He feels it's all his father's fault that he is treated so carefully, and the
violin is the latest example of overprotection and injustice. . . .

2. *Addition of ominous people, ghosts, animals, objects, or qualities.*
Besides illustrating the projection of negative feelings and intentions, the
previous two stories also illustrate another component of projection: the
addition of an ominous quality to the story. This occurs in the first story
when the setting is stated to be an insane asylum; in the second story the
boy is described as being a hemophiliac. It is important, of course, that
there is nothing in either picture to possibly suggest these ominous additions.

Another example of ominous additions is seen in the following story
told in response to TAT card 17BM (man on a rope) by a 4½-year-old boy:

That man is on the rope. Because he is trying to get away. Because he
doesn't want to get hurt, by the guards. The guards are bad. The
guards have long, sharp things. . .'.

In this story, we see first the addition of guards who are bad, and then
the further addition of the "long, sharp things." Although in creating a
story it is often necessary for the storyteller to make additions to the rather
sparse picture, we score only ominous additions as instances of projection,
in keeping with our definition of projection as involving the placing of *neg-*
ative feelings outside of the self.

As a special subgroup of this category, we score references to people,
animals, or objects as being decrepit, falling apart, or deteriorating. The
assumption is that such a reference, when made without justification in
reality, represents some (unacceptable) aspect of the storyteller's experience of himself. Sometimes this occurs with TAT Card 1 in references to
the violin, or its strings, being broken, without explanation, but it may
occur on any card, as in the following examples for CAT Card 5 (a room
with a large bed and lamp in the background and a crib in the foreground, in which there are two baby bears): "The crib looks like it's going to fall over" (age 9 years); "The lamp looks like it's all cracked" (age
5 years).

The most striking example I have encountered supporting the assumption that references to objects or people being damaged or defective are actually projections of feelings about oneself as damaged came from a story
told by a 5½-year-old boy. This young fellow had already twice undergone
eye surgery to correct a muscle imbalance; at the time of storytelling, he

was again about to travel to the hospital for further surgery. In response to TAT Card 1 (the boy and the violin), he said:

I think he is putting his arm like that (gestures). *And he's—is he, um, is he blind, or could he see?*

Descriptions of the boy in the picture as blind are extremely rare. It seems highly likely that this description is related to the child's concern about his own eyes.

3. *Magical or circumstantial thinking.* A person's use of magical or circumstantial thinking is often related to her projection of responsibility onto causes external to the self. By maintaining that events occur as a result of magical, illogical, and uncontrollable external forces, the individual is absolved from any personal responsibility and therefore from experiencing shame or guilt. Related to magical thinking is the use of animism, in which human thoughts or emotions are attributed to objects other than animals or people. Such attribution often serves the purpose of locating responsibility outside of the (human) individual. At the same time, an individual's belief that she is controlled from without is often associated with a hyper-alertness to the environment, in which the person is on the lookout for events that may have a negative effect on her. This suspicious stance is an attempt to protect the self from felt external control. The circularity of this process—the person's attempt to protect the self against her own projections—may result in thinking that is peculiar, personalized, or overly circumstantial. The projection of responsibility is seen clearly in the story of a 14-year-old boy told in response to TAT Card 1:

This boy of less than ten years is pondering over how such an inanimate object could cause him such grief. . . .

In this example the responsibility for the boy's frustration is attributed to the inanimate violin, rather than being acknowledged as due to his own difficulties in playing the instrument.

The projection of responsibility is also seen in stories in which one character hypnotizes another or displays other unusual powers of control over others. It is not unusual that a story about a hypnotist is told in response to Card 12M of the TAT; the picture of a prone man and another standing over him with an outstretched arm easily evokes this theme. It is important to note, however, that stories focusing on the benign concern of one man for another are also frequently given to this picture. Only when one character assumes control over the other is this projection category scored.

The following story told in response to Card 12M by a 12-year-old boy illustrates the concern over being controlled by another:

> *Once upon a time there was a great hypnotist . . . he had to get somebody he could really practice on. So, he was out walking on this street, and he went into an alley, and he pulled this kid in with him. And then he jumped into his little car, and he took off for the woods. And when they got into the cave . . . he turned him into a little green thing. . . .*

The presence of animism in TAT stories occurs primarily with very young children. Its occurrence in older individuals is generally an indication of defensive weakness, although occasionally a person may consciously use animism as a literary technique. Examples from preschoolers include a story in which "canes are talking" (CAT Card 3) and "rifles are feeling sorry" (TAT Card 8BM: Adolescent boy looks straight out of picture; surgical operation in background; a rifle at one side of picture). An example from an adolescent—"an idiotic violin" (TAT Card l, the boy and the violin)—is more indicative of defensive weakness.

Some stories, rather than portraying a feeling of external control directly, express a hypervigilant focusing on flaws in the environment that are perceived as being guileful or misleading. This concern may take the form of searching for "tricks" in the task itself, noting, for example, inadequacies in the drawings or hidden ambiguities, the presence of which is assumed to make the task more difficult. For the person who adopts this point of view the responsibility for one's performance in the storytelling task lies with the inadequate picture (and its creator), rather than with the person telling the story. Thinking of this sort is often circumstantial and may have a paranoid flavor.

Examples of this category occur in statements made by the storyteller about the task—"There's probably a trick to this"—or about the picture—"Is the rope supposed to suggest a hanging?" They may also occur in the attempt to justify hostile themes through the use of circumstantial or illogical reasoning—"It must have been a murder he committed, because he isn't carrying any valuables or money," referring to the partially clad man clinging to the rope on TAT Card 17BM. A similar use of circumstantial reasoning to justify the idea of someone chasing the hero appears in the following story of a 16-year-old adolescent boy to the same card:

> *The man on the rope seems either angry or excited to get down the rope. I would think that there is someone chasing him down the rope since he is in the process of climbing down. . . .*

In fact, there could be many reasons that a man would be climbing down a rope. Further, it is not clear from the picture whether the man is climbing down or up. To use the rope climbing as a *justification* for assuming that someone is chasing him—he is climbing down; therefore someone is chasing him—involves circumstantial reasoning. The use of this kind of reasoning must be differentiated from the expression of a similar theme, in which the storyteller takes responsibility for the idea of the chase.

4. *Concern for protection against external threat.* The projection of negative feelings and intentions onto others, although ridding the individual of one kind of anxiety may produce a new source of stress. The effect of such projection is to change the environment into a dangerous place, in which other people are seen as threatening; it then becomes necessary to find ways to protect oneself against this threat. The protective stance may be seen in an attitude of suspiciousness, of being on the lookout for expected danger or expected persecution. In the discussion of magical or circumstantial thinking, this protective stance appeared directly in the story-teller's comment, "There's probably a trick to this," but it may also appear in the story itself. The following story, told by a 16-year-old adolescent boy in response to TAT Card 17BM (man clinging to a rope), illustrates this concern for protection from external threat:

> *The criminal has taken many precautions before he is shown in the picture. He has checked to see if people are coming and he has other people on the lookout for him. . . .*

The self-protective attitude sometimes appears as the storyteller's defensive need for self-justification. For example, some individuals are disturbed by TAT Card 8BM, a picture of a prone man being operated on and with a rifle standing near the boy in the front of the picture. Storytellers sometimes handle this disturbance by omitting any mention of the rifle; such an omission is scored under denial. Other storytellers mention the rifle and add a personal justification for doing so: "I say it is a gun because it looks like one we had at home." Such self-justification is scored under category 4.

The concern for protection may also take the form of creating physical barriers (e.g., constructing walls, locking doors) in the story, or by references to hiding or the use of disguises that protect one from being discovered. A dramatic example of assuming a disguise occurs in the following story by a 15-year-old girl:

> *The person in this story is a 35-year-old con man. . . . The policeman recognizes him . . . he is taken to prison. But he escapes and after a*

plastic surgeon changes his face, he cuts his fingers and toes to change his fingerprints. . . .

References to hiding may be of two sorts. In one case, the character may hide himself, so as not to be found, or he may believe that others are hiding (lying in wait). In the other case, the character hides something he knows, has produced, or has seen, so that he may not be blamed or harmed. Examples of hiding oneself are often quite straightforward: in response to TAT Card 17BM, an 8-year-old girl told this succinct story:

A man is climbing a rope. Because he was afraid of something. He was trying to hide.

Somewhat more complex is the theme that someone *else* is hiding or lying in wait. A 10-year-old girl expresses this concern in response to the same TAT card:

He's thinking that when he gets down, he thinks that man is hiding somewhere and he's not sure whether he should get down or not.

The need to hide something one knows or has done appears in the story of a 16-year-old boy, responding to TAT Card 1 (the boy and the violin): "He does not reveal his discovery to anyone."

5. *Apprehensiveness about death, injury, or assault.* Related to the concern for protection against external threat are themes involving the overt occurrence of physical harm, or even death, to characters in the story. In the preceding category, the emphasis is on the need for *protection* against threat. To score the present category, events involving death, physical attack, or injury must actually occur, or have occurred, in the story.

Examples of this category occur frequently at every developmental level. A 4½-year-old boy told the following story in response to TAT Card 17BM:

A giant is climbing a rope. . . . The rope breaks and the building falls down. The giant is dead.

A 7-year-old boy portrayed his apprehensiveness of external attack by adding some animals to the situation. The ominous addition of alligators as a vehicle for carrying out the projection of oral aggressive impulses occurs with some frequency in this age group.

That's a guy climbing a rope. . . . He's climbing down and I wonder what's going to be under him. Maybe there'll be alligators under there. . . . He's going to get eaten up by the alligators.

In contrast, a 10-year-old boy told a story in which the external attack occurs from the ominous addition of sharp, pointed spikes—vehicles for carrying the projection of phallic aggressive impulses.

This man is [sic] just got in trouble and is climbing down the rope. . . . But down here are some spikes; and I think when he gets down to the bottom his feet are going to get holes [in them] and starting bleeding to death.

An example of injury and death comes from a 15-year-old boy:

A person rescuing someone. . . . The person being rescued [not shown] is moaning of a broken leg. He and the rescuer are hated enemies. . . . The rescuer dies saving his enemy. . . .

This example is interesting not only for the two incidents of injury and death, but also because it illustrates the process of projection in two other ways. First, the addition of the person moaning with the broken leg is entirely of the storyteller's own creation; there is nothing in the picture to suggest another person, and thus category 2 is scored. Second, having created a second person to whom physical injury is attributed, the storyteller additionally projects feelings of animosity between the two individuals, which earns a score in category 1.

Sometimes the projection of aggressive feelings takes the form of the attack being turned back on the self, so that a character hurts himself or commits suicide. Although this theme is quite rare with younger children, it does occur in the stories of adolescents. Thus, a 16-year-old girl told the following story in response to TAT Card 1:

A small boy is sitting at a desk, concentrating on the thing that is on his desk. . . . The object on the desk is a gun. It has just killed someone he loves very much. . . . Finally he is so overcome by the death he picks up the heavy gun and shoots himself. . . .

The first example of projection in this story occurs when the storyteller misperceives the violin and turns it into a gun. Although benign misperceptions are scored as denial, those in which the content is clearly ominous are scored as projection. As the story unfolds, we see that this misperception is used as the vehicle to carry the projection of two murders. In the first case, "it" (the gun) has killed someone; the responsibility for the murder is attributed to the gun. The storyteller is unable to connect the murderous impulse with a person. The likely reason for this—extreme guilt experienced in connection with the existence of hostile feelings—becomes apparent in the second murder, in which the boy uses the gun to kill himself.

6. *Themes of pursuit, entrapment, and escape.* This category includes another kind of manifestation of the fear of being controlled by others. Included here are themes involving one character being pursued by another or the mention of being trapped or kidnapped or put in prison without legal justification. Also included are themes of escape from physical imprisonment or physical danger or the threat thereof.

A story told in response to TAT Card 17BM by a 7-year-old boy illustrates the theme of being pursued: "A man's sliding down the rope and someone was after him."

A more vivid example comes from a 17-year-old boy:

> *The man is looking back to see where his pursuers are. . . . The soldiers throw spears at the man. He is pierced by one. He falls to the ground and dies.*

This story also includes ominous additions and the theme of phallic aggression and would also be scored for projection under categories 2 and 5. Sometimes the emphasis is on being trapped rather than on the pursuit or the escape. Such is the case in the following story from a 6-year-old boy:

> *He's trying to climb the rope and he's going up from where the alligators were and he's trying to get away from them so he won't get killed. Then there's an alligator up at the top, so he's trapped. He'll just have to stay there.*

Although many of these examples have come from boys, and the empirical research suggests that projection is used more frequently by boys, girls also tell stories in which the use of projection is prominent. The following story was told by an 11-year-old girl; the numerous incidents that may be scored as projection are underlined.

> *He was in jail and he's climbing down the rope to get out of jail, <u>to break out of prison</u>. He's climbing down and he's <u>looking around to see if anyone sees him</u> and then somebody sees him and he starts climbing back up the rope and there's somebody up above the rope. He has a <u>gun</u> with him, but <u>it's hidden</u> right between the rope and his leg and*

he's going to <u>try to shoot the man</u> at the bottom but he misses him. And the <u>man at the bottom shoots him</u> and he falls off the rope and <u>kills himself.</u>

7. *Bizarre or very unusual story or theme.* This category depends heavily on the subjective judgment of the scorer, who must determine the limits of bizarreness. It includes negative themes that occur very rarely, especially if they have a peculiar twist. An example comes from a 12-year-old boy in response to TAT Card 17BM:

> *It looks like a sick chimpanzee swinging from a potato vine and right now he's feeling like he's about to die. And he goes to a circus and he's a super chimpanzee. He rips out the bars and he hangs himself with it.*

The following story, although it contains a number of elements that may be scored as projection, does not qualify as bizarre until the very end. It was told by a 16-year-old girl:

> *He is a man being chased by others. He has escaped from them since he was unjustly accused of a crime. The people feel he should be put to death for this and will not believe his story of innocence. . . . The crowd has just realized that he has escaped and is pursuing him. . . . The crowd cuts the rope and the prisoner falls and after a long time he hits water. This water is not as ordinary water, so the man keeps sinking and finally he is dissolved by this strange water. . . .*

Also included in this category are instances of unusual punishment, including unusual self-punishment. An example follows of an unusual story that ends with an unusual self-punishment, which was told by a 17-year-old girl in response to TAT Card 1:

> *Mark hasn't been adopted yet and will be lucky if he is. He was found in a city slum. Some say it was lucky he was found, others say it was to his misfortune. Mark is handicapped in that he was born with nubs where his legs should have been. The reason is because of the birth control pill his mother had been given at the free clinic. Mark is trying to do difficult work; intellectually, however, he is unable to do that either. He rolls his wheelchair over to the top of the stairs and pushes it over and he falls down the stairs and lies still at the bottom.*

The portrayal of the boy in this story as an abandoned, discarded child is extremely unusual. This idiosyncratic response is immediately followed by an assumption that the boy is physically defective; the "nubs" that replace his legs are ominous additions, again highly unusual, and indicate the projection of the storyteller's concerns around being defective, damaged, and unwanted. In explaining how this damage occurred, the storyteller attributes responsibility to the mother, and especially to the mother's sexual activity; if mother had not engaged in sex, the damage would not have occurred. There is also, in the reference to the birth control pill, the suggestion that mother did not want the child, and in this way too has rejected the boy. Clearly, the responsibility for his infirmity and aloneness are placed squarely on the mother. The object that might help replace his lost mobility— namely, the wheelchair—is then turned into an agent of self-destruction.

ASSESSMENT OF IDENTIFICATION WITH THE DMM

The assessment of the last of the three defenses to be discussed—identification— is also based on scoring categories derived from the components of the defense. In Chapter 5 we noted several different ways in which identification may be manifest. Some of these components involve the person being similar to, or like, another individual; this aim for "likeness" may be expressed through imitation, learning from a model, or assuming the characteristics of the other. The counterpart to being alike is differentiation between self and other and differentiation among others. This differentiation, which is also a part of the developmental process of identification, creates the possibility for the development of new objects of identification.

Other components of identification relate to the change that comes about in the structure of the ego as a result of internalizing the rules, sanctions, and interests of the significant adults in the child's life. This aspect of identification is seen especially in the development of internal controls, the ability to delay gratification, and the capacity to work. It is also seen in the development of conscience and, in the more extreme form, the expression of moralism.

Additional components of identification relate to the internalization of the values of the significant other. The changes in the ego that result from this internalization enable the child to maintain a positive emotional state through preserving an emotional attachment to the significant other and contributing to the development of self-esteem.

In this section we see how these components can be expressed in stories told in response to the TAT. As with denial and projection, seven scoring categories have been developed to represent the different components of identification. Two of these categories focus on the theme of becoming like someone else by acquiring either her skills or psychological attributes. Two other categories focus on a change in behavior that comes about as a result of the internalization of the mores of others. Another category relates to the capacity to differentiate among others, and another to the experience of self-esteem that comes from identifying with those outside of the family. The final category covers instances in which internalized beliefs regarding goodness, truth, and justice are expressed by way of a moralistic aphorism.

Scoring Categories for Identification

The following is a summary of the seven scoring categories for identification:

1. Emulation of skills
2. Emulation of characteristics
3. Regulation of motives or behavior
4. Self-esteem through affiliation
5. Work; delay of gratification
6. Role differentiation
7. Moralism

Using the Scoring Categories for Identification

1. *Emulation of skills.* This category includes references to one character imitating, taking over, or otherwise acquiring a skill or talent of another character, or trying to do so. This theme is often expressed by a younger character trying to be like an older one. In some cases, the desire to acquire the skill of another remains at the level of a wish. In response to TAT Card 1, an 11-year-old boy said the following:

> *Once upon a time there was this boy, and his father was a great violin player. . . . He thought, "Maybe if I could be as great as my father. . . ."*

In other cases, the skill is actually acquired, as in the story of a 9-year-old boy:

> *There was this little boy. . . . His father was a violin player. He liked to play the violin too, because his father used to teach him. . . . When he got grown up he was a fine musician.*

Occasionally, the acquisition of another person's skill as a means to maintain an emotional bond with that person is made especially clear. Thus an 11th-grade girl wrote this story:

> *I loved my grandfather. . . . He always brought this fiddle wherever we went, and played it. . . . I'm going to play it! I'm going to make my grandfather proud of me.*

In these examples, it is important to note that the hero wants to acquire the skill of the other—that is, the wish or action derives from his own initiative, not from the insistence of someone else.

2. *Emulation of characteristics.* This category includes references to one character imitating, taking over, or otherwise acquiring a characteristic, quality, or attitude of another character, or trying to do so. It also includes examples of "identification with the aggressor."

An example of emulating a distinctive characteristic of a youthful hero is seen in the story of a 5-year-old boy responding to TAT Card 17BM (the man on the rope): "The boy is playing . . . the bad guy came. . . . The boy gave his Tarzan call [the storyteller gives a clear imitation of the call] . . . "

Sometimes the emulated characteristic is more general, as in the following story from a 9-year-old boy: "He's feeling he is like Robin Hood or something"; or from a late-adolescent girl: "He longs to be like his father, perhaps to be loved as he is."

In other examples emulation is expressed through one character becoming the *same as* another, or, in the extreme case, *merging with* another. A 6-year-old girl expressed this idea by saying "He's trying to be Tarzan"; a 10-year-old boy provided the example "He is going to play the fiddle. . . . And he comes to be Wagner." These examples are differentiated from the earlier ones by the absence of the adjective *like*. Rather than becoming similar to, or *like*, another person through sharing some common feature, these characters *become* the other person.

Among college students, for whom the defense of identification is more highly developed, we often see this category expressed in a reversed manner, in which the parent is described as being like the child. A college man told the following story in response to TAT Card 7BM (older man looking at younger man):

A father and son, sitting in their church pew during Christmas season. The father looks over at his son, seeing much of himself in his own son.

3. *Regulation of motives or behavior.* The rationale underlying this category is based on the storyteller's internalization of certain rules, codes, or mores governing behavior. That is, these rules, codes, or mores, originally derived from parents or other authority figures, have been taken in and integrated, to greater or lesser degree, into the storyteller's ego. Within the context of the storytelling task, these regulatory mechanisms are expressed by assigning them to one of the characters in the story; a second character may then be regulated or influenced by these demands or prohibitions, or may rebel against the constraints. The conflict between the regu-

lating character and the character who is being regulated reflects an intrapsychic conflict between internalized prohibitions and the pleasure-seeking ego. In some stories, the conflict is fairly straightforward. An 11th-grade adolescent girl wrote, in response to TAT Card 1:

> *Maybe this boy has been given a job to do by his mother. . . . He's deciding if he'll do it or not. He may do it, although he doesn't want to.*

In other instances, there is an additional focus on how the regulated character would feel if the regulator's dictates were violated. Thus an 11th-grade boy wrote:

> *The kid tries to make his parents happy or do what they tell him to but he can't. Now he feels that he's bad, or a failure. . . .*

Sometimes the consequences of what would happen if the regulator's demands were not met are made quite explicit. To qualify as a component of identification, it is important that these negative consequences are presented in such a way that they appear as justified. An 11th-grade boy wrote the following:

> *He has just been told to read some boring literature. . . . He tries to act like he is done. The teacher gives him a test on it and he flunks so he must go back to reading.*

Another way in which the internalized regulation of motives or behavior is expressed in TAT stories is through the occurrence of self-criticism, or self-reflection, on the part of either the storyteller or a character in the story. For example, the storyteller may interject "This isn't a very good story," or a character may demonstrate a critical attitude toward his or her own behavior. Thus in response to TAT Card 1, an 11th-grade girl wrote:

> *He has tried to learn how to play but can't do it. . . . He is very angry at himself because he can't live up to his own and others' expectations of his playing.*

Self-reflection is expressed in a final example of this category, from an 11th-grade girl:

> *He is wondering why his parents are making him do something he doesn't want to do. . . . As he gets older he will realize that his parents were trying to help him. He will see that what they were doing was for his own good.*

In addition to providing a good example of self-reflection, the last sentence of the story borders on moralistic and might qualify to be scored under identification category 7 (moralism).

4. *Self-esteem through affiliation.* This category includes instances of success or satisfaction that come about as a result of a character's association with peers or extrafamilial adults, as well as references to the *need* for this kind of affiliation. A story told by an 11th-grade girl, responding to TAT Card 1, exemplifies the theme of emotional support derived from identification with a peer:

> *He knows not which way to turn.... His roommate discovers him.... Talking to his roommate, Tom realizes that they are both in exactly the same situation. Before the night is over they have become very close and comforted themselves.*

The need for identification with others is expressed in the story of an 11th-grade boy in response to TAT Card 17BM (the man on a rope):

> *This is a guy who is troubled by society.... As he pulls himself farther and farther away from reality he realizes that he cannot survive on his own.*

Sometimes this category is expressed through a character's affiliation with a special group, from which some special pleasure or help derives. In the following story from a ninth-grade girl in response to TAT Card 17BM, pleasure is associated with being part of a national group:

> *This man is . . . a Russian gymnast who is trying to help his country.... He feels very proud of himself. Everything seems to be going okay and soon he will be back with his people.*

5. *Work; delay of gratification.* In this category there is a recognition that the acquisition of skills is a slow process that requires considerable expenditure of effort. This recognition indicates a developmental advance over the wish to acquire skills through "being like" someone else (category 1). Examples of this category are seen in references to a character working or in implications that a character is about to work or has been working, where this is not clearly suggested by the picture.

Sometimes references to work focus on a specific situation, as in the story of an 11-year-old boy in response to TAT Card 17BM:

> *They're going to hold a mountain climbing race.... Mark started to get ready for the climb.... Mark works so hard that he had huge muscles.*

In other cases, the reference to work is more general, as with this 11th-grade boy: "The man is one who has worked hard all of his life at achieving a specific goal. . . . " References to work may also include the recognition that success will not be immediate, and that some delay must be tolerated to attain future gratification. Thus a ninth-grade boy wrote the following in response to TAT Card 1:

> *This is a young man trying to master the difficult skill of playing a violin. He has tried and tried. . . . After many hours of practice and failure he finally succeeds.*

6. *Role differentiation.* This category is meant to reflect the individual's ability to differentiate among others, a capacity that follows the ability to differentiate between self and others. In the TAT this category is scored for the mention of characters occupying specific adult roles other than parents or relatives.

Thus, for TAT Card 17BM, the man on the rope may be specifically designated as a "gymnast," a "criminal," a "warrior," a "fireman," or an "officer in army training." For TAT Card 1, the young boy may be thinking of future roles for himself: "Maybe he wants to be an *inventor* when he grows up" or "Maybe he feels like all the big *composers.*" Or, the boy may be thinking of adults who occupy specific roles: "It looks like he's waiting for his *teacher*"; "He has to go to the *doctor*"; "He's thinking about some kind of *princess*" These references to specific roles or occupations reflect a recognition of the differences among people in the world outside of the family. This recognition is related, in turn, to the opportunity to choose among various options in forming one's own identity.

7. *Moralism.* Included in this category are stories that have a moralistic outcome, in which goodness begets goodness, or good conquers evil, or a moral lesson is learned. The story of an 11th-grade girl in response to TAT Card 17BM contains the latter two themes:

> *The criminal makes it over the wall but is caught. . . . He knows it is best, however, because he must pay for his mistakes fully.*

An 11th-grade boy portrays good winning out over evil in his story:

> *The convict . . . succeeds in escaping, and, realizing he has a fresh start in life, goes straight, and lives a quiet, but honest life!!!*

Moralism may also be expressed by themes in which wrongdoing is punished by an extrafamilial authority figure. In this case, the intervention of society's guardians of justice (policemen, judges, etc.) ensures that "justice triumphs." A 10-year-old boy's story is typical of many schoolage children: "This man was a robber. . . . He's going to be put in jail." An early-adolescent boy expresses the same idea in a more elaborated form: "Ted is part of a smuggling ring. . . . He is caught with the goods and brought to justice."

Stories from older adolescents may express the need for punishment by an authority and the negative consequences of the absence of such administration of justice. Thus an 11th-grade boy wrote a story in response to TAT Card 1 that ends with moral indignation:

> *This boy will casually glance over at the answers the other children have on their papers. He won't get caught. . . . In the long run, this incident will hurt him. He'll cheat more and more and study less and less because it seemed so easy to cheat. Dummy.*

The need for the intervention of a moral authority is also expressed in this story from an 11th-grade girl:

> *He gets away from the people, but nothing is solved. As long as he continues to do what he does without being stopped, he won't change.*

Occasionally, the punishment for wrongdoing may be self-inflicted, as in the story of this 11th-grade boy:

> *The young man had committed a crime. . . . He completes the escape. . . . Upon his arrival in England he works towards ending world hunger as a self-punishment to make up for the sin he has committed.*

CONCLUDING REMARKS

This chapter has shown how the various components of the three defenses of denial, projection, and identification are used to establish a scoring system to assess the presence of these defenses in narrative stories. Through the use of multiple examples, we have discussed each of the components and how they can be revealed in projective stories. We also have seen how the same component may be manifest at different age levels with different dynamic content.

Since the original publication of the DMM (Cramer, 1991a), a great deal of further information has been gathered concerning the psychometric properties, validity, and reliability of the measures. Throughout this book, I have presented extensive evidence for the validity of this approach to assessing defenses; I have shown that empirical data support the theory that different defenses emerge and become predominant at different developmental periods, and that such defense change can be observed within individual children (Chapter 2). We have seen that, as would be expected, experimentally induced stress increases DMM defense mechanism scores,[5] as does real-life stress and the presence of psychopathology (Chapters 6, 7, 11, and 12). Further DMM studies have demonstrated meaningful relations between defense use and gender, and between defense use and different aspects of personality (Chapters 8, 9, and 10). Finally, research with the DMM has shown that the intervention of psychotherapy with seriously disturbed patients results in a decreased use of defenses (Chapter 13). In all these ways, the validity of the DMM has been demonstrated.

For any assessment method that relies on observation, it is important to demonstrate that the method is reliable—that is, that two (or more) observers reach the same conclusions (scores) when observing the same individuals. In each of the DMM studies reported in this book, two, and sometimes more, observers have coded a substantial number of the TAT stories, and their ratings have been compared to determine interrater reliability. As reported in Cramer (1998a), information on interrater reliability from 17 different samples that were studied prior to 1998 yielded median Pearson correlations for denial of .81, for projection of .80, and for identification of .64. In published studies conducted since 1997 with 8 different samples, interrater reliability, based on either Pearson or intraclass correlations, yielded reliability median coefficients for denial of .78 (range .71–.95), for projection of .84 (range .71–.88), and for identification of .82 (range .74–.93).[6] Similar findings for interrater reliability have been reported in 9 unpublished Ph.D. dissertations from different institutions with different samples. The median value for denial was .78; excluding one highly anomalous finding ($r = .04$), the range was from .66 to .87. For projection, the median value was .85, with a range from .81 to .95. For identification, the median correlation was .85, with a range from .67 to .96. In sum, these more recent findings, coming from a number of different laboratories, consistently demonstrate that the interrater reliability of the DMM is high.

Further investigation of the psychometric properties of the DMM, from a different laboratory (Hibbard et al., 1994), supported its reliability, internal consistency, and three-factor structure, as well as the criterion and divergent validity of the three defense measures. Additional study by Hibbard and Porcerelli (1998) investigated the characteristics of the distribution of DMM defense scores. The results indicated that the three defense score distributions were unimodal, and indices of kurtosis and skewness showed that the distribution of scores was adequate for applying most inferential statistics. A factor analysis of these data showed that the three defenses are distinct, with mature and immature aspects of each defense loading on the same factor—that is, a denial factor, a projection factor, and an identification factor. These findings are consistent with a previous factor analysis reported in Cramer (1991a).

The detailed coding rules for the DMM may be freely downloaded from www.williams.edu/Psychology/Faculty/Cramer/cramer.html.

CHAPTER 16

Other Approaches to Assessing Defense Mechanisms

*I*n this chapter I review other defense measures that have been discussed throughout the book, to make it clear which defenses are studied by each measure and how the assessment is carried out. The Defense Style Questionnaire (DSQ) and the Defense Mechanism Rating Scales (DMRS) are discussed at greater length, because these are the primary measures, along with the DMM, that are used in the research studies reviewed in this book.

DEFENSE STYLE QUESTIONNAIRE

There are several different versions of the DSQ. Throughout the book, I have indicated which version of the DSQ has been used in each research study. Because the DSQ is used so frequently in research studies, it is important to be aware of the differences among the several versions. In the following material, the various versions of the DSQ are explained in the chronological order of their appearance.

1983: DSQ-81

In a 1983 report (Bond et al., 1983), the DSQ was described as consisting of 81 items, based on a previous factor analysis. Beginning with 24 defenses, the results of a further factor analysis reduced this to 14 defenses

323

and four defense styles. *Style 1* was designated "Maladaptive Action Pattern" and included acting out, passive–aggression, regression, withdrawal, inhibition, and projection. *Style 2*, labeled "Image Distorting," included omnipotence/devaluation, primitive idealization, and splitting. *Style 3*, "Self-Sacrificing," included pseudoaltruism and reaction formation. (Denial also loaded on this factor for a combined patient/nonpatient group, and for patients alone. However, it loaded negatively for nonpatients alone and so was eliminated. As is discussed later, factor structure of the DSQ often changes, depending on the sample.) *Style 4* was considered "Adaptive" and included humor, suppression, and sublimation.

1989: DSQ-88

The original 81-item questionnaire was modified by Bond et al. (1989); 14 statements were omitted and 21 new statements were added, resulting in 88 items that measured 20 defenses and four defense styles. Ten of the items are "lie" items—that is, not defenses. The new statements were designed to measure six additional defenses: the mature defense/coping styles of anticipation, task orientation, and affiliation, as well as isolation, undoing, and help-rejecting/complaining (hypochondriasis). Four defenses—sublimation, pseudoaltruism, fantasy, and projective identification—were measured by only one item. Six defenses—suppression, anticipation, idealization, regression, somatization, and affiliation—were measured by two items.

Test–retest reliability for the four defense styles, based on 39 individuals tested over a period of 6 months, indicated considerable stability in scores, with correlations ranging from .68 to .73 (Bond et al., 1989).

1989: DSQ-72; DSQ-36

Andrews et al. (1989) were concerned that the defenses from the 88-item version of the DSQ did not match those used by Bond (or Vaillant) in previous work. In order to establish a correspondence and to develop a shorter form of the DSQ, Bond's 88-item version was modified. From the 88-item version, the 78 items that assessed defense mechanisms were relabeled to correspond to Bond's defenses. Six of the items could not be relabeled and were dropped, leaving 72 items, plus the 10 "lie" items. Bond's original items and the new relabeled items were factor analyzed separately. Both yielded three factors (vs. Bond's four-factor solution) designated *immature* (12 defenses), *neurotic* (4 defenses), and *mature* (4 defenses). In the 72-item version, repression and intellectualization were dropped; anticipation, as a mature defense, was added.

Internal consistency reliability (coefficient alpha) for the 72-item version, based on 712 individuals, ranged from .59 to .89 for the three defense factors, and from .07 to .82 for the 20 individual defenses (Andrews et al., 1993).

This 72-plus-10-item version was then reduced to 36 items. A factor analysis yielded three factors. Factor 1 (Immature) was described as "immature defenses wherein the very occurrence of the threat is denied or the responsibility is transferred" (Andrews et al., 1989, p. 460). Factor 2 (Neurotic) defenses were described as being "characteristic of the neurotic or superego type of defenses wherein the event is recognized, responsibility is accepted, but the meaning is inverted" (Andrews et al., 1989, p. 460). Factor 3 (Mature Coping) mechanisms were described as "the threat being recognized but the pain is being controlled until the threat can be dealt with" (Andrews et al., 1989, p. 460).

Items were kept or dropped on the basis of item–total-defense-score correlations. As a result, factor 1 (Immature) and factor 3 (Mature Coping) were emphasized. Factor 1 consisted of projection (6 items), passive–aggression (1 item), acting out (2 items), isolation (2 items), devaluation (3 items), autistic fantasy (1 item), denial (2 items), splitting (2 items), rationalization (1 item), and somatization (2 items), for a total of 22 items. Factor 3 consisted of sublimation (3 items), humor (2 items), anticipation (2 items), and suppression (3 items), for a total of 10 items. In contrast, factor 2 (neurotic) consisted of undoing (3 items), idealization (1 item) and reaction formation (1 item), for a total of 5 items. Several defenses that appeared in Bond's 1989 version (altruism, displacement, and dissociation) were dropped from the 36-item version. Note also that several defenses are represented by only 1 item.

Retest reliability, based on 56 individuals over an 18-month period, was reported as .60 for factor 1 (immature) and .71 for factor 3 (mature) (Andrews et al., 1993).[1]

1993: DSQ-40

Noting the problem of having one defense represented by 10 items, whereas another is represented by only 1 item, Andrews et al. (1993) decided to create a version of the DSQ in which each defense would be represented by 2 items. The data for this project came from 712 individuals (both patients and nonpatients) and included 413 persons who were part of the Andrews et al. (1989) study. All of this group took the DSQ-72.

Criteria used to select the final items for this new version of the DSQ included item–total-defense-score correlation, item–factor-score correlation, unique factor loading, adequate retest reliability, face validity, capacity to discriminate between nonpatients and patients with anxiety and to differentiate among specific anxiety diagnoses. Several new items were created or reworded. The final version of the DSQ-40 includes 20 defenses, each represented by 2 items. A factor analysis of this version yielded three factors (Immature, Neurotic, Mature) that correlated highly (.93–.97) with the factor scores from the DSQ-72. As compared with the DSQ-36, the DSQ-40 adds the defense of pseudoaltruism to the Neurotic scale, and displacement and dissociation to the Immature scale.

Test–retest reliability for the three defense factors, based on 89 individuals tested over a period of 4 weeks, ranged from .75 to .85. For the individual defenses, retest reliability ranged from .38 to .80. Measures of internal consistency (coefficient alpha), based on 712 individuals, ranged from .58 to .80 for the three defense factors, and from –.01 to .89 for the individual defenses (Andrews, Singh, & Bond, 1992).

1996: DSQ-78

A downward extension of the DSQ for use with adolescents was created through a series of studies by Steiner and colleagues (Nasserbakht et al., 1996). In this study the DSQ-78 (DSQ-72 + 6 items that had been dropped from the DSQ-88) was given to a group of adolescents composed of 260 control subjects, 371 psychiatric patients, and 106 juvenile offenders (456 females, 281 males). Regardless of whether a revised DSQ, consisting of 26 defenses relabeled by Steiner and colleagues, or Bond's DSQ-88, or Andrews' DSQ-72 were used, a factor analysis of the items on each version yielded a factor structure that differed from that found with adults. This difference was not due to the different defenses constituting the three DSQ measures.

A fourth factor analysis, including only those defenses for which there was agreement across all three measures for the coding of defenses, was carried out. Again, the factor structure obtained was different from that found with adults. Factor 1, which might be considered "Immature," consisted of passive–aggression, projection, acting out, somatization, splitting, fantasy, and devaluation. Factor 2 (which might be considered "Mature"), consisted of altruism, sublimation, and anticipation. Factor 3 (an alternative variety of "Mature") consisted of suppression and humor. Factor 4 (which I might consider "Adolescent") consisted of idealization, reaction formation, projection (a typical adolescent defense, when assessed using the DMM), and somatization, all of which load positively on this factor. Information on reliability was not provided.

2001: REM-71

Further revision of the DSQ-78 by Steiner et al. (2001) resulted in the Response Evaluation Measure (REM-71). Initially based on the DSQ-78, items were reworded and several defenses were dropped, resulting in a final list of 21 defenses, each represented by 3 or 4 items, for a total of 66 items. An additional lie item and four neutral items were added. Factor analyses of these defense scores yielded either two factors (unrotated solution) or three factors (rotated solution). The authors appear to prefer the two-factor solution, with factor 1 consisting primarily of immature and neurotic defenses, but also including sublimation. Factor 2 includes mature defenses, but also includes denial. These cross-loadings of sublimation and denial make the theoretical conceptualization of the two factors difficult. Measures of internal consistency (coefficient alpha) were above .40 for 20 of the 21 defenses, with a mean of .58.[2] Additional defense measures for use with children are discussed at the end of this chapter.

Discussion of the DSQ

As becomes apparent from the above information, there may be some difficulty in interpreting the results from the various DSQ studies, in that they use different versions of the measure. In turn, this means that different items, and different numbers of items, are used in different studies. Also, there are different defenses, and different numbers of defenses, in the various versions. Further, although the reliability of the three defense factors is acceptable, there is considerable variability across the individual defenses. For example, using a minimal criterion of coefficient alpha = .50, 13 of the 20 defenses measured on the DSQ-40 failed to meet an acceptable level (Andrews et al., 1993).

An additional problem for interpreting the DSQ studies is that different reported studies used the same samples of participants or a previous sample with new participants added to the previous sample. In that the results reported in separate papers are not always based on new or independent samples, it is difficult to determine if the new results are *confirming* earlier results or are being *determined* by those earlier results.

Another issue to keep in mind when considering the DSQ is that the nature of the factor scales has been found to vary across different samples. Even when using the same version of the DSQ, in different samples the factor scores are comprised of different defenses. Thus, across studies, correlations between defense factors and outcome variables are based on defense factors that are defined in different ways. The solution to this problem would be to look at the correlation of individual defense scales with outcome variables, but these correlations are often nonsignificant and/or not provided.

As examples of the different composition of factor scales, consider the factor structure for two studies using the DSQ-40. In the original study by Andrews et al. (1993), with 712 persons equally divided between patients and nonpatients, a factor analysis of the 20 defenses yielded three factors. The Mature scale consisted of the defenses of sublimation, humor, suppression, and anticipation. The Neurotic scale consisted of undoing, idealization, reaction formation, and pseudoaltruism. The Immature scale consisted of the remaining 12 defenses.

A second study with the DSQ-40 was based on 437 adolescents (Muris et al., 2003). A factor analysis of their responses again yielded three factors, but these differed from those of the Andrews et al. study. The Mature factor included the defenses of acting out and dissociation—defenses that loaded on the Immature factor in the Andrews study. The Neurotic factor included the defense of anticipation, which previously loaded on the Mature factor, and the defense of idealization, which loaded equally on both the Neurotic and Immature factors. The authors of the second study suggest that the results may be due to adolescents not reading the DSQ items in the ways that the authors presume they will. There is some support for this possibility in the data; there was a strong correlation between the Mature and Neurotic scales, and between the Mature and Immature scales, suggesting that response style—that is, the tendency to favor responding either "Very true" or "Not true"—may influence defense scores. Alternatively, the authors suggest that defense style organization in adolescents may be still developing, and so may be different from that found in adults.

Differences in factor structure have also been found in studies with the DSQ-81. In the original study (Bond et al., 1983) with 209 persons (evenly divided between patients and nonpatients), the 14 defense scales yielded a four-factor solution: (1) The Mature factor consisted of suppression, sublimation, and humor; (2) the Self-Sacrificing factor consisted of reaction formation and pseudoaltruism; (3) the Image-Distorting factor was comprised of omnipotence, splitting, and primitive idealization; and (4) the Immature factor was made up of repression, acting out, withdrawal, inhibition, passive–aggression, and projection.

A subsequent study with the DSQ-81, based on 113 adults attending evening college classes, also yielded four similarly named factors, but the composition of these factors differed from those of the original study. The Mature factor did not include the defenses of suppression or humor, but did include primitive idealization, previously an image-distorting defense. The Self-Sacrificing factor included suppression, and the Image-Distorting factor included humor, both previously part of the Mature defense factor. Only the Immature factor was consistent with the earlier study (Flannery & Perry, 1990).

Similar differences have been found across studies using the DSQ-88. Based on the same 113 evening college adults, the 20 defenses yielded four factors (Flannery & Perry, 1990): The first factor was the same as the Immature factor found with the DSQ-81, plus the added scales of Undoing,

Help-Rejecting/Complaining, and Consummatory Behavior. Factors 2, 3, and 4 also consisted of a mixture of defense levels. Factor 2 consisted of isolation, omnipotence, and task orientation. Factor 3 included the mature defenses of affiliation and humor, as well as the image-distorting defenses of splitting and primitive idealization. Factor 4 consisted of the mature defenses of sublimation and suppression as well as the neurotic defenses of reaction formation and pseudoaltruism.

Another study with the DSQ-88 was carried out with a Finnish sample of 426 individuals. Of the total sample, 17% were psychiatric outpatients and the remainder were nonpatient city employees (Sammallahti & Aalberg, 1995). Factor analysis yielded four factors. The first factor, Immature, included the same defenses found by Flannery and Perry (1990), plus the defenses of autistic fantasy, somatization, consumption, and help-rejecting/complaining. The Mature factor included sublimation, humor, and task orientation. The Neurotic factor included reaction formation, undoing, pseudoaltruism, idealization, suppression, anticipation, and affiliation. the fourth factor was different from the earlier analysis; labeled "Borderline," it included omnipotence, isolation, denial, splitting, and projective identification. These factors are quite different from those found by Flannery and Perry (1990).

We might be tempted to think that the difference in factor structure was due to the presence of psychiatric patients in the sample and/or to a different culture. A further study shows that this is not the case (Sammallahti et al., 1994). This investigation used 101 of the outpatients from the previous sample and 50 of the city employees, thus weighting the sample more heavily with patients (66% of the current sample). Analysis of the responses of this group yielded four factors, but these are not identical to the factors obtained with the larger number of participants. For example, splitting, which was part of the previous Borderline factor, was located on the Immature factor in this present study. Suppression, which was part of the Neurotic factor, was now located on the Mature factor. Denial, which was on the Borderline factor, was now part of the Neurotic scale. Notably, the previous Borderline factor did not appear, despite the larger number of patients in the group. Rather, the fourth factor was characterized as Inhibition and included isolation, withdrawal, and inhibition.

Thus, even within the same group of individuals using the same version of the DSQ, the resulting factor structure depends on the number of persons included and the ratio of patients to nonpatients. In the previous study, 17% of the group participants were patients; in the present study, 66% were patients.

A further study with the DSQ-88 yielded yet a different factor structure (Soldz et al., 1995). Factor analysis of outpatients' responses yielded three factors, two of which were quite similar (Mature, Immature) to those of Andrews et al. (1989), who used the DSQ-72. The third factor, designated "Withdrawal," was unique to this sample. Yet another study with the DSQ-88, using only the 57 items that showed sufficient response variability across respondents, yielded five factors: two Immature, one Neurotic, and one Mature (Wastell, 1999). The two Immature and two Neurotic factors differed on the basis of whether the defenses were affect- or content-focused.

In sum, whereas the original DSQ-81 was characterized by four-factor scales, subsequent versions (DSQ-88, DSQ-72, DSQ-40, DSQ-36) have been found to represent three-, four-, or even five-factor scales. Further, there is evidence that the factor structure of the DSQ may vary when given to special groups. Thus, when the DSQ is used with different samples, the factor structure for that sample should be determined prior to using summary defense scales. Factor scales developed from other, different samples should not be applied. In turn, these limitations mean that the DSQ defense factors in one study may be based on different defense scales than similarly named factors in another study. It is thus difficult to compare results across studies in order to determine if findings have or have not been replicated.

DEFENSE MECHANISM RATING SCALES

In recent years, the DMRS (Perry, 1990) is one of the most frequently used approaches to assessing defense use. On the basis of recorded clinical interviews, 27 defenses are rated on a 3-point scale (*absent to definite*) for frequency of use. From this information, three different scores may be calculated. To obtain *individual defense scores*, the number of times each individual defense occurs is divided by the total instances of all defenses. To obtain *defense level scores*, the proportional scores of each individual defense that have been assigned to one of seven defense levels are added together. To obtain an *overall defensive functioning* (ODF score), the occurrence of each individual defense is multiplied by the level at which it is placed (1–7). The average of these weighted scores results in an ODF value, which could range from 1 to 7.

As with any measure based on observer ratings, the question of interrater reliability is critical. According to Perry and Ianni (1998), the interrater reliability of the individual defense scales, when based on the consensus scores from several different raters, ranges from .37 to .79, with a median of .57. The reliability for the seven defense levels is better, with a median of .74. The reliability for the single ODF score has been reported as high as .89.

In another report on DMRS reliability (Bond, 1992), the range for individual defense scales was .04–.80, with a median of .41. For the six summary defense levels,[3] the reliabilities ranged from .30 to .66, with a median of .57.

Another study of reliability (Perry & Cooper, 1992) compared the ratings of nonprofessional raters with those of professional raters. For nonprofessional raters, reliability for 22 of the *individual defenses* (mature defenses were not rated) varied from .11 to .59, with a median of .36. When the scores of individual raters were combined into "consensus" scores, the reliabilities varied from .35 to .79, with a median of .57. For professional raters, the reliability for 27 individual defenses ranged from .02 to .99, with a median of .46. When 10 defenses that occurred infrequently were removed, the reliability estimates ranged from .19 to .87, with a median of .53.

For nonprofessional raters, the reliability of six of the seven *defense levels* (Mature was omitted) ranged from .39 to .65, with a median of .53. Using consensus ratings, the range was .57–.78, with a median of .74. For the professional raters, reliability for the seven levels ranged from .65 to .80, with a median of .69. Based on these findings, the authors concluded that only "Summary Level" scales that are used by professional raters reach acceptable levels of reliability. For nonprofessional raters, there should be six raters, and consensus ratings should be used.

A COMPARISON OF THE DSQ AND THE DMRS

Although the DSQ and DMRS are likely assessing defensive functioning at different psychological levels, it is interesting to see how the two measures relate to each other. For this purpose, the defense scores of 156 psychiatric outpatients (mean age = 36 years, range = 16–73 years) were compared for the DSQ-88 and the DMRS (Bond, 1992; Bond et al., 1989). The results showed that two of the seven defense levels of the DMRS were significantly correlated with DSQ-88 scores. The DMRS Action scale (level 1) was positively correlated with the DSQ-88 Maladaptive, Image-Distorting, and Self-Sacrificing scales. None of the other five DMRS levels were related to DSQ-88 styles, and the DSQ Adaptive scale did not relate to any DMRS defense levels. Bond (1992) also reports that scores for certain individual defenses on the two measures were in agreement, including splitting, omnipotence/devaluation, neurotic denial, projection, and identification.

Vaillant's Clinical Vignette Ratings

An extensive discussion of Vaillant's long-term study of defense mechanisms (Vaillant, 1975, 1976, 1990, 1993) and the methods he used appear in my earlier book. Briefly, Vaillant's observer-rating method takes vignettes from clinical interviews in which the interviewee describes reactions to situations of conflict and crisis. Each vignette is then coded for the occurrence of any of 15 defenses (18, if three psychotic defenses are included). These defenses are then grouped into three categories: Mature (altruism, humor, suppression, anticipation, and sublimation), Neurotic (repression, displacement, reaction formation, intellectualization), and Immature (dissociation/neurotic denial, projection, passive–aggression, hypochondriasis, and schizoid fantasy). A fourth category, Psychotic (delusional projection, psychotic denial, and distortion), can be included when assessing clinical patients. Scores for each of the three (or four) levels are expressed as a proportion of total defense use. In turn, using a predetermined formula, each of the three levels is then given a score representing the relative strength of that level. The difference between these scores for the Immature and Mature levels is then used to create a 9-point scale that indicates overall maturity of defense style (Vaillant & Vaillant, 1992).

An alternative scoring method, based on the assessment of individual defense use in the clinical vignette, takes into account the frequency with which each individual defense is used. In some investigations (e.g., Soldz & Vaillant, 1998; Vaillant, Bond, & Vaillant, 1986), a 3-point scale was used to indicate defense frequency. In other studies (e.g., Vaillant & Gerber, 1996), a 4-point scale has been used.

Earlier reports on interrater reliability (Vaillant, 1976) for the 18 defenses varied from a low of –.01 (dissociation) to a high of .95 (projection), with a median of .54. These values were improved when consensus scores from two raters were used (median = .75, range = .53–.96).

DEFENSE AXIS OF DSM-IV

This defense scale (Appendix B, DSM-IV) consists of a seven-level hierarchy of 27 defenses and generally corresponds to the DMRS, from which it was derived (Perry et al., 1998), and to Valliant's vignette rating method (Vaillant, 2000). Different from the DMRS, the defense axis includes a very low defense level (defensive dysregulation) that includes psychotic defenses. Also, levels 5 and 6 of the DMRS have been combined into a single level in the DSM-IV model. Another important difference with the DMRS is that the rater codes only seven individual defenses from the list of 27 provided. Defenses that are coded are arranged in descending order of prominence. These ratings may be further collapsed into three predominant "defensive styles" or levels. Research carried out with this defense rating scale at three different clinical sites yielded findings generally consistent with those for the DMRS (Perry et al., 1998).

DEFENSE MECHANISM INVENTORY

The DMI (Gleser & Ihilevich, 1969) consists of 10 stories read by the individual, who then checks the provided response alternatives as being characteristic, or not, of his or her own behavior. Reactions to these alternatives provide the basis for scoring five defense clusters: turning against the object (TAO), projection, turning against the self (TAS), reversal (REV), and principalization (PRN).[4] In addition to the psychometric problem that the TAO and projection, and the REV and PRN response scales are strongly intercorrelated, the main limitation of this measure is the ipsative scoring method, which requires that a high score on one cluster necessitates a low score on another. In turn, this scoring method results in all individuals being assessed as equally defensive; the total of the five scales must always equal 200. Although some of the scales have been shown to be meaningfully related to other personality and clinical variables, contradictory results have also been obtained. An extensive discussion of this measure appears in my earlier book (Cramer, 1991a) and in Cramer (1988).

DEFENSE-Q

The Defense-Q (Davidson et al., 2004) assesses 25 defenses, including those of the defense axis of the DSM-IV and those identified in other measures (e.g., the DMI, DMRS). Each defense is represented by one card. Raters use the 25 Q-cards to assess the defense use of an individual that occurs during recorded clinical interviews or other behavioral situations that may be observed. Cards are sorted into a seven-step fixed distribution (1, 2, 5, 9, 5, 2, 1), ranging from "*Most Characteristic*" to "*Least Characteristic*" of the individual being evaluated. The value assigned to each defense card is then used to plot a profile that represents the relative strength of each defense for that individual. This profile is then compared to an Adaptive Defense Profile (ADP), which was created by having eight clinical and personality psychologists sort the 25 cards to represent a continuum of adaptive defense use.

Sorters showed high agreement (average correlation = .92) for the placement of the defenses on the adaptive continuum. These ratings were composited to form the ADP prototype. The correlation between an individual's Defense-Q profile and the ADP prototype provides a score for adaptive defense use. A strong positive correlation between the individual's profile and the prototype ADP indicates greater use of adaptive, as compared to nonadaptive, defenses. The method also allows for future development of other profiles such as, for example, a defense profile that would characterize the BPD.

The Defense-Q is based on the rationale that the profile or pattern of use of multiple defenses is more important than the overall level, or frequency, of total defense use (Davidson et al., 2004). As with the DMI, due to the ipsative nature of this method, it is not possible to assess differences across individuals in the overall level or intensity of defense use. Also, because *all* 25 defenses must be placed in the seven-step distribution, for an individual who manifests only three defenses, these three would be ranked in the top two categories ("*Most Characteristic*" and "*Quite Characteristic*"), leaving the remaining 22 defenses to be placed in the other five categories. This means that five defenses the individual has never used will be given a rank of "*Somewhat Characteristic*." Given the low incidence of occurrence of certain defenses that has been found repeatedly with the DMRS, this is a problem for the Defense-Q: If a significant number of defenses never occurs, the requirement that all defenses be sorted into categories based on differential frequency of occurrence is clearly problematic.

LIFE STYLE INDEX

The Life Style Index (Plutchik et al., 1979) is a 97-item questionnaire with statements to which the test-taker responds "*usually true*" or "*usually not true*." From these responses, scores for eight defense mechanisms are derived, including compensation, denial, displacement, intellectualization, projection, reaction formation, regression, and repression. Four of these are combinations of several other defenses. For example, scores for the defense of compensation include identification and fantasy; scores for intellectualization consist of responses to items assessing rationalization, undoing, and sublimation. Reliability (inter-item consistency, coefficient alpha) is reported as ranging from .30 (intellectualization, student sample) to .86 (projection, inpatient sample) (Conte & Plutchik, 1993). As with the DSQ and the DMI, this measure requires the respondent to self-report on mental mechanisms (defenses) that are, by definition, operating outside of awareness.

OTHER MEASURES FOR ASSESSING CHILDREN'S DEFENSES

In addition to the REM-71, discussed earlier in this chapter, two other measures have been designed to assess defense use among children and adolescents.

Comprehensive Assessment of Defense Style

The CADS (Laor et al., 2001) relies on parents' report of their children's use of defense-related behaviors. Each defense is assessed from two questions. When the data for all 28 defenses were factor analyzed, three factors emerged. For the first factor, labeled "Other-Oriented" by the authors, projection is the defining defense—that is, the defense with the highest loading on the factor. The second factor is labeled "Self-Oriented"; reaction formation had the highest loading, and denial had the second highest loading. The third factor is labeled "Mature"; humor had the highest loading (.58), closely followed by identification (.57).

It is noteworthy that the three dimensions that are found to underlie the 28 individual defense scales represent the three defenses assessed by the DMM. Factor 1, "Other-Oriented," is defined by projection; indeed, the authors of the CADS validated this scale by demonstrating its significant correlation with DMM Projection. Factor 3, "Mature," is strongly defined by identification; again, the correlation between this factor and DMM Identification was significant. Additionally, the factor analysis showed that factor 2, "Self-Oriented," is strongly defined by denial. In essence, then, the 28 defense scales reduce down to three factors, and these factors are conceptually defined by the three defenses represented in the DMM.

Internal consistency reliability (coefficient alpha; $n = 81$) for factor 1 was reported as .73; for factor 2, alpha = .80; for factor 3, alpha = .56 (Wolmer et al., 2001). In a second study ($n = 243$; Laor et al., 2001), alphas were reported as .84 (factor 1), .79 (factor 2), and .66 (factor 3). Test–retest reliability (intraclass correlation) for factor 1 = .90, factor 2 = .86, and factor 3 = .87. For individual defenses, test–retest reliability (weighted kappa) ranged from .28 to .83, with all but three defenses having values above .50.

Ego-Defense Scale

The Ego-Defense Scale (Pfeffer, 1986) is one of the Child Suicide Potential Scales, and is based on ratings derived from semistructured interviews. The defenses assessed include compensation, denial, displacement, intellectualization, introjection, projection, reaction formation, regression, repression, sublimation, and undoing. Defenses are rated for frequency of use on a 3-point scale. A total defense score is based on the sum of scores from the individual defenses. Interrater reliability for the individual defenses has been reported as ranging from .15 to .82, with a median of .35 (Pfeffer et al., 1995); for the total defense score, interrater reliability was reported as .44.

CONCLUDING REMARKS

This chapter has reviewed the most commonly used methods to assess defense mechanisms. The various versions of the DSQ are compared, noting that the factor structure and scales vary with version and sample assessed. Observational methods, including the DMRS and Vaillant's vignette rating method, are reviewed, noting the difficulties in obtaining reliable ratings for individual defenses; combining the individual defenses into four or seven defense levels produces better reliability. The defense axis of the DSM-IV is based on these two observational methods. Two self-report measures in addition to the DSQ—the DMI and the Life Style Index—are summarized. Finally, three approaches to assessing defense in children and adolescents—the REM-71, the CADS, and the Ego Defense Scale, are discussed.

Notes

PREFACE

1. These chapters were published in my earlier book. The current chapters include some revisions and updating.
2. The earlier psychoanalytic theories have been discussed at some length in Cramer (1991a).
3. Further details of the early experimental studies and the replies of critics may be found in Cramer (2000).

CHAPTER 1

1. An extensive discussion of contemporary defense mechanism theory has been provided by Cooper (1998).
2. Material in the following sections originally appeared in Cramer (1998c); adapted with permission from the *Journal of Personality*.
3. Some qualifications to this statement are discussed in Cramer (1998c).
4. A comprehensive discussion of self-report measures and their limitation is provided in Davidson and MacGregor (1998).
5. For a comparison of results obtained using the DMRS and DSQ, see Chapter 16.
6. Other observer-based approaches are discussed by Perry and Ianni (1998).
7. See Perry and Ianni (1998) and Cramer (1991a) for an extended discussion of these rating scales.
8. It is possible to administer the TAT in a group format.
9. See also Bond et al. (1989).

10. As explained in the Preface, research published since 1990 is included; prior studies were reviewed in Cramer (1991a).
11. Varimax rotation; the unrotated analysis yielded two factors.

CHAPTER 2

1. The idea that defenses have their origin in infant behaviors is discussed more fully by Lichtenberg and Slap (1971), Mahler and McDevitt (1968), and Spitz (1957, 1961), and reviewed by Cramer (1991a).
2. A number of examples of these innate neurophysiological reactions are discussed in Cramer (1991a).
3. A similar distinction, with regard to the use of coping strategies, was proposed by Folkman and Lazarus (1980, 1985). They suggested that older adults use less "escapism" or avoidance of stressful situations, but did not differ from other adults in their use of problem-solving coping.
4. The authors were still in the process of naming these factors.
5. Costa et al. (1991) state that "for adults over 30, it appears that maturity of defense reflects psychological adjustment rather than continuing adult development" (p. 286).

CHAPTER 3

1. We will see that denial is also used to ward off unpleasant perceptions of the inner world.
2. Negation, sometimes considered as a separate defense, is included here as a variety of denial. For a discussion of the relationship between denial and negation, see Weinshel (1977).
3. "The Emperor's New Clothes," version by Hans Christian Andersen, *Andersen's Fairy Tales* (E. V. Lucas & H. B. Paull, Trans.). New York: Grosset & Dunlap (1945).
4. In a Spanish version of this tale, he who cannot see the cloth is an illegitimate son. The wish to preserve the personal belief of legitimacy is stronger than the wish to perceive reality.
5. "Red Riding Hood," from *Grimms' Fairy Tales* (E. V. Lucas, L. Crane, & M. Edwardes, Trans.). New York: Grosset & Dunlap (1945).
6. The tales of Cinderella and Snow White are taken from *Grimms' Fairy Tales* (E. V. Lucas, L. Crane, & M. Edwardes, Trans.). New York: Grosset & Dunlap (1945).
7. In the original Grimms' version, when the shoe does not fit, the stepsisters attempt to alter reality by lopping off part of their feet, but the ploy is discovered.
8. The use of denial by the terminally ill and their families has been investigated by Aitken-Swan and Easson (1959); Croog, Shapiro, and Levine (1971); Hackett, Cassem, and Wishnie (1968); Shady (1978); and Weisman (1972), among others.

9. Perhaps these psychological factors are important in understanding the finding that the mothers of father–daughter incest victims are heavily invested in the use of denial as a primary defense mechanism (cf. Weiner, 1962).

10. Basch (1983) has also distinguished between the defense that operates on the perceptual level, which he calls "denial," and that which involves higher level mental process, which he terms "disavowal."

11. Freud (1940) spoke of the stimulus barrier as serving a primitive defense function that precedes the ego's more elaborate and highly developed protective mechanisms.

12. Bridger (1962) noted that a strong stimulus produces sleep in the neonate, and Cameron (1963) described the phenomenon of adults falling asleep in the midst of excessive sensory bombardment. The general issue of sleep as an *anlage* of defense has been discussed by Wallerstein (1967).

13. For example, *Grief: A Peril in Infancy* (1947, New York University).

14. These results have been questioned by Caron, Caron, and Myers (1985) on the basis of their study of 4- to 7-month-old infants. However, their study used a different experimental paradigm (habituation/novelty), in which the tendency to avoid may have been confounded with the novelty issue.

15. A small proportion of 4-year-olds can voluntarily shift from one image to the alternative image; the ability steadily increases at ages 5 and 6, and by age 7 most children are capable of perceptual reversal (Elkind, 1964; Elkind & Scott, 1962; Elkind, Koegler, & Go, 1964; see also Vurpillot, 1976).

16. *Candide* (1759) by F. M. A. deVoltaire. New York: Appleton-Century-Crofts (1946).

17. The use of this fantasy to deny aspects of reality that are both disappointing and painful has been discussed by Freud (1909) and Rank (1914).

18. Disavowal may also be manifest in the compulsive doubting of reality, perception, or memories (cf. Fenichel, 1945).

19. See also Moore and Rubinfine (1969, p. 32) for a discussion of hallucinatory wish fulfillment as the earliest form of denial through fantasy.

20. "The Snow Queen," from *Andersen's Fairy Tales* (E. V. Lucas & H. B. Paull, Trans.). New York: Grosset & Dunlap (1945).

21. For a further discussion of how this fantasy of omnipotence influences development and becomes the basis for a sadomasochistic personality structure, see Novick and Novick (1996a, 2002).

22. Basch (1983) suggested that dreams are the earliest form of denial through fantasy.

23. In my analysis of the tale, the "bad mirror" is understood as a metaphor for the failure of adequate psychological "mirroring" by the mother or significant other.

CHAPTER 4

1. Mahler and McDevitt (1968, p. 12) have stated that the splitting of objects into "good" and "bad" is the precursor of projection and remains an essential part of the mechanism.

2. Other varieties of projective identification are discussed by Kernberg (1987).
3. This discussion is based in part on the work of Novick and Novick (1996b).
4. "The Castle of No Return" appears in S. Thompson, *One Hundred Favorite Folk Tales*. Bloomington, IN: Indiana University Press (1968, pp. 14–19).
5. "The Giant Who Had No Heart in His Body" appears in Thompson (1968, pp. 13–14).
6. "The Maiden in the Tower" appears in Thompson (1968, pp. 21–23). It is a variation on the story of "Rapunzel." The element of projection is not found in "Rapunzel," who herself tells the witch what the parrot is made to say in the "Maiden" tale.
7. "Little Claus and Big Claus" appears in Thompson (1968, pp. 397–407).
8. "Lord Peter" appears in Thompson (1968, pp. 226–230). The cat is actually a princess in disguise.
9. The Homeric "Hymn to Demeter" appears in *The Homeric Hymns* (C. Boer, Trans.). Chicago: Swallow Press (1970).
10. The tale of "Anpu and Bata" appears in M. Rugoff (Ed.), *A Harvest of World Folk Tales*. New York: Viking Press (1949).
11. The organization of this section has been significantly influenced by the work of Novick and Kelly (1970) and Novick and Novick (1996b). However, the present work deviates in some respects from theirs and is the responsibility of the author.
12. Karl Abraham (1924) considered defecation and urination to be the prototype of projection. This idea was explicitly rejected by René Spitz, whose observations of infants during the first year of life led him to believe that they were not much aware of what went on in the anal region. "In contrast to Abraham, we believe that the prototype available for projection at the three-month level is regurgitation and vomiting" (Spitz, 1961, p. 641).
13. Mahler and McDevitt (1968, p. 12) have pointed to the toddler's alternating behaviors of holding on and letting go, or of kissing and biting, which they term *ambitendencies*, as being surface manifestations of splitting.
14. However, splitting may continue for some time longer for other inhabitants of the child's psychological world. In a study of children's conceptions of God, for example, it was found that 4-year-olds tend to create two coexisting gods, one all good and the other all bad (Heller, 1986). Rizzuto (1979) has suggested that the splitting of the God concept is the result of the child projecting good and bad internal representations of parents onto the God concept.
15. The process for other object representations is assumed to follow a similar course.
16. This has also been demonstrated in the work of Loevinger (1966) and Kohlberg (1969).
17. As is discussed in Chapter 5, this is a precursor of identification as well.
18. "The Goose Girl" appears in *Grimms' Fairy Tales* (E. V. Lucas, L. Crane, & M. Edwardes, Trans.). New York: Grosset & Dunlap (1945).
19. Projection, as well as other defenses, may be assessed from other projective assessment methods. See, for example, Schafer (1954).

CHAPTER 5

1. Internalization is another term that has sometimes been used interchangeably with identification. Behrends and Blatt (1985) discussed the developmental course of internalization, a process ultimately responsible for psychological growth. Their use of this term and their developmental approach are somewhat similar to the current conception of "identification," especially to its adaptive, structure-building aspects. However, their determination of what is being internalized—namely, a "gratifying involvement" (p. 19) with another person followed by "experienced incompatibilities" (p. 20)—differs in its emphasis on the *relationships* with significant others as being internalized rather than (as in the present conception) the *qualities* of those significant others.

2. From R. Graves, *The Greek Myths* (Vol. 1). New York: George Braziller (1955, p. 46).

3. From S. Fox, *The Mythology of All Races: Greek and Roman* (Vol. 1). Boston: Marshall Jones Co. (1916, p. 156).

4. From J. A. MacCulloch, *The Mythology of All Races: Celtic* (Vol. 3). Boston: Marshall Jones Co. (1918).

5. From MacCulloch (1918, pp. 109–110).

6. In S. Thompson (Ed.), *One hundred favorite folk tales*. Bloomington, IN: University Press (1968, pp. 303–306).

7. From Sir J. G. Frazer, *The Golden Bough*. New York: Macmillan (1963, p. 573).

8. This version of the Grimms' tale is offered by Thompson (1968, p. 328).

9. "Snow White and the Seven Dwarfs," from *Grimms' Fairy Tales* (E. V. Lucas, L. Crane, & M. Edwardes, Trans.). New York: Grosset & Dunlap (1945, p. 168).

10. From E. E. Clark, *Indian Legends from the Northern Rockies*. Norman, OK: University of Oklahoma Press (1966, pp. 329–330).

11. The version of this well-known story discussed here is taken from "The Three Bears," in *Great Children's Stories: The Classic Volland Edition*. Northbrook, IL: Hubbard Press (1972).

12. From T. P. Cross and C. H. Stover (Eds.), *Ancient Irish Tales*. New York: Holt (1936).

13. It is interesting to note how remnants of incorporation may be manifest at later stages of development. Freud's "Wolfman," as a small child, would hold his breath when he passed cripples or beggars on the street, so as to not breathe in their infirmity (Compton, 1985; Menaker, 1979, p. 217). Among today's schoolchildren, a group of 9-year-olds was observed to ritualistically refuse to breathe or speak when passing any cemetery, to protect themselves from taking in the dead spirits.

14. This behavior has been described by Erikson (1950) as an alternation between "holding on and letting go."

15. In considering the point that identification requires the integration of introjections, I suggest an alternative view of the relationship between the "clinging

and cleaving" crisis and the development of identification. Rather than assuming that identification makes possible the resolution of the crisis, it may be that the crisis makes possible the development of identification. This latter conception is based on the idea that for true identification to occur, object constancy— the integration of the introjects "good mother" and "bad mother" into a single concept—must have been attained. In turn, the integration of the two "mothers" requires giving up the introjects. As long as the good mother and bad mother remain as internal introjects, separated by the mechanism of splitting, it is difficult or impossible to integrate them. However, if the relationships with the two introjects can be externalized, the child's advance in the capacity for reality testing enables him to recognize the two mothers as one. Thus the alternating behaviors of clinging and fighting with the mother may be understood as an attempt to externalize the good and bad introjects and the relationships with them. From this point of view, we can see the crisis as an attempt to consolidate the conflicting introjects into one representation, thereby making *possible* the process of identification. In other words, the crisis is seen as an attempt to give up the process of introjection to make identification possible.

16. In a patriarchal family the identifications that lead to superego development are more likely to be with father than with mother, because father is more often the source of frustrations and prohibitions (Fenichel, 1945, p. 104).

17. The introjection of the parents' prohibitions, which has occurred during an earlier phase of development, thus serves as a forerunner of the superego.

18. This process has been described by Blos (1979) as follows: "Adolescent individuation is the reflection of those structural changes that accompany the emotional disengagement from internalized infantile objects" (p. 143).

19. According to classical psychoanalytic theory, the ego-ideal is the heir of (the adolescent resolution of) the negative Oedipus complex (Blos, 1979, p. 329), just as the superego is the heir of the positive Oedipus complex.

20. Bios (1979) mentions Martin Luther, at the Diet of Worms, as an example of this kind of heroism. Joan of Arc also comes to mind.

21. From "Andrea Del Sarto" (1855), by Robert Browning, in *Poems and Plays*. New York: Charles Scribner's Sons (1922, p. 161). A similar sentiment was expressed by Browning in "The Statue and the Bust" (1855):

> Do your best, whether winning or losing it,
> If you choose to play!—is my principle.
> Let a man contend to the uttermost
> For his life's set prize, be it what it will! (p. 129)

22. Prince Hal, in *Henry IV*, has been the subject of psychological study by Aarons (1970) and by Lichtenberg and Lichtenberg (1969), among others. The views of the present author are independent of these earlier analyses.

23. As in *Henry IV*, there is an element of comedy throughout. However, in Shakespeare's drama the comedy is carried out through one character, whereas the issue of identification is portrayed in another. In Cervantes' story, the issue of identification and humor are combined into a single character.

The use of humor in *Henry IV* has been discussed by Lichtenberg and Lichtenberg (1969). Humor in *Don Quijote* has been discussed by Freud (1905) as follows:

> The ingenious knight Don Quijote de la Mancha is a figure who possesses no humour himself but who with his seriousness offers us a pleasure which could be called humorous, though its mechanism shows an important divergence from that of humour. Don Quijote is originally a purely comic figure, a big child; the phantasies from his books of chivalry have gone to his head. It is well known that to begin with the author intended nothing else of him and that his creation gradually grew far beyond its creator's first intentions. But after the author had equipped this ridiculous figure with the deepest wisdom and the noblest purposes and had made him into the symbolic representative of an idealism which believes in the realization of its aims and takes duties seriously and takes promises literally, this figure ceased to have a comic effect. (p. 232)

24. From Miguel de Cervantes Saavedra, *Don Quijote de la Mancha* (P. Motteux, Trans.). New York: Random House (1941).

CHAPTER 6

1. The following material originally appeared in Dollinger and Cramer (1990); adapted with permission from Lawrence Erlbaum Associates, Inc.
2. However, males reported more delinquent symptoms, and females reported more thought problems than found in the normative data.
3. The CADS is a 50-item questionnaire that, based on an observer's report, evaluates 25 individual defenses and three defense styles.
4. Interestingly, these findings are consistent with Brody's suggestion (Brody, Muderrisoglu, & Nakash-Eisikovits, 2002) that defenses and emotions are "matched"—that is, externalizing defenses such as projection are matched with externalizing emotions such as anger, whereas internalizing defenses such as reaction formation are matched with internalizing emotions such as anxiety. These ideas are discussed further in Chapter 8.
5. Aspects of this study were also reported in Feldman et al. (1996).
6. Interrater reliabilities for the 11 defense scales had been reported as satisfactory in a previous study (Pfeffer, Zuckerman, Plutchik, & Mizruchi, 1984).

CHAPTER 7

1. The following material originally appeared in Cramer (2003a); adapted with permission from the *Journal of Personality*.
2. The original study was conducted by Shedler and Block at the University of California, Berkeley. The study of defense mechanisms was undertaken by Cramer (2003a).

CHAPTER 8

1. Extensive information on their development was systematically collected over the years by Jack and Jeanne Block. See Block and Block (1980) for a full description of the sample and study.
2. The following material originally appeared in Cramer (2002a); adapted with permission from the *Journal of Personality*.
3. This is the intergenerational study from the Institute of Human Development, University of California, Berkeley.
4. Actual ages for the two groups were 40 and 47, and then 54 and 61.
5. The withdrawal factor, which includes the defenses of inhibition, withdrawal, and affiliation (negative loading), differs from the neurotic factor found in other studies.
6. Gender differences were not studied.
7. The Q-sort ratings were converted to identity status scores by comparing each participant's Q-sort with an identity status template constructed from the judgments of experts in the study of identity. In this way each of the participants had a score indicating his or her standing on each of the identity statuses.
8. The preceding six paragraphs originally appeared in Cramer (1997a); copyright 1997; adapted with permission from Elsevier.
9. Interestingly, these students who advanced to the achieved status during their senior year were already using less denial and projection at the beginning of their freshman year, as compared to those students who remained in moratorium. This finding suggests that the transition to the achieved status may have already begun at the earlier period.
10. The following study originally appeared in Cramer (1990c); adapted with permission from the *Journal of Personality*.
11. One earlier stage is assumed to be nonverbal and thus not easily assessed.
12. The perception may be of an external or internal event.
13. The relationship is curvilinear.
14. The preceding paragraph originally appeared in Cramer (1990c); adapted with permission from the *Journal of Personality*.
15. See Chapter 10 for a description of these samples.

CHAPTER 9

1. Parts of this chapter originally appeared in Cramer (2002b); copyright 2002 by the American Psychological Association; adapted with permission.
2. The intergenerational sample from the Institute of Human Development, Berkeley.
3. See Chapter 8 and Block and Block (1980) for a description of this study.
4. The authors concluded that DSQ-40 "scores are unaffected by the sex of the respondent" (Andrews et al., 1993, p. 246).
5. Examples of inappropriate externalizing emotions include those that imply a demeaning attitude toward others, such as contempt, disgust, or boredom. Ex-

amples of appropriate externalizing emotions are those that do not imply a demeaning attitude, such as anger, annoyance, or surprise. Inappropriate internalizing emotions in response to rejection are those that imply a negative judgment about the self, such as guilt and shame. Appropriate internalizing emotions include disappointment, sadness, and hurt.

6. Portions of the following discussion originally appeared in Cramer (2002a); adapted with permission from the *Journal of Personality*.

CHAPTER 10

1. Studies reported in this chapter represent longitudinal relations where there has been no planned intervention such as psychotherapy. Longitudinal studies in which such intervention has occurred are discussed in Chapter 13.
2. The DSQ-72 was translated into Finnish.
3. The preceding paragraph originally appeared in Cramer and Tracy (2005); copyright 2005; adapted with permission from Elsevier.
4. These young men had originally been selected to act as a control group for a study of juvenile delinquents.
5. The idea that personality does not change after age 30 was presented by Costa and McCrae (1994). However, myriad research has provided evidence of considerable personality change in adulthood (e.g., Aldwin & Levenson, 1994; Caspi & Roberts, 1999; Cramer, 2003b; Haan et al., 1986; Helson & Stewart, 1994; Helson & Wink, 1992; Roberts, 1997; Roberts & DelVecchio, 2000; Srivastava et al., 2003).
6. The interaction between denial and IQ was significant; at low levels of IQ, denial was unrelated to openness.
7. The interaction between projection and IQ was significant; at high levels of IQ, projection was unrelated to conscientiousness.
8. The interaction between identification and IQ was significant; at low levels of IQ, identification was unrelated to neuroticism and predicted a decrease in openness.
9. The interaction between projection and IQ was significant; at high levels of IQ, projection predicted a decrease in conscientiousness.
10. The preceding four paragraphs originally appeared in Cramer (2003b); copyright 2003; adapted with permission from Elsevier.
11. See Chapter 5 for an explanation of these prototypes.
12. The preceding paragraph originally appeared in Cramer (2004); copyright 2004; adapted with permission from Elsevier.
13. Preliminary examination of the results indicated that there were no differences attributable to gender; thus men and women were combined into one group.
14. Due to the strong negative correlation between the diffused and achieved identity style measures, analyses with these variables produced a replicated but reversed set of results. For this reason, the findings for the diffused identity are not reported.

15. The preceding three paragraphs originally appeared in Cramer (2003b); copyright 2003; adapted with permission from Elsevier.
16. This investigation also studied the role of life experiences in this identity change; these findings are reported in Cramer (2004).

PART IV

1. These ideas were discussed further in Cramer (1999b).

CHAPTER 11

1. Evidence of this salience is seen in the inclusion of a proposed axis in the DSM-IV in which defenses would be arranged in a seven-step hierarchical continuum from "defensive dysregulation" to "high adaptive."
2. Parts of the following discussion originally appeared in Cramer (1999b); adapted with permission from the *Journal of Personality*.
3. For denial, categories 1–5 are considered immature; 6 and 7, mature. For projection, categories 1–3 are considered immature; 4–7, mature. For identification, categories 1 and 2 are considered immature; 3–7, mature.
4. Two of the three measures of histrionic personality disorder did not correlate with any of the three defense scales.
5. Individuals could be rated as using more than one defense.

CHAPTER 12

1. Defenses and psychiatric disturbance in children and adolescents are discussed in Chapter 6.
2. The following discussion originally appeared in Cramer (1999a); adapted with permission from Lawrence Erlbaum Associates, Inc.
3. The introjective concern with self-definition might be expected to be reflected in a greater use of identification.
4. In later versions of the DMRS, the Obsessional scale was weighted as level 6.

CHAPTER 13

1. Portions of the following material originally appeared in Cramer (1999a); adapted with permission from Lawrence Erlbaum Associates, Inc.
2. These findings differ from those of Busch, Shear, Cooper, Shapiro, and Leon (1995).
3. The DSQ-ODF was calculated using the same weighting procedure as used for the DMRS.

4. This measure (Derogatis, 1983) provides an indicator of the current level of global symptom distress, combining information on the number of symptoms and the intensity of the perceived distress.
5. The Working Alliance Inventory, short form (12 items, 7-point Likert scales; Hovarth & Greenberg, 1994).
6. The authors indicate that the "intermediate" level defenses are similar to Vaillant's (1971) "neurotic" defenses.
7. Dropout status was not related to BPD diagnosis.

CHAPTER 14

1. Throughout this chapter, pseudonyms are used.
2. The preceding two TAT stories originally appeared in Porcerelli, Abramsky, Hibbard, and Kamoo (2001); reprinted with permission from Lawrence Erlbaum Associates, Inc.
3. These cases were presented at the Society for Personality Assessment meetings, San Antonio, Texas, March 2002. The case history, description of the treatment, outcome status, as well as the coding of defense mechanisms have been provided by these three psychologists. The overall discussion and interpretation of the findings are the responsibility of the present author.
4. The case history and TAT stories were provided by Dr. Kelly.
5. The case history and TAT stories were provided by Dr. Hibbard.
6. These data are based on the Berkeley Guidance Study and the Oakland Growth Study from the Institute of Human Development, University of California, Berkeley.
7. The case history and TAT stories were provided by Dr. Porcerelli.
8. This case is taken from Colarusso (1991, 2000). The defense analysis of the treatment is presented in greater detail in Cramer (2000b); copyright 2000; adapted with permission from Elsevier.
9. The following material originally appeared in Cramer (2000b); copyright 2000; adapted with permission from Elsevier.

CHAPTER 15

1. This chapter originally appeared in Cramer (1991a).
2. The interest of these stories is not restricted to the single scoring category being discussed. Many of the stories include additional themes that may be of defense or psychodynamic interest to the reader but are not taken up in the discussion.
3. In folk art, this idea is portrayed in the three monkeys who "see no evil, hear no evil, and speak no evil."
4. See David Rapaport (1967, p. 92) for a discussion of the projective hypothesis.
5. In contrast to the DSQ and the DMRS, only the DMM has demonstrated the effects of experimentally induced stress.

6. Intraclass correlations fell in the middle of each range—that is, they were not different from Pearson correlations.

CHAPTER 16

1. Reliability for factor 2 was not reported.
2. For the passive–aggression defense, alpha was less than .40.
3. Levels 5 and 6 were combined in this version.
4. The latter two scales consist of several response styles that are usually identified as separate defenses.

References

Aarons, Z. A. (1970). Normality and abnormality in adolescence: With a digression on Prince Hal—"The sowing of wild oats." *Psychoanalytic Study of the Child, 25,* 309–339.

Abraham, K. (1924). A short study of the development of the libido. *Selected Papers on Psycho-Analysis.* London: Hogarth Press, 1927.

Achenbach, T. M. (1991). *The manual for the Youth Self Report.* Burlington: University of Vermont.

Achenbach, T. M., & Edelbrock, C. (1983). The classification of child psychopathology: A review and analysis of empirical efforts. *Psychological Bulletin, 58,* 1275–1301.

Ainsworth, M., Blehar, M., Waters, E., & Wall, S. (1978). *Patterns of attachment: A psychological study of the strange situation.* Hillsdale, NJ: Erlbaum.

Ainsworth, M. D. S., & Bell, S. M. (1970). Attachment, exploration, and separation: Illustrated by the behavior of one-year-olds in a strange situation. *Child Development, 41,* 49–67.

Ainsworth, M. D. S., Bell, S. M., & Stayton, D. J. (1971). Individual differences in strange situation behaviour of one-year-olds. In H. R. Schaffer (Ed.), *The origins of human social relations* (pp. 17–57). Oxford, UK: Academic Press.

Ainsworth, M. D. S., & Witting, B. A. (1969). Attachment and exploratory behavior of one-year-olds in a strange situation. In B. M. Foss (Ed.), *Determinants of infant behavior IV* (pp. 111–126). London: Methuen.

Aitken-Swan, J., & Easson, E. C. (1959). Reactions of cancer patients on being told their diagnosis. *British Medical Journal, 1,* 779–783.

Akkerman, K., Carr, V., & Lewin, T. (1992). Changes in ego defenses with recovery from depression. *Journal of Nervous and Mental Disease, 180,* 634–638.

Albucher, R. C., Abelson, J. L., & Ness, R. M. (1998). Defense mechanism changes in successfully treated patients with obsessive–compulsive disorder. *American Journal of Psychiatry, 155,* 558–559.

Aldwin, C. M., & Levenson, M. R. (1994). Aging and personality assessment. In M. P. Lawton & J. A. Terisi (Eds.), *Annual review of gerontology and geriatrics* (pp. 182–209). New York: Springer.

Aldwin, C. M., Sutton, K. J., & Lackman, M. (1996). The development of coping resources in adulthood. *Journal of Personality and Social Psychology, 64,* 837–872.

Alexander, F. (1939). Emotional factors in essential hypertension: Presentation of a tentative hypothesis. *Psychosomatic Medicine, 1,* 173–179.

American Psychiatric Association. (1980). *Diagnostic and statistical manual of mental disorders* (3rd ed.). Washington, DC: Author.

American Psychiatric Association. (1994). *Diagnostic and statistical manual of mental disorders* (4th ed.). Washington, DC: Author.

Amsterdam, B. (1972). Mirror self-image reactions before age two. *Developmental Psychobiology, 5,* 297–305.

Andrews, G., Pollock, C, & Stewart, G. (1989). The determination of defense style by questionnaire. *American Journal of Psychiatry, 46,* 455–460.

Andrews, G., Singh, M., & Bond, M. (1993). The Defense Style Questionnaire. *Journal of Nervous and Mental Disease, 181,* 246–256.

Apter, A., Plutchik, R., Sevy, S., Korn, M., Brown, S., & van Praag, H. (1989). Defense mechanisms in risk of suicide and risk of violence. *American Journal of Psychiatry, 146,* 1027–1031.

Assor, A., Aronoff, J., & Messe, L. A. (1986). An experimental test of defensive processes in impression formation. *Journal of Personality and Social Psychology, 50,* 644–650.

Avery, R. R. (1985). *The place of self and object representations in personality organization and social behavior.* Unpublished doctoral dissertation, University of Rochester, NY.

Bartek, S. E., Krebs, D. L., & Taylor, M. C. (1993). Coping, defending, and the relations between moral judgment and moral behavior in prostitutes and other female juvenile delinquents. *Journal of Abnormal Psychology, 102,* 66–73.

Basch, M. F. (1983). The perception of reality and the disavowal of meaning. *Annual of Psychoanalysis, 11,* 125–153.

Behrends, R. S., & Blatt, S. J. (1985). Internalization and psychological development throughout the life style. *Psychoanalytic Study of the Child, 40,* 11–39.

Bem, S. (1974). The measurement of psychological androgyny. *Journal of Consulting and Clinical Psychology, 42,* 155–162.

Bergman, P., & Escalona, S. (1949). Unusual sensitivities in very young children. *Psychoanalytic Study of the Child, 3–4,* 333–352.

Berman, S. (1970). Alienation: An essential process of the psychology of adolescence. *Journal of the American Academy of Child Psychiatry, 9,* 233–250.

Bertenthal, B. I., & Fischer, K. W. (1978). Development of self-recognition in the infant. *Developmental Psychology, 14,* 44–50.

Bettelheim, B. (1976). *The uses of enchantment.* New York: Knopf.

Bibring, G., Dwyer, T., Huntington, D. F., & Valenstein, A. F. (1961). A study of the psychological processes in pregnancy and of the earliest mother–child relationship. *Psychoanalytic Study of the Child, 16,* 9–72.

Blaess, D. R. (1998). *The relationships among defense mechanisms, psychological and physical health symptoms, and electrodermal response to emotionally evo-*

cative stimuli. Unpublished doctoral dissertation, California School of Professional Psychology, San Diego, CA.

Blatt, S. J. (1990). Interpersonal relatedness and self-definition: Two personality configurations and their implications for psychopathology and psychotherapy. In J. L. Singer (Ed.), *Repression and dissociation* (pp. 299–335). Chicago: University of Chicago Press.

Blatt, S. J., D'Affitti, J. P., & Quinlan, D. M. (1976). Experiences of depression in normal young adults. *Journal of Abnormal Psychology, 85,* 383–389.

Blatt, S. J., & Ford, R. Q. (1994). *Therapeutic change: An object relations perspective.* New York: Plenum Press.

Bloch, A. L., Shear, K., Markowitz, J. C., Leon, A. C., & Perry, J. C. (1993). An empirical study of defense mechanisms. *American Journal of Psychiatry, 150,* 1194–1198.

Block, J. H., & Block, J. (1980). The role of ego-control and ego-resiliency in the organization of behavior. In W. A. Collins (Ed.), *Development of cognition, affect and social relations: Minnesota symposia on child psychology* (pp. 39–101). Hillsdale, NJ: Erlbaum.

Blos, P. (1962). *On adolescence.* New York: Free Press.

Blos, P. (1979). *The adolescent passage: Developmental issues.* New York: International Universities Press.

Bond, M. (1990). Are "borderline defenses" specific for borderline personality disorders? *Journal of Personality Disorders, 4,* 251–256.

Bond, M. (1992). An empirical study of defensive styles: The Defense Style Questionnaire. In G. E. Vaillant (Ed.), *Ego mechanisms of defense: A guide for clinicians and researchers* (pp. 127–158). Washington, DC: American Psychiatric Association.

Bond, M. (2004). Empirical studies of defense style: Relationships with psychopathology and change. *Harvard Review of Psychiatry, 12,* 263–278.

Bond, M., Gardner, S. R., Christian, J., & Sigal, J. J. (1983). Empirical study of self-rated defense styles. *Archives of General Psychiatry, 40,* 333–338.

Bond, M., Paris, J., & Zweig-Frank, H. (1994). Defense styles and borderline personality disorder. *Journal of Personality Disorders, 8,* 28–31.

Bond, M., Perry, J. C., Gautier, M., Goldenberg, M., Oppenheimer, J., & Simand, J. (1989). Validating the self-report of defense styles. *Journal of Personality Disorders, 3,* 101–112.

Bond, M. P., & Vaillant, J. S. (1986) An empirical study of the relationship between diagnosis and defense style. *American Journal of Psychiatry, 43,* 285–288.

Borst, S. R., & Noam, G. G. (1993). Developmental psychopathology in suicidal and nonsuicidal adolescent girls. *Journal of the American Academy of Child and Adolescent Psychiatry, 32,* 501–508.

Brennan, J., Andrews, G., Morris-Yates, A., & Pollock, C. (1990). An examination of defense style in parents who abuse children. *Journal of Nervous and Mental Disease, 178,* 592–595.

Bridger, W. (1962). Panel discussion: Symposium on research in infancy and early childhood. *Journal of the American Academy of Child Psychiatry, 1,* 92–107.

Brody, L. R., Mudderrisoglu, S., & Nakash-Eisikovits, O. (2002). Emotions, defenses, and gender. In R. F. Bornstein & J. M. Masling (Eds.), *The psychodynamics of gender and gender role.* Washington, DC: American Psychological Association.

Brody, L. R., Rozek, M. K., & Muten, E. O. (1985). Age, sex, and individual differences in children's defensive styles. *Journal of Child Clinical Psychology, 14,* 132–138.

Bronfenbrenner, U. (1960). Freudian theories of identification and their derivatives. *Child Development, 31,* 15–40.

Brunstein, J. C., & Schultheiss, O. C. (1998). Personal goals and emotional well-being: The moderation role of motive dispositions. *Journal of Personality and Social Psychology, 75,* 494–508.

Bulik, C. M., Sullivan, P. F., Carter, F. A., & Joyce, P. R. (1997). Lifetime comorbidity of alcohol dependence in women with bulimia nervosa. *Addictive Behaviors, 22,* 437–446.

Busch, F. N., Shear, M. K., Cooper, A. M., Shapiro, T., & Leon, A. C. (1995). An empirical study of defense mechanisms in panic disorder. *Journal of Nervous and Mental Disease, 183,* 299–303.

Bushnell, I. W. R., Sai, F., & Mullen, J. T. (1989). Neonatal recognition of the mother's face. *British Journal of Developmental Psychology, 7,* 3–15.

Byrne, D. (1961). The repression–sensitization scale: Rationale, reliability, and validity. *Journal of Personality, 29,* 334–349.

Cameron, N. (1963). *Personality development and psychopathology.* Boston: Houghton-Mifflin.

Caron, R. F., Caron, A. J., & Myers, R. S. (1985). Do infants see emotional expressions in static faces? *Child Development, 56,* 1552–1560.

Carver, C. S., & Scheier, M. F. (1994). Situational coping and coping dispositions in a stressful transaction. *Journal of Personality and Social Psychology, 66,* 184–195.

Caspi, A., & Roberts, B. (1999). Personality continuity and change across the life course. In L. A. Pervin & O. P. John (Eds.), *Handbook of personality* (2nd ed., pp. 300–326). New York: Guilford Press.

Cassidy, J., & Kobak, R. R. (1988). Avoidance and its relation to other defensive processes. In J. Belsky & T. Nezworski (Eds.), *Clinical implications of attachment* (pp. 300–323). Hillsdale, NJ: Erlbaum.

Chandler, M. J., Paget, K. F., & Koch, D. A. (1978). The child's demystification of psychological defense mechanisms: A structural developmental analysis. *Developmental Psychology, 14,* 197–205.

Cohen, D. J., Dibble, E., & Grawe, J. M. (1977). Fathers' and mothers' perceptions of children's personality. *Archives of General Psychiatry, 34,* 480–487.

Cohn, L. D. (1991). Sex differences in the course of personality development: A meta analysis. *Journal of Personality and Social Psychology, 109,* 252–266.

Colarusso, C. (1991). The analysis of a neurotic boy. In J. Glenn & P. Sholenar (Eds.), *Psychoanalytic case studies* (pp. 199–238). Boston: Little, Brown.

Colarusso, C. (2000). A child-analytic case report: A 17-year follow-up. In J. Cohen & B. J. Cohler (Eds.), *The psychoanalytic study of lives over time* (pp. 49–65). New York: Academic Press.

Colby, A., & Kohlberg, L. (1987). *The measurement of moral judgment* (Vol. II). New York: Cambridge University Press.

Compton, A. (1985). The concept of identification in the work of Freud, Ferenczi, and Abraham: A review and commentary. *Psychoanalytic Quarterly, 54,* 200–233.

Connell, J. P. (1985). A new multidimensional measure of children's perceptions of control. *Child Development, 56,* 1018–1041.

Conte, H. R., & Plutchik, R. (1993). The measurement of ego defenses in clinical research. In U. Hentschel, G. J. W. Smith, W. Ehlers, & J. G. Draguns (Eds.), *The concept of defense mechanisms in contemporary psychology: Theoretical, research, and clinical perspectives* (pp. 275–289). New York: Springer-Verlag.

Conte, H. R., Plutchik, R., Karasu, T. B., & Jerrett, I. (1980). A self-report Borderline scale: Discriminative validity and preliminary norms. *Journal of Nervous and Mental Disease, 168*, 428–435.

Cooper, S. H. (1998). Changing notions of defense within psychoanalytic theory. *Journal of Personality, 66*, 947–964.

Cooper, S. H., Perry, J. C., & Arnow, D. (1988). An empirical approach to the study of defense mechanisms: I. Reliability and preliminary validity of the Rorschach Defense Scales. *Journal of Personality Assessment, 52*, 187–203.

Corruble, E., Hatem, N., Damy, C., Falissard, B., Guelfi, J.-D., Reynaud, M., et al. (2003). Defense styles, impulsivity and suicide attempts in major depression. *Psychopathology, 36*, 279–284.

Costa, P. T., & McCrae, R. R. (1994). Set like plaster? Evidence for the stability of adult personality. In T. F. Heatherton & J. L. Weinberger (Eds.), *Can personality change?* (pp. 21–40). Washington, DC: American Psychological Association.

Costa, P. T., Somerfield, M. R., & McCrae, R. R. (1996). Personality and coping: A reconceptualization. In M. Zeidner & N. S. Endler (Eds.), *Handbook of coping: Theory, research, applications*. Oxford, UK: Wiley.

Costa, P. T., Zonderman, A. B., & McCrae, R. R. (1991). Personality, defense, coping and adaptation in older adulthood. In E. M. Cummings, A. L. Greene, & K. H. Karraker (Eds.), *Life-span developmental psychology* (pp. 277–293). Hillsdale, NJ: Erlbaum.

Cramer, P. (1979). Defense mechanisms in adolescence. *Developmental Psychology, 15*, 476–477.

Cramer, P. (1983). Children's use of defense mechanisms in reaction to displeasure caused by others. *Journal of Personality, 51*, 78–94.

Cramer, P. (1987). The development of defense mechanisms. *Journal of Personality, 55*, 597–614.

Cramer, P. (1988). The Defense Mechanism Inventory: A review of research and discussion of the scales. *Journal of Personality Assessment, 52*, 142–164.

Cramer, P. (1991a). *The development of defense mechanisms: Theory, research and assessment*. New York: Springer-Verlag.

Cramer, P. (1991b). Anger and the use of defense mechanisms in college students. *Journal of Personality, 59*, 39–55.

Cramer, P. (1995). Identity, narcissism and defense mechanisms in late adolescence. *Journal of Research in Personality, 29*, 341–361.

Cramer, P. (1997a). Identity, personality and defense mechanisms: An observer-based study. *Journal of Research in Personality, 31*, 58–77.

Cramer, P. (1997b). Evidence for change in children's use of defense mechanisms. *Journal of Personality, 65*, 233–247.

Cramer, P. (1998a). Threat to gender representation: Identity and identification. *Journal of Personality, 66*, 335–357.

Cramer, P. (1998b). Freshman to senior year: A follow-up study of identity, narcissism and defense mechanisms. *Journal of Research in Personality, 32*, 156–172.

Cramer, P. (1998c). Coping and defense mechanisms: What's the difference? *Journal of Personality, 66,* 919–946.

Cramer, P. (1999a). Future directions for the Thematic Apperception Test. *Journal of Personality Assessment, 72,* 74–92.

Cramer, P. (1999b). Personality, personality disorders, and defense mechanisms. *Journal of Personality, 67,* 535–554.

Cramer, P. (1999c). Ego functions and ego development: Defense mechanisms and intelligence as predictors of ego level. *Journal of Personality, 67,* 735–760.

Cramer, P. (2000a). Defense mechanisms in psychology today: Further processes for adaptation. *American Psychologist, 55,* 637–646.

Cramer, P. (2000b). Change in defense mechanisms during psychoanalysis and psychotherapy: A case study. In J. Cohen & B. Cohler (Eds.), *The psychoanalytic study of lives over time: Clinical and research perspectives on children who return to treatment in adulthood* (pp. 309–330). New York: Academic Press.

Cramer, P. (2001). Identification and its relation to identity development. *Journal of Personality, 69,* 667–688.

Cramer, P. (2002a). Defense mechanisms, behavior and affect in young adulthood. *Journal of Personality, 70,* 103–126.

Cramer, P. (2002b). The study of defense mechanisms: Gender implications. In R. F. Bornstein & J. M. Masling (Eds.), *The psychodynamics of gender and gender role* (pp. 81–127). Washington, DC: American Psychological Association.

Cramer, P. (2003a). Defense mechanisms and physiological reactivity to stress. *Journal of Personality, 71,* 221–244.

Cramer, P. (2003b). Personality change in later adulthood is predicted by defense mechanism use in early adulthood. *Journal of Research in Personality, 37,* 76–104.

Cramer, P. (2004). Identity change in adulthood: The contribution of defense mechanisms and life experiences. *Journal of Research in Personality, 38,* 280–316.

Cramer, P. (2005). Another "lens" for understanding therapeutic change: The interaction of IQ with defense mechanisms. In J. S. Auerbach, K. N. Levy, & C. E. Schaffer (Eds.), *Relatedness, self-definition and mental representation: Essays in honor of Sidney J. Blatt* (pp. 120–133). New York: Brunner-Routledge.

Cramer, P., & Blatt, S. J. (1990). Use of the TAT to measure change in defense mechanisms following intensive psychotherapy. *Journal of Personality Assessment, 54,* 236–251.

Cramer, P., & Blatt, S. J. (1993). Change in defense mechanisms following intensive treatment, as related to personality organization and gender. In W. Ehlers, U. Hentshel, G. Smith, & J. G. Draguns (Eds.), *The concept of defense mechanisms in contemporary psychology* (pp. 310–320). New York: Springer-Verlag.

Cramer, P., Blatt, S. J., & Ford, R. Q. (1988). Defense mechanisms in the anaclitic and introjective personality configuration. *Journal of Consulting and Clinical Psychology, 56,* 610–616.

Cramer, P., & Block, J. (1998). Preschool antecedents of defense mechanism use in young adults. *Journal of Personality and Social Psychology, 74,* 159–169.

Cramer, P., & Brilliant, M. (2001). Defense use and defense understanding in children. *Journal of Personality, 69,* 291–321.

Cramer, P., & Carter, T. (1978). The relationship between sexual identification and the use of defense mechanisms. *Journal of Personality Assessment, 42,* 63–73.

Cramer, P., & Gaul, R. (1988). The effects of success and failure on children's use of defense mechanisms. *Journal of Personality, 56,* 729–742.

Cramer, P., & Kelly, F. D. (2004). Defense mechanisms in adolescent conduct disorder and adjustment reaction. *Journal of Nervous and Mental Disease, 192,* 139–145.

Cramer, P., & Tracy, A. (2005). The pathway from child personality to adult adjustment: The road is not straight. *Journal of Research in Personality, 39,* 369–394.

Crandall, V. C., Katkovsky, W., & Crandall, V. J. (1965). Children's beliefs in their control of reinforcements in intellectual academic achievement situations. *Child Development, 36,* 91–109.

Crick, N. R. (1997). Engagement in gender normative versus nonnormative forms of aggression: Links to social-psychological adjustment. *Developmental Psychology, 33,* 610–617.

Crick, N. R., & Dodge, K. A. (1994). A review and reformulation of social information- processing mechanisms in children's social adjustment. *Psychological Bulletin, 115,* 74–101.

Croog, S. H., Shapiro, D. S., & Levine, S. (1971). Denial among male heart patients. *Psychosomatic Medicine, 33,* 385–397.

Davidson, K., & MacGregor, M. W. (1997). Reliability of an idiographic Q-sort measure of defense mechanisms. *Journal of Personality Assessment, 66,* 624–639.

Davidson, K., & MacGregor, M. W. (1998). A critical appraisal of self-report defense mechanism measures. *Journal of Personality, 66,* 965–992.

Davidson, K. W., MacGregor, M. W., Johnson, E. A., Woody, E. Z., & Chaplin, W. F. (2004). The relation between defense use and adaptive behavior. *Journal of Research in Personality, 38,* 105–129.

DeCasper, A. L., & Fifer, W. P. (1980). Of human bonding: Newborns prefer their mothers' voices. *Science, 208,* 1174–1176.

Derogatis, L. R. (1983). The Brief Symptom Inventory: An introductory report. *Psychological Medicine, 13,* 595–605.

Derogatis, L. R. (1989). *Description and bibliography for the SCL-90-R and other instruments of the psychopathology rating scale series.* Riderwood, MD: Clinical Psychometric Research.

Derogatis, L. R., & Cleary, P. A. (1977). Confirmation of the dimensional structure of the SCL-90: A study in construct validation. *Journal of Clinical Psychology, 33,* 981–989.

Despland, J.-N., de Roten, Y., Despars, J., Stigler, M., & Perry, J. C. (2001). Contribution of patient defense mechanisms and therapist interventions to the development of early therapeutic alliance in a brief psychodynamic investigation. *Journal of Psychotherapy Practice and Research, 10,* 155–164.

Deutsch, H. (1944). *The psychology of women* (Vol. 1). New York: Grune & Stratton.

Devens, M., & Erickson, M. T. (1998). The relationship between defense styles and personality disorders. *Journal of Personality Disorders, 12,* 86–93.

Diehl, M., Coyle, N., & Labouvie-Vief, G. (1996). Age and sex differences in strategies of coping and defense across the life span. *Psychology and Aging, 11,* 127–139.

Dollinger, S. J., & Cramer, P. (1990). Children's defensive responses and emotional upset following a disaster: A projective assessment. *Journal of Personality Assessment, 54,* 116–127.

Dollinger, S. J., & McGuire, B. (1981). The child as psychologist: Attributions and evaluations of defensive strategies. *Child Development, 52,* 1084–1086.

Dorpat, T. L. (1985). *Denial and defense in the therapeutic situation.* New York: Aronson.

Dozier, M., & Kobak, R. R. (1992). Psychophysiology in attachment interviews: Converging evidence for deactivating strategies. *Child Development, 63,* 1473–1480.

Drapeau, M., De Roten, Y., Perry, J. C., & Despland, J.-N. (2003). A study of stability and change in defense mechanisms during a brief psychodynamic investigation. *Journal of Nervous and Mental Disease, 191,* 496–502.

Eichorn, D. H., Clausen, J. A., Haan, N., Honzik, M. P., & Mussen, P. H. (1981). *Present and past in middle life.* New York: Academic Press.

Elkind, D. (1964). Ambiguous pictures for study of perceptual development and learning. *Child Development 35,* 1391–1396.

Elkind, D., Koegler, R. R., & Go, E. (1964). Studies in perceptual development: II. Part–whole perception. *Child Development, 35,* 81–90.

Elkind, D., & Scott, L. (1962). Studies in perceptual development: I. The decentering of perception. *Child Development, 33,* 619–630.

Erickson, S., Feldman, S. S., & Steiner, H. (1997). Defense reactions and coping strategies in normal adolescents. *Child Psychiatry and Human Development, 28,* 45–56.

Erikson, E. (1950). *Childhood and society.* New York: Norton.

Erikson, E. H. (1964). Inner and outer space: Reflections on womanhood. In R. J. Lifton (Ed.), *The woman in America* (pp. 1–26). Boston: Beacon Press.

Erikson, E. H. (1968). *Identity: Youth and crisis.* New York: Norton.

Evans, D. W., & Seaman, J. L. (2000). Developmental aspects of psychological defenses: Their relation to self-complexity, self-perception, and symptomatology in adolescents. *Child Psychiatry and Human Development, 30,* 237–254.

Evans, R. G. (1979). The relationship of the Marlowe–Crowne Scale and its components to defensive preferences. *Journal of Personality Assessment, 43,* 406–410.

Evans, R. G. (1982). Defense mechanisms in females as a function of sex-role orientation. *Journal of Clinical Psychology, 38,* 816–817.

Eysenck, H. (1998). *Dimensions of personality.* New Brunswick, NJ: Transaction.

Feather, N. T. (1967). Some personality correlates of external control. *American Journal of Psychology, 19,* 253–260.

Feldman, S. S., Araujo, K. B., & Steiner, H. (1996). Defense mechanisms in adolescence as a function of age, sex, and mental health status. *Journal of the Academy of Child and Adolescent Psychiatry, 34,* 1344–1354.

Fenichel, O. (1945). *The psychoanalytic theory of neurosis.* New York: Norton.

Finzi, R., Har-Even, D., & Weizman, A. (2003). Comparison of ego defenses among physically abused children, neglected, and non-maltreated children. *Comprehensive Psychiatry, 44,* 388–395.

Fiske, S. T., & Stevens, L. E. (1993). What's so special about sex?: Gender stereotyping and discrimination. In S. Oskamp & M. Costanzo (Eds.), *Gender issues in contemporary society* (pp. 173–196). Newbury Park, CA: Sage.

Flannery, R. B., & Perry, J. C. (1990). Self-rated defense style, life stress, and health status. *Psychosomatics, 31,* 313–320.

Folkman, S., & Lazarus, R. S. (1980). An analysis of coping in a middle-aged community sample. *Journal of Health and Social Behavior, 21,* 219–239.

Folkman, S., & Lazarus, R. S. (1985). If it changes it must be a process: Study of emotion and coping during three stages of a college examination. *Journal of Personality and Social Psychology, 46,* 839–852.

Fraiberg, S. (1982). Pathological defenses in infancy. *Psychoanalytic Quarterly, 51,* 612–635.

Frank, S. J., McLaughlin, A. M., & Crusco, A. (1984). Sex role attributes, symptom distress, and defensive style among college men and women. *Journal of Personality and Social Psychology, 47,* 182–192.

Freud, A. (1936). *The ego and the mechanisms of defense.* New York: International Universities Press. (Revised edition published 1966)

Freud, A. (1965). *Normality and pathology in childhood.* New York: International Universities Press.

Freud, A. (1973). Infants without families. Reports on the Hamstead Nurseries: 1939–1945. In *The writings of Anna Freud, Vol. III.* New York: International Universities Press.

Freud, S. (1894). The neuro-psychoses of defence. *Standard Edition, 3,* 45–61. London: Hogarth Press, 1962.

Freud, S. (1895). Draft H. Paranoia. *Standard Edition, 1,* 206–212. London: Hogarth Press, 1966.

Freud. S. (1896). Further remarks on the neuro-psychoses of defense. *Standard Edition, 3,* 161–185. London: Hogarth Press, 1966.

Freud, S. (1905). Three essays on the theory of sexuality. *Standard Edition, 7,* 125–248. London: Hogarth Press, 1959.

Freud, S. (1909). Family romance. *Standard Edition, 9,* 235–244. London: Hogarth Press, 1959.

Freud, S. (1911). Formulations regarding the two principles in mental functioning. *Standard Edition, 12,* 213–226. London: Hogarth Press, 1958.

Freud, S. (1915). Instincts and their vicissitudes. *Standard Edition, 14,* 117–140. London: Hogarth Press, 1957.

Freud, S. (1920). Beyond the pleasure principle. *Standard Edition, 18,* 1–64. London: Hogarth Press, 1955.

Freud, S. (1923). The ego and the id. *Standard Edition, 19,* 12–66. London: Hogarth Press, 1961.

Freud, S. (1924). The loss of reality in neurosis and psychosis. *Standard Edition, 19,* 183–187. London: Hogarth Press, 1961.

Freud, S. (1925). Negation. *Standard Edition, 19,* 234–239. London: Hogarth Press, 1961.

Freud, S. (1926). Inhibition, symptoms and anxiety. *Standard Edition, 20,* 77–174. London: Hogarth Press, 1959.

Freud, S. (1932). The psychology of women. *Standard Edition, 22,* 112–135. London: Hogarth Press, 1964.

Freud, S. (1937). Analysis terminable and interminable. *Standard Edition, 23,* 216–253. London: Hogarth Press, 1964.

Freud, S. (1940). An outline of psychoanalysis. *Standard Edition, 23,* 144–207. London: Hogarth Press, 1940.

Gaddini, E. (1969). On imitation. *International Journal of Psychoanalysis, 50,* 475–484.

Geleerd, E. R. (1965). Two kinds of denial: Neurotic denial and denial in the service of the need to survive. In M. Schur (Ed.), *Drives, affects and behavior* (Vol. 2, pp. 118–127). New York: International Universities Press.

Gillieron, E. (1989). Short psychotherapy interventions (4 sessions). *Psychotherapy and Psychosomatics, 51,* 32–37.

Gladstone, L. R. (1976). *A study of the relationship between ego defense style preferences and experimental pain tolerance and attitudes toward physical disability.* Unpublished doctoral dissertation, New York University, New York, NY.

Glasberg, R., & Aboud, F. (1982). Keeping one's distance from sadness: Children's self-reports of emotional experience. *Developmental Psychology, 18,* 287–293.

Gleser, G. C., & Ihilevich, D. (1969). An objective instrument for measuring defense mechanisms. *Journal of Consulting and Clinical Psychology, 33,* 51–60.

Glueck, S., & Glueck, E. (1966). *Criminal careers in retrospect.* New York: Kraus Reprint Corp.

Goldberg, D. (1972). *The detection of psychiatric illness by questionnaire.* London: Oxford University Press.

Goldschmid, M. (1968). The relation of conservation to emotional and environmental aspects of development. *Child Development, 39,* 597–589.

Gothelf, D., Apter, A., Ratzoni, G., Orbach, I., Weiaman, R., Tyano, S., et al. (1995). Defense mechanisms in severe adolescent anorexia nervosa. *Journal of the American Academy of Child and Adolescent Psychiatry, 34,* 1648–1654.

Gray, J. A. (1975). *Elements of a two-process theory of learning.* New York: Academic Press.

Grzegolowska-Klarkowska, H., & Zolnierczyk, D. (1988). Defense of self-esteem, defense of self-consistency: A new voice in an old controversy. *Journal of Social and Clinical Psychology, 6,* 171–179.

Grzegolowska-Klarkowska, H., & Zolnierczyk, D. (1990). Predictors of defense mechanisms under conditions of threat to the objective self: Empirical testing of a theoretical model. *Polish Psychological Bulletin, 21,* 129–155.

Gutmann, D. L. (1964). An exploration of ego configurations in middle and later life. In B. L. Neugarten (Ed.), *Personality in middle and late life* (pp. 114–148). New York: Atherton Press.

Haan, N. (1965). Coping and defense mechanisms related to personality inventories. *Journal of Consulting Psychology, 29,* 373–378.

Haan, N. (1977). *Coping and defending.* New York: Academic Press.

Haan, N., Millsap, R., & Hartka, E. (1986). As time goes by: Change and stability in personality over fifty years. *Psychology and Aging, 1,* 220–232.

Haan, N., Stroud, J., & Holstein, C. (1973). Moral and ego stages in relationship to ego processes: A study of "hippies." *Journal of Personality, 41,* 596–612.

Hackett, T. P., & Cassem, N. H. (1974). Development of a quantitative rating scale to assess denial. *Journal of Psychosomatic Research, 18,* 93–100.

Hackett, T. P., Cassem, N. H., & Wishnie, H. A. (1968). The coronary care unit: An appraisal of its psychological hazards. *New England Journal of Medicine, 279,* 1365.

Hart, D., & Chmiel, S. (1992). Influence of defense mechanisms on moral judgment development: A longitudinal study. *Developmental Psychology, 28,* 722–730.

Harter, S. (1982). The Perceived Competence Scales for children. *Child Development, 53,* 7–97.

Hartman, C. A., Hox, J., Mellenbergh, G. J., Boyle, M. H., Offord, D. R., Racine, Y., et al. (2001). DSM-IV internal construct validity: When a taxonomy meets data. *Journal of Child Psychology and Psychiatry, 42,* 817–836.

Heldt, E., Manfro, G. G., Kipper, L., Blaya, C., Maltz, S., Isolan, L., et al. (2003). Treating medication-resistant panic disorder: Predictors and outcome of cognitive-behavior therapy in a Brazilian public hospital. *Psychotherapy and Psychosomatics, 72,* 43–48.

Heller, D. (1986). *The children's God.* Chicago: University of Chicago Press.

Helms, J. E. (1984). Toward a theoretical explanation of the effects of race on counseling: A black and white model. *Counseling Psychologist, 12,* 153–165.

Helms, J. E. (1990) *Black and white racial identity: Theory, research, and practice.* Westport, CT: Greenwood Press.

Helson, R., Kwan,V. S. Y., John, O. P., & Jones, C. (2002). The growing evidence for personality change in adulthood: Findings from research with personality inventories. *Journal of Research in Personality, 36,* 287–306.

Helson, R., Pals, J., & Solomon, M. (1997). Is there adult development distinctive to women? In R. Hogan, J. Johnson, & S. Briggs (Eds.), *Handbook of personality psychology* (pp. 291–314). New York: Academic Press.

Helson, R., & Stewart, A. (1994). Personality change in adulthood. In T. F. Heatherton & J. L. Weinberger (Eds.), *Can personality change?* (pp. 201–226). Washington, DC: American Psychological Association.

Helson, R., & Wink, P. (1992). Personality change in women from the early 40s to the early 50s. *Psychology and Aging, 7,* 46–55.

Hernandez, W. (1999). *The use of defense mechanisms among adolescent boys diagnosed as conduct disordered, depressed and normal.* Unpublished doctoral dissertation, City University of New York, New York, NY.

Hersoug, A. G., Sexton, H. C., & Hoglend, P. (2002). Contribution of defensive functioning to the quality of working alliance and psychotherapy outcome. *American Journal of Psychotherapy, 56,* 539–554.

Hibbard, S., Farmer, L., Wells, C., Difillipo, E., Barry, W., Korman, R., & Sloan, P. (1994). Validation of Cramer's Defense Mechanism Manual for the TAT. *Journal of Personality Assessment, 63,* 197–210.

Hibbard, S., & Porcerelli, J. (1998). Further validation for the Cramer Defense Mechanism Manual. *Journal of Personality Assessment, 70,* 460–483.

Hibbard, S., Tang, P. C.-Y., Latko, R., Park, J.-H., Munn, S., Bolz, S., et al. (2000). Differential validity of the Defense Mechanism Manual for the TAT between Asian Americans and whites. *Journal of Personality Assessment, 75,* 351–372.

Hill, K. T., & Sarason, S. B. (1966). The relation of test anxiety and defensiveness to test and school performance over the elementary-school years. *Monographs of the Society for Research in Child Development, 31*(2), 1–76.

Hoglend, P., & Perry, J. C. (1998). Defensive functioning predicts improvement in major depressive episodes. *Journal of Nervous and Mental Disease, 186,* 238–243.

Horner, A. J. (1983). Refusal to identify: Developmental impasse. *Dynamic Psychotherapy, 1,* 111–121.

Hovarth, A. O., & Greenberg, L. S. (Eds.). (1994). *The working alliance: Theory, research and practice.* New York: Wiley.

Hyler, S. E., Skodol, A. E., Kellman, H. D., Oldham, J. M., & Rosnick, L. (1990). Validity of the Personality Diagnostic Questionnaire—Revised: Comparison with two structured interviews. *American Journal of Psychiatry, 147,* 1043–1048.

Ihilevich, D., & Gleser, G. C. (1986). *Defense mechanisms: Their classification, correlates, and measurement with the Defense Mechanisms Inventory.* Owosso, MI: DMI Associates.

Jacobson, A. M., Beardslee, W., Hauser, S. T., Noam, G. G., & Powers, S. I. (1986). An approach to evaluating adolescent ego defense mechanisms using clinical interviews. In G. E. Vaillant (Ed.), *Empirical studies of ego mechanisms of defense* (pp. 47–59). Washington, DC: American Psychiatric Association.

Jacobson, E. (1954). The self and the object world. *Psychoanalytic Study of the Child, 9,* 75–127.

Jacobson, E. (1957). Denial and repression. *Journal of the American Psychoanalytic Association, 5,* 61–92.

Joffee, P., & Naditch, M. P. (1977). Paper and pencil measures of coping and defense processes. In N. Haan (Ed.), *Coping and defending.* New York: Academic Press.

John, O. P., & Srivastava, S. (1999). The Big Five trait taxonomy: History, measurement, and theoretical perspectives. In L. A. Pervin & O. P. John (Eds.), *Handbook of personality* (pp. 102–138.) New York: Guilford Press.

Johnson, J. G., Bornstein, R. F., & Krukonis, A. B. (1992). Defense styles as predictors of personality disorder symptomatology. *Journal of Personality Disorders, 6,* 408–416.

Kavanaugh, R. D., Eizenman, D. R., & Harris, P. L. (1997). Young children's understanding of pretense expressions of independent agency. *Developmental Psychology, 33,* 764–770.

Kelly, F. D. (2003, March). *Changes in object relations and defensive functioning after four years of psychotherapy: SCORS and Cramer Defense Mechanism (DMM) scale measures in a 14-year-old male adolescent.* Paper presented at the Society for Personality Assessment, San Francisco, CA.

Kernberg, O. (1967). Borderline personality organization. *Journal of the American Psychoanalytic Association, 15,* 641–684.

Kernberg, O. (1975). *Borderline conditions and pathological narcissism.* New York: Aronson.

Kernberg, O. (1987). Projection and projective identification. In J. Sandler (Ed.), *Projection, identification and projective identification* (pp. 93–115). Madison, CT: International Universities Press.

Kernberg, O. (1989). The narcissistic personality disorder and the differential diagnosis of antisocial behavior. *Psychiatric Clinics of North America, 12,* 553–570.

Kernberg, P. (1994). Mechanisms of defense: Development and research perspectives. *Bulletin of the Menninger Clinic, 58,* 55–87.

Kim, M. W. (2001). *Defense mechanisms of stranger violent college student men.* Unpublished doctoral dissertation, Texas Tech University, Lubbock, TX.

Kneepkens, R. G., & Oakley, L. D. (1996). Rapid improvement in the defense style of depressed women and men. *Journal of Nervous and Mental Disease, 184,* 358–361.

Knight, R. P. (1940). Introjection, projection, and identification. *Psychoanalytic Quarterly, 9,* 334–341.

Kohlberg, L. (1969). *Stages in the development of moral thought and action.* New York: Holt.

Kohut, H. (1977). *The restoration of the self.* New York: International Universities Press.

Kwon, P. (1999). Attributional style and psychodynamic defense mechanisms: Toward an integrative model of depression. *Journal of Personality, 67,* 645–658.

Kwon, P. (2000). Hope and dysphoria: The moderating role of defense mechanisms. *Journal of Personality, 68,* 199–223.

Kwon, P. (2002). Hope, defense mechanisms, and adjustment: Implications for false hope and defensive hopelessness. *Journal of Personality, 70,* 207–231.

Kwon, P., & Lemon, K. E. (2000). Attributional style and defense mechanisms: A synthesis of cognitive and psychodynamic factors in depression. *Journal of Clinical Psychology, 56,* 723–735.

LaBarbera, J. D., Izard, C. R., Vietze, P., & Parisi, S. A. (1976). Four- and six-month-old infants' visual responses to joy, anger, and neutral expressions. *Child Development, 47,* 535–538.

Lacey, J. I. (1967). Somatic response patterning and stress: Some revisions of activation theory. In M. H. Appley & R. Trumbull (Eds.), *Psychological stress* (pp. 14–42). New York: Appleton-Century-Crofts.

Lampl-de Groot, J. (1957.) On defense and development: Normal and pathological. *Psychoanalytic Study of the Child, 12,* 114–126.

Laor, N., Wolmer, L., & Cicchetti, D. C. (2001). The Comprehensive Assessment of Defense Style: Measuring defense mechanisms in children and adolescents. *Journal of Nervous and Mental Disease, 189,* 360–368.

Laplanche, J., & Pontalis, J. B. (1973). *The language of psychoanalysis.* London: Hogarth Press.

Lerner, P. M., & Lerner, H. D. (1980). Rorschach assessment of primitive defenses in borderline personality structure. In J. S. Kwawer, H. Lerner, P. Lerner, & A. Sugarman (Eds.), *Borderline phenomena and the Rorschach test* (pp. 257–274). New York: International Universities Press.

Levit, D. B. (1991). Gender differences in ego defenses in adolescence: Sex roles as one way to understand the differences. *Journal of Personality and Social Psychology, 61,* 992–999.

Levit, D. B. (1993). The development of ego defenses in adolescence. *Journal of Youth and Adolescence, 22,* 493–512.

Lewis, H. B. (1985). Depression vs. paranoia: Why are there sex differences in mental illness? *Journal of Personality, 53,* 151–177.

Lewis, M., & Brooks, J. (1975). Infants' social perception: A constructivist view. In L. B. Cohen & P. Salapatek (Eds.), *Infant perception: From sensation to cognition* (Vol. 2, pp. 101–148). New York: Academic Press.

Lewis, M., & Ramsay, D. (2004). Development of self-recognition, personal pronoun use, and pretend play during the 2nd year. *Child Development, 75*, 1821–1831.

Lichtenberg, J. D., & Lichtenberg, C. (1969). Prince Hal's conflict, adolescent idealism, and buffoonery. *Journal of the American Psychoanalytic Association, 17*, 873–887.

Lichtenberg, J. D., & Slap, J. W. (1971). On the defensive organization. *International Journal of Psychoanalysis, 52*, 451–457.

Lichtenberg, J. D., & Slap, J. W. (1972). On the defense mechanism: A survey and synthesis. *Journal of the American Psychoanalytic Association, 20*, 776–792.

Lingiardi, V., Lonati, C., Delucchi, F., Fossati, A., Vanzulli, L., & Maffei, C. (1999). Defense mechanisms and personality disorders. *Journal of Nervous and Mental Disease, 187*, 224–228.

Little, S. A. (1998). *Defense functioning in depressed patients treated with medication and group psychotherapy.* Unpublished doctoral dissertation, The City University of New York, New York, NY.

Lobel, T. E., & Winch, G. L. (1986). Different defense mechanisms among men with different sex role orientations. *Sex Roles, 15*, 215–220.

Loevinger, J. (1966). The meaning and measurement of ego development. *American Psychologist, 21*, 195–206.

Loevinger, J. (1976). *Ego development.* San Francisco: Jossey-Bass.

Loevinger, J., & Hy, L. X. R. (1970). *Measuring ego development.* Mahwah, NJ: Erlbaum.

Loevinger, J., & Wessler, R. (1970). *Measuring ego development: Scoring manual for women and girls.* San Francisco: Jossey-Bass.

Loewenstein, R. M. (1967). Defensive organization and autonomous ego functions. *Journal of the American Psychoanalytic Association, 15*, 795–809.

Lorr, M., & Manning, T. T. (1978). Measurement of ego development by sentence completion and personality test. *Journal of Clinical Psychology, 34*, 354–360.

Luciano, J. (1997). *A measure of defense mechanisms in gay and heterosexual men from Thematic Apperception Test narratives.* Unpublished manuscript, Gallaudet University, Washington, DC.

Luciano, J. (1999). *Examining the cultural specificity of the Thematic Apperception Test through ego defense measurement.* Unpublished doctoral dissertation, Gallaudet University, Washington, DC.

MacGregor, M. W., Davidson, K. W., Barksdale, C., Black, S., & MacLean, D. (2003). Adaptive defense use and resting blood pressure in a population-based sample. *Journal of Psychosomatic Research, 55*, 531–541.

MacGregor, M. W., Davidson, K. W., Rowan, P., Barksdale, C., & MacLean, D. (2003). The use of defenses and physician health care costs: Are physician health care costs lower in persons with more adaptive defense profiles? *Psychotherapy and Psychosomatics, 72*, 315–323.

Maffei, C., Fossati, A., Lingiardi, V., Madeddu, F., Borellini, C., & Petrachi, M. (1995). Personality maladjustment, defenses and psychopathological symptoms in nonclinical subjects. *Journal of Personality Disorders, 9*, 330–345.

Mahalik, J. R., Cournoyer, R. J., de Franc, W., Cherry, J., & Napolitano, J. M. (1998). Men's gender role conflict and use of psychological defenses. *Journal of Counseling Psychology, 45*, 247–255.

Mahler, M., Pine, F., & Bergman, A. (1975). *The psychological birth of the human infant.* New York: Basic Books.

Mahler, M. S., & McDevitt, J. B. (1968). Observations on adaptation and defense *in statu nascendi. Psychoanalytic Quarterly, 37,* 1–21.

Main, M. (1981). Avoidance in the service of attachment: A working paper. In K. Immelman, G. Barlow, M. Main, & L. Petrinovitch (Eds.), *Behavioral development: The Bielefeld interdisciplinary project* (pp. 651–693). New York: Cambridge University Press.

Main, M. (1995). Attachment: Overview, with implications for clinical work. In S. Goldberg, R. Muir, & J. Kerr (Eds.), *Attachment theory: Social, developmental and clinical perspectives* (pp. 407–474). Hillsdale, NJ: Analytic Press.

Main, M. (2000). The organized categories of infant, child, and adult attachment: Flexible vs. inflexible attention under attachment-related stress. *Journal of the American Psychoanalytic Association, 48,* 1055–1096.

Mallory, M. E., (1989). Q-sort definition of ego identity status. *Journal of Youth and Adolescence, 18,* 399–411.

Maner, J. K., Kenrick, D. T., Becker, D. V., Robertson, T. E., Hofer, B., Neuberg, S. L., et al. (2005). Functional projection: How fundamental social motives can bias interpersonal perception. *Journal of Personality and Social Psychology, 88,* 63–78.

Marcia, J. E. (1966). Development and validation of ego-identity status. *Journal of Personality and Social Psychology, 3,* 551–558.

Margo, G. M., Greenberg, R. P., Fisher, S., & Dewan, M. (1993). A direct comparison of the defense mechanisms of nondepressed people and depressed psychiatric inpatients. *Comprehensive psychiatry, 34,* 65–69.

Massong, S. R., Dickson, A. I., Ritzler, B. A., & Layne, C. C. (1982). Assertion and defense mechanism preference. *Journal of Counseling Psychology, 29,* 591–596.

Masterson, J. F. (1985). *Treatment of the borderline adolescent.* New York: Brunner/Mazel.

Matsuba, M. K., & Walker, L. J. (1998). Moral reasoning in the context of ego functioning. *Merrill–Palmer Quarterly, 44,* 464–483.

McAdams, D. P. (1993). *The stories we live by: Personal myths and the making of the self.* New York: Guilford Press.

McClelland, D. C. (1963). The Harlequin complex. In R. W. White (Ed.), *The study of lives* (pp. 94–119). New York: Atherton Press.

McCrae, R. R. (1984). Situational determinants of coping responses, loss, threat, and challenge. *Journal of Personality and Social Psychology, 46,* 919–928.

McCrae, R. R., & Costa, P. T. (1999). A five-factor theory of personality. In L. A. Pervin & O. P. John (Eds.), *Handbook of personality* (pp. 139–153). New York: Guilford Press.

McDevitt, J. B. (1979). The role of internalization in the development of object relations during the separation–individuation phase. *Journal of the American Psychoanalytic Association, 27,* 327–343.

McLeod, J. D., & Kessler, R. C. (1990). Socioeconomic status differences in vulnerability to undesirable life events. *Journal of Health and Social Behaviour, 31,* 162–172.

Meissner, W. W. (1974). The role of imitative social learning in identificatory processes. *Journal of the American Psychoanalytic Association, 22,* 512–536.

Meltzoff, A. N., & Moore, M. K. (1977). Imitation of facial and manual gestures by human neonates. *Science, 198,* 75–78.

Meltzoff, A. N., & Moore, M. K. (1983). Newborn infants imitate adult facial gestures. *Child Development, 54,* 702–709.

Menaker, E. (1979). *Masochism and the emergent ego.* New York: Human Sciences Press.

Miller, A. (1981). *Prisoners of childhood: The drama of the gifted child and the search for the true self.* New York: Basic Books.

Miller, D. R., & Swanson, G. E. (1960). *Inner conflict and defense.* New York: Holt, Rinehart & Winston.

Miller, L. C., Barrett, C. L., Hampe, E., & Noble, H. (1972). Factor structure of childhood fears. *Journal of Consulting and Clinical Psychology, 39,* 264–268.

Millon, T. (1996). *Disorders of personality: DSM-IV and beyond* (2nd ed.). New York: Wiley.

Moore, B. E., & Rubinfine, D. L. (1969). The mechanism of denial. In B. D. Fine, E. D. Joseph, & H. F. Waldhorn (Eds.), *The Kris study group of the New York Psychoanalytic Institute, Monograph III* (pp. 3–57). New York: International Universities Press.

Mulder, R. T., Joyce, P. R., Sellman, J. D., Sullivan, P. F., & Cloninger, C. R. (1996). Towards an understanding of defense style in terms of temperament and character. *Acta Psychiatrica Scandinavica, 93,* 99–104.

Muris, P., & Merckelbach, H. (1996). The short version of the Defense Style Questionnaire: Factor structure and psychopathological correlates. *Personality and Individual Differences, 20,* 123–126.

Muris, P., Winands, D., & Horselenberg, R. (2003). Defense styles, personality traits, and psychopathological symptoms in nonclinical adolescents. *Journal of Nervous and Mental Disease, 191,* 771–780.

Nasserbakht, A., Araujo, K., & Steiner, H. (1996). A comparison of adolescent and adult defense styles. *Child Psychiatry and Human Development, 27,* 3–14.

Newman, L. S., Duff, K. J., & Baumeister, R. F. (1997). A new look at defensive projection: Thought suppression, accessibility, and biased person perception. *Journal of Personality and Social Psychology, 72,* 980–1001.

Nghe, L. T., & Mahalik, J. R. (2001). Examining racial identity statuses as predictors of psychological defenses in African American college students. *Journal of Counseling Psychology, 48,* 10–16.

Nishimura, R. (1998). Study of the measurement of defense style using Bond's Defense Style Questionnaire. *Psychiatry and Clinical Neurosciences, 52,* 419–424.

Noam, G. G., & Recklitis, C. J. (1990). The relationship between defenses and symptoms in adolescent psychopathology. *Journal of Personality Assessment, 54,* 311–327.

Noam, G. G., Recklitis, C. J., & Paget, K. F. (1991). Pathways of ego development: Contributions to maladaptation and adjustment. *Development and Psychopathology, 3,* 311–328.

Novick, J., & Kelly, K. (1970). Projection and externalization. *Psychoanalytic Study of the Child, 25,* 69–95.

Novick, J., & Novick, K. K. (1996a). A developmental perspective on omnipotence. *Journal of Clinical Psychoanalysis, 5*, 129–173.

Novick, J., & Novick, K. K. (1996b). *Fearful symmetry: The development and treatment of sadomasochism.* Northvale, NJ: Aronson.

Novick, J., & Novick, K. K. (2002). Two systems of self-regulation. *Psychoanalytic approaches to the treatment of children and adolescents* [Special Issue]. *Journal of Psychoanalytic Social Work, 8*, 95–122.

Novick, K. K., & Novick, J. (1998). An application of the concept of the therapeutic alliance to sadomasochistic pathology. *Journal of the American Psychoanalytic Association, 46*, 813–846.

O'Brien, M. L. (1988). Further evidence of the validity of the O'Brien Multiphasic Narcissism Inventory. *Psychological Reports, 62*, 879–882.

Obrist, P. A. (1981). *Cardiovascular psychophysiology: A perspective.* New York: Plenum Press.

Offer, R., Lavie, R., Gothelf, D., & Apter, A. (2000). Defense mechanisms, negative emotions, and psychopathology in adolescent inpatients. *Comprehensive Psychiatry, 41*, 35–41.

Pennebaker, J. W., Barger, S. D., & Tiebout, J. (1989). Disclosure of traumas and health among Holocaust survivors. *Psychosomatic Medicine, 51*, 577–589.

Pennebaker, J. W., & Chew, C. H. (1985). Behavioral inhibition and electrodermal activity during deception. *Journal of Personality and Social Psychology, 49*, 1427–1433.

Perry, J. C. (1988). A prospective study of life stress, defenses, psychotic symptoms, and depression in borderline and antisocial personality disorders and bipolar type II affective disorder. *Journal of Personality Disorders, 2*, 49–59.

Perry, J. C. (1990). *Defense mechanism rating scales (DMRS)* (5th ed.). Cambridge, MA: Author.

Perry, J. C. (1992). Perry's Defense Mechanism Rating Scale. In G. E. Vaillant (Ed.), *Ego mechanisms of defense: A guide for clinicians and researchers* (pp. 253–259). Washington, DC: American Psychiatric Association.

Perry, J. C. (2001). A pilot study of defenses in adults with personality disorders entering psychotherapy. *Journal of Nervous and Mental Disease, 189*, 651–660.

Perry, J. C., & Cooper, S. H. (1986). A preliminary report on defenses and conflicts associated with borderline personality disorder. *Journal of the American Psychoanalytic Association, 34*, 863–893.

Perry, J. C., & Cooper, S. H. (1989). An empirical study of defense mechanisms. *Archives of General Psychiatry, 46*, 444–452.

Perry, J. C., & Cooper, S. H. (1992). What do cross-sectional measures of defense mechanisms predict? In G. E. Vaillant (Ed.), *Ego mechanisms of defense: A guide for clinicians and researchers* (pp. 195–216). Washington, DC: American Psychiatric Association.

Perry, J. C., Hoglend, P., Shear, K., Vaillant, G. E., Horowitz, M., Kardos, M. E., et al. (1998). Field trial of a diagnostic axis for defense mechanisms for DSM-IV. *Journal of Personality Disorders, 12*, 56–68.

Perry, J. C., & Ianni, F. F. (1998). Observer-rated measures of defense mechanisms. *Journal of Personality, 66*, 993–1024.

Pfeffer, C. R. (1986). *The suicidal child.* New York: Guilford Press.

Pfeffer, C. R., Hart, S. W., Peskin, J. R., & Siefker, C. A. (1995). Suicidal children grow up: Ego functions associated with suicide attempts. *Journal of the American Academy of Child and Adolescent Psychiatry, 34,* 1318–1325.

Pfeffer, C. R., Plutchik, R., & Mizruchi, M. S. (1986). A comparison of psychopathology in child psychiatric inpatients, outpatients, and nonpatients. *Journal of Nervous and Mental Disease, 174,* 529–535.

Pfeffer, C. R., Zuckerman, S., Plutchik, R., & Mizruchi, M. S. (1984). Suicidal behavior in normal school children: A comparison with child psychiatric inpatients. *Journal of the American Academy of Child Psychiatry, 23,* 416–423.

Pfohl, B., Blum, N., & Zimmerman, M. (1994). *Structured Interview for DSM-IV Personality Disorders.* Iowa City, IA: University of Iowa Press.

Piaget, J. (1929). *The child's conception of the world.* New York: Harcourt Brace

Piaget, J. (1952). *The origins of intelligence in children.* New York: International Universities Press.

Pickens, M. S. (2002). *MMPI-2 scales of defensiveness: Are they measuring defensiveness?* Unpublished doctoral dissertation, Biola University, La Mirada, CA.

Plutchik, R., Kellerman, H., & Conte, H. R. (1979). A structural theory of ego defenses and emotions. In C. E. Izard (Ed.), *Emotions in personality and psychopathology* (pp. 229–257). New York: Plenum Press.

Poikolainen, K., Kanerva, R., & Lonnqvist, J. (1995). Social class and defence styles among adolescents. *Journal of Adolescence, 18,* 669–677.

Pollock, C., & Andrews, G. (1989). Defense styles associated with specific anxiety. *American Journal of Psychiatry, 146,* 1500–1502.

Porcerelli, J. H., Abramsky, M. F., Hibbard, S., & Kamoo, R. (2001). Object relations and defense mechanisms of a psychopathic serial sexual homicide perpetrator. *Journal of Personality Assessment, 77,* 87–104.

Porcerelli, J. H., Cogan, R., Kamoo, R., & Leitman, S. (2004). Defense mechanisms and self-reported violence toward partners and strangers. *Journal of Personality Assessment, 82,* 317–320.

Porcerelli, J. H., Thomas, S., Hibbard, S., & Cogan, R. (1998). Defense mechanism development in children, adolescents, and late adolescents. *Journal of Personality Assessment, 71,* 411–420.

Porter, R. H., Makin, J. W., Davis, L. B., & Christensen, K. M. (1992). Breast-fed infants respond to olfactory cues from their own mother and unfamiliar lactating females. *Infant Behavior and Development, 15,* 85–93.

Potter, A. E., & Williams, D. E. (1991). Development of a measure examining children's roles in alcoholic families. *Journal of Studies on Alcohol, 52,* 70–77.

Pulkkinen, L., & Kokko, K. (2000). Identity development in adulthood: A longitudinal study. *Journal of Research in Personality, 34,* 445–470.

Radloff, L. S. (1977). The CES-D Scale: A new self-report depression scale for research in the general population. *Applied Psychological Measures, 1,* 385–401.

Randolph, D. L., Anderson, C. E., Smith, P. L., & Shipley-Clark, M. (2003). Social desirability, defense styles, and the children's role inventory. *Psychological Reports, 92,* 842–846.

Rank, O. (1914). *The myth of the birth of the hero.* New York: Vintage.

Rapaport, D. (1967). Principles underlying projective techniques. In M. M. Gill (Ed.), *The collected papers of David Rapaport* (pp. 91–97). New York: Basic Books.

Raskin, R., & Terry, H. (1988). A principal-components analysis of the Narcissistic Personality Inventory and further evidence of its construct validity. *Journal of Personality and Social Psychology, 54*, 890–902.

Raush, S. L. (1994). *The role of defense mechanism development in children's peer relationships.* Unpublished doctoral dissertation, Long Island University, Brookville, NY.

Recklitis, C. J., Noam, G. G., & Borst, S. R. (1992). Adolescent suicide and defensive style. *Suicide and Life-Threatening Behavior, 22*, 374–387.

Richert, A. J., & Ketterling, R. (1978). Psychological defense as a moderator variable. *Psychological Reports, 42*, 291–294.

Rizzuto, A. M. (1979). *The birth of the living God.* Chicago: University of Chicago Press.

Roberts, B. W. (1997). Plaster or plasticity: Are adult work experiences associated with personality change in women? *Journal of Personality, 65*, 205–232.

Roberts, B. W., & DelVecchio, W. F. (2000). The rank-order consistency of personality traits from childhood to old age: A quantitative review of longitudinal studies. *Psychological Bulletin, 126*, 3–25.

Romans, S. E., Martin, J. L., Morris, E., & Herbison, G. P. (1999). Psychological defense styles in women who report childhood sexual abuse: A controlled community study. *American Journal of Psychiatry, 156*, 1080–1085.

Rozsnafazky, J. (1981). The relationship of level of ego development to Q-sort personality ratings. *Journal of Personality and Social Psychology, 41*, 99–120.

Rump, E. E., & Court, J. (1971). The Eysenck Personality Inventory and social desirability response set with student and clinical groups. *British Journal of Social and Clinical Psychology, 10*, 42–54.

Sammallahti, P., & Aalberg, V. (1995). Defense style in personality disorders: An empirical study. *Journal of Nervous and Mental Disease, 183*, 516–521.

Sammallahti, P., Aalberg, V., & Pentinsaari, J.-P. (1994). Does defense style vary with severity of mental disorder? *Acta Psychiatric Scandinavica, 90*, 290–294.

Sandler, J. (1960). On the concept of the superego. *Psychoanalytic Study of the Child, 18*, 139–158.

Sandler, J., & Freud, A. (1985). *The analysis of defense: The ego mechanisms of defense revisited.* New York: International Universities Press.

Sandler, J., & Joffe, W. G. (1967). On the psychoanalytic theory of autonomy and the autonomy of psychoanalytic theory. *International Journal of Psychiatry, 3*, 512–515.

Sandstrom, M., & Cramer, P. (2003a). Girls' use of defense mechanisms following peer rejection. *Journal of Personality, 71*, 605–627.

Sandstrom, M., & Cramer, P. (2003b). Defense mechanisms and psychological adjustment in childhood. *Journal of Nervous and Mental Disease, 191*, 487–495.

Sanford, N. (1955). The dynamics of identification. *Psychological Review, 62*, 106–118.

Schafer, R. (1954). *Psychoanalytic interpretation in Rorschach testing.* New York: Grune & Stratton.

Schafer, R. (1968). *Aspects of internalization.* New York: International Universities Press.

Schimel, J., Greenberg, J., & Martens, A. (2003). Evidence that projection of a feared trait can serve a defensive function. *Personality and Social Psychology Bulletin,* *29,* 969–979.

Scholz, J. A. (1973). Defense styles in suicide attempters. *Journal of Consulting and Clinical Psychology, 40,* 70–73.

Schultheiss, O. C., & Brunstein, J. C. (2001). Assessment of implicit motives with a research version of the TAT: Picture profiles, gender differences, and relations to other personality measures. *Journal of Personality Assessment, 77,* 71–86.

Schwartz, L., & Eagle, C. J. (1986). *Psychological portraits of children.* New York: Lexington Books.

Shabad, P., Worland, J., Lander, H., & Deitrich, D. (1979). A retrospective analysis of the TATs of children at risk who subsequently broke down. *Child Psychiatry and Human Development, 10,* 49–59.

Shady, G. (1978). Coping styles of patients with life-threatening illness: A literature review. *Essence, 2,* 149–154.

Shaw, R. J., Ryst, E., & Steiner, H. (1996). Temperament as a correlate of adolescent defense mechanisms. *Child Psychiatry and Human Development, 27,* 105–114.

Shelder, J., Karliner, R., & Katz, E. (2003). Cloning the clinician: A method for assessing illusory mental health. *Journal of Clinical Psychology, 59,* 635–650.

Silverman, D. K. (2003). Cutting the symbiotic bond: A challenge to some current female mythology. In J. Reppen, M. A. Schulman, & J. Tucker (Eds.), *Way beyond Freud: Postmodern psychoanalysis observed* (pp. 238–263). London: Open Gates Press.

Silverman, D. K. (2005). Early developmental issues reconsidered: Commentary on Pine's ideas on symbiosis. *Journal of the American Psychoanalytic Association,* *53,* 239–251.

Silverman, L. R. (1999). *Defense and adaptation in uninfected "affected" siblings of HIV-positive children.* Unpublished doctoral dissertation, The City University of New York, New York, NY.

Simeon, D., Guralnik, O., Knutelska, M., Schmeidler, J. (2002). Personality factors associated with dissociation: Temperament, defenses, and cognitive schemata. *American Journal of Psychiatry, 159,* 489–491.

Sinha, B. K., & Watson, D. C. (1999). Predicting personality disorder traits with the Defense Style Questionnaire in a normal sample. *Journal of Personality Disorders, 13,* 281–286.

Sjoback, H. (1973). *The psychoanalytic theory of defensive processes.* New York: Wiley.

Skodol, A. E., & Perry, J. C. (1993). *Should* an axis for defense mechanisms be included in DSM-IV? *Comprehensive Psychiatry, 34,* 108–119.

Smith, C., Feldman, S. S., Nasserbakht, A., & Steiner, J. (1993). Psychological characteristics and DSM-III-R diagnoses at 6-year follow-up of adolescent anorexia nervosa. *Journal of the American Academy of Child and Adolescent Psychiatry, 32,* 1237–1245.

Smith, G. J., & Danielsson, A. (1982). *Anxiety and defense strategies in childhood and adolescence.* New York: International Universities Press.

Smith, W. P., & Rossman, B. B. R. (1986). Developmental changes in trait and situational denial under stress during childhood. *Journal of Child Psychiatry, 27,* 227–235.

Soldz, S., Budman, S., Demby, A., & Merry, J. (1995). The relation of defensive style to personality pathology and the Big Five personality factors. *Journal of Personality Disorders, 9,* 356–370.

Soldz, S., & Vaillant, G. E. (1998). A 50-year longitudinal study of defense use among inner city men: A validation of the DSM-IV defense axis. *Journal of Nervous and Mental Disease, 186,* 104–111.

Soldz, S., & Vaillant, G. E. (1999). The Big Five personality traits and the life course: A 45-year longitudinal study. *Journal of Research in Personality, 33,* 208–232.

Spinhoven, P., & Kooiman, C. G. (1997). Defense style in depressed and anxious psychiatric outpatients: An explorative study. *Journal of Nervous and Mental Disease, 185,* 87–94.

Spitz, R. (1957). *No and yes: On the beginning of human communication.* New York: International Universities Press.

Spitz, R. (1958). On the genesis of superego components. *Psychoanalytic Study of the Child, 13,* 375–404.

Spitz, R. (1961). Some early prototypes of ego defenses. *Journal of the American Psychoanalytic Association, 9,* 626–651.

Spitz, R. (1966). Metapsychology and direct infant observation. In R. Loewenstein, L. Newman, M. Schur, & A. Solnit (Eds.), *Psychoanalysis—A general psychology: Essays in honor of Heinz Hartmann* (pp. 123–151). New York: International Universities Press.

Spitz, R. S. (1965). *The first year of life: A psychoanalytic study of normal and deviant development of object relations.* New York: International Universities Press.

Srivastava, S., John, O. P., Gosling, S. D., & Potter, J. (2003). Development of personality in early and middle adulthood: Set like plaster or persistent change? *Journal of Personality and Social Psychology, 84,* 1041–1053.

Starrett, R. H. (1983). The conceptual commonality between impulsiveness as a personality trait and as an ego development stage. *Personality and Individual Differences, 4,* 265–274.

Steiner, H. (1990). Defense styles in eating disorders. *International Journal of Eating Disorders, 9,* 141–151.

Steiner, H., Araujo, K. B., & Koopman, C. (2001). The Response Evaluation Measure (REM-71): A new instrument for the measurement of defenses in adults and adolescents. *American Journal of Psychiatry, 158,* 467–473.

Steiner, H., & Feldman S. S. (1995). Two approaches to the measurement of adaptive style: Comparison of normal, psychosomatically ill, and delinquent adolescents. *Journal of the American Academy of Child and Adolescent Psychiatry, 34,* 180–190.

Stern, D. (2000). The relevance of empirical infant research to psychoanalytic theory and practice. In J. Sandler, A.-M. Sandler, & R. Davies (Eds.), *Clinical and observational psychoanalytic research: Roots of a controversy* (pp. 73–90). London: Karmac Books.

Stewart, A. J., Ostrove, J. M., & Helson, R. (2001). Middle aging in women: Patterns of personality change from the 30s to the 50s. *Journal of Adult Development, 8,* 23–37.

Stolorow, R. D., & Lachmann, F. M. (1978). The developmental prestages of defenses: Diagnostic and therapeutic implications. *Psychoanalytic Quarterly, 47*, 73–102.

Strauss, J. S., & Harder, D. W. (1981). The Case Record Rating Scale: A method for rating symptom and social function data from case records. *Psychology Research, 4*, 333–345.

Suinn, R. M., Acuna, C., & Khoo, G. (1992). The Suinn–Lew Asian Self-Identity Acculturation Scale: Concurrent and factorial validity. *Educational and Psychological Measurement, 52*, 1041–1046.

Svrakic, D. M., & McCallum, K. (1991). Antisocial behavior and personality disorders. *American Journal of Psychotherapy, 45*, 181–197.

Svrakic, D. M., & McCallum, K., & Milan, P. (1991). Developmental, structural, and clinical approach to narcissistic and antisocial personalities. *American Journal of Psychoanalysis, 51*, 413–432.

Tang, P. (2002). *The effect of exposure to erotic images on defense mechanisms.* Unpublished doctoral dissertation, Pacific Graduate School of Psychology, Palo Alto, CA.

Taylor, J. A. (1953). A personality scale of manifest anxiety. *Journal of Abnormal and Social Psychology, 48*, 285–290.

Taylor, S. E., & Armor, D. A. (1996). Positive illusions and coping with adversity. *Journal of Personality, 64*, 873–898.

Tennes, K. H., & Lampl, E. E. (1969). Defensive reactions to infantile separation anxiety. *Journal of the American Psychoanalytic Association, 17*, 1142–1162.

Terman, L. M. (1959). *Genetic studies of genius: Vol. I. Mental and physical traits of a thousand gifted children.* Stanford, CA: Stanford University Press.

Thelen, M. H. (1965). Similarities of defense preferences within families and within sex groups. *Journal of Projective Techniques and Personality Assessment, 29*, 461–464.

Thienemann, M., Shaw, R. J., & Steiner, H. (1998). Defense style and family environment. *Child Psychiatry and Human Development, 28*, 189–198.

Thomas, A., & Chess, S. (1980). *The dynamics of psychological development.* New York: Brunner/Mazel.

Tuller, O. V. (2002). *The use of the TAT in measuring defense mechanisms.* Unpublished doctoral dissertation, Biola University, La Mirada, CA.

Tuulio-Henriksson, A., Poikolainen, K., Aalto-Setala, T., & Lonnqvist, J. (1997). Psychological defense styles in late adolescence and young adulthood: A follow- up study. *Journal of the American Academy of Child and Adolescent Psychiatry, 36*, 1148–1153.

Ungerer, J. A., Waters, B., Barnett, B., & Dolby, R. (1997). Defense style and adjustment in interpersonal relationships. *Journal of Research in Personality, 31*, 375–384.

Vaillant, G. E. (1971). Theoretical hierarchy of adaptive ego mechanisms. *Archives of General Psychiatry, 24*, 107–118.

Vaillant, G. E. (1975). Natural history of male psychological health: III. Empirical dimensions of mental health. *Archives of General Psychiatry, 32*, 420–426.

Vaillant, G. E. (1976). Natural history of male psychological health: V. The relation of choice of ego mechanisms of defense to adult adjustment. *Archives of General Psychiatry, 33*, 535–545.

Vaillant, G. E. (1977). *Adaptation to life.* Boston: Little, Brown.

Vaillant, G. E. (1983). Childhood environment and maturity of defense mechanisms. In D. Magnusson & V. L. Allen (Eds.), *Human development: An interactional perspective* (pp. 343–352). New York: Academic Press.

Vaillant, G. E. (1990). Repression in college men followed for half a century. In J. L. Singer (Ed.), *Repression and dissociation* (pp. 259–273). Chicago: University of Chicago Press.

Vaillant, G. E. (1992). *Ego mechanisms of defense: A guide for clinicians and researchers*. Washington, DC: American Psychiatric Association.

Vaillant, G. E. (1993). *The wisdom of the ego*. Cambridge, MA: Harvard University Press.

Vaillant, G. E. (1994). Ego mechanisms of defense and personality psychopathology. *Journal of Abnormal Psychology, 103*, 44–50.

Vaillant, G. E. (2000). Adaptive mental mechanisms. *American Psychologist, 55*, 89–98.

Vaillant, G. E., Bond, M., & Vaillant, C. O. (1986). An empirically validated hierarchy of defense mechanisms. *Archives of General Psychiatry, 43*, 786–794.

Vaillant, G. E., & Drake, R. E. (1985). Maturity of ego defenses in relation to DSM-III Axis II personality disorder. *Archives of General Psychiatry, 42*, 597–601.

Vaillant, G. E., & Gerber, P. D. (1996). Natural history of male psychological health: XIII. Who develops higher blood pressure and who responds to treatment. *American Journal of Psychiatry, 153*, 24–29.

Vaillant, G. E., & McCullough, L. (1987). The Washington University Sentence Completion Test compared with other measures of adult ego development. *American Journal of Psychiatry, 144*, 1189–1194.

Vaillant, G. E., & McCullough, L. (1998). The role of ego mechanisms of defense in the diagnosis of personality disorders. In J. W. Barren (Ed.), *Making diagnosis meaningful: Enhancing evaluation and treatment of psychological disorders* (pp. 161–195). Washington, DC: American Psychological Association.

Vaillant, G. E., & Mukamal, K. (2001). Successful aging. *American Journal of Psychiatry, 158*, 839–847.

Vaillant, G. E., & Vaillant, C. O. (1990). Determinants and consequences of creativity in a cohort of gifted women. *Psychology of Women Quarterly, 14*, 607–616.

Vaillant, G. E., & Vaillant, C. O. (1992). A cross validation of two methods of investigating defenses. In G. E. Vaillant (Ed.), *Ego mechanisms of defense: A guide for clinicians and researchers* (pp. 159–170). Washington, DC: American Psychiatric Association.

Van der Leeuw, P. J. (1971). On the development of the concept of defense. *International Journal of Psychoanalysis, 52*, 51–58.

Vurpillot, E. (1976). *The visual world of the child*. New York: International Universities Press.

Wallerstein, R. S. (1967). Development and metapsychology of the defense organization of the ego. *Journal of the American Psychoanalytic Association, 15*, 130–149.

Wastell, C. A. (1999). Defensive focus and the Defense Style Questionnaire. *Journal of Nervous and Mental Disease, 187*, 217–223.

Watson, D. C., & Hubbard, B. (1996). Adaptational style and dispositional structure: Coping in the context of the five-factor model. *Journal of Personality, 64*, 737–774.

Watson, D. C., & Sinha, B. K. (1998). Gender, age, and cultural differences in the Defense Style Questionnaire-40. *Journal of Clinical Psychology, 54*, 67–75.

Wechsler, D. (1955). *Manual for the Wechsler Adult Intelligence Scale.* Oxford, UK: Psychological Corporation.

Weiner, I. B. (1962). Father–daughter incest: A clinical report. *Psychiatric Quarterly, 36*, 607–632.

Weinshel, E. M. (1977). "I didn't mean it": Negation as a character trait. *Psychoanalytic Study of the Child, 32*, 387–419.

Weisman, A. D. (1972). *On dying and denying.* New York: Behavioral Publications.

Westen, D., Lohr, N., Silk, K. R., Gold, L., & Kerber, K. (1989). *Measuring object relations and social cognition using the TAT: A scoring manual.* Unpublished manuscript, University of Michigan, Ann Arbor.

Westenberg, P. M., & Block, J. (1993). Ego development and individual differences in personality. *Journal of Personality and Social Psychology, 65*, 792–800.

White, R. W. (1961). Ego and reality in psychoanalytic theory. *Psychological Issues, 3*(3), 1–210.

Whiteman, M. (1967). Children's conceptions of psychological causality. *Child Development, 38*, 143–156.

Whitty, M. T. (2003). Coping and defending: Age differences in maturity of defence and coping strategies. *Aging and Mental Health, 7*, 123–132.

Wilson, J. F. (1982). Recovery from surgery and scores on the Defense Mechanism Inventory. *Journal of Personality Assessment, 46*, 312–319.

Winnicott, D. (1965). Ego distortion in terms of true and false self. In *Maturational processes and the facilitating environment* (pp. 140–152). New York: International Universities Press.

Winston, B., Winston, A., Samstage, L. W., & Muran, J. C. (1994). Patient defense/therapist intervention. *Psychotherapy, 31*, 478–660.

Wolff, P. H. (1959). Observations on newborn infants. *Psychosomatic Medicine, 21*, 110–118.

Wolmer, L., Laor, N., & Cicchetti, D. (2001). Validation of the Comprehensive Assessment of Defense Style (CADS): Mothers' and children's responses to the stresses of missile attacks. *Journal of Nervous and Mental Disease, 189*, 369–376.

Worth, B. (1998). *A psychoanalytic investigation of the presumed link between paranoia and projection.* Unpublished doctoral dissertation, University of Detroit Mercy, Detroit, MI.

Yasnovsky, J., Araujo, K., King, M., Mason, M., Pavelski, R., Shaw, R., et al. (2003). Defenses in school age children: Children's versus parents' report. *Child Psychiatry and Human Development, 33*, 307–323.

Index

"f" following a page number indicates a figure; "n" following a page number indicates a note; "t" following a page number indicates a table.

373